HIKING DEATH VALLEY

A Guide to its Natural Wonders and Mining Past

Michel Digonnet

First printing, October 1997
Fourth printing, May 2007

Maps, illustrations and book design by the author
Photographs by the author, unless otherwise specified
Volume Editor: Susan Cole
Copy Editor: Kathleen Hallam
Cover Designer: Lucija Hadziselimovic, Design Site, California

Published in Palo Alto, California
Printed and bound in the United States of America

Front Cover: - Narrows in Fall Canyon, Grapevine Mountains
Back Cover: (left to right)
- Beavertail cactus, Panamint Mountains
- Eureka Dunes, Eureka Valley
- Ore bin, Inyo Mine, Funeral Mountains

Publisher's Cataloging-in-Publication
(Provided by Quality Books, Inc.)

Digonnet, Michel.
    Hiking Death Valley : a guide to its natural wonders and
mining past / Michel Digonnet -- 1st ed.
    p. cm.
    Includes bibliographical references and index.
    Preassigned LCCN: 97-92255
    ISBN: 0-9659178-0-0

    1. Hiking--Death Valley (Calif. and Nev.) 2. Death Valley
(Calif. and Nev.)--Guidebooks.   I. Title.

GV199.42.A175D54 1997   796.5'1'0979487
                                         QBI97-40833

To Elea

WARNING

Many of the hikes suggested in this book are potentially very dangerous. They involve hours of strenuous physical activity across often rugged terrain, with no water, little to no shade, in one of the hottest deserts on Earth. They should be attempted only by hikers in excellent physical condition, with prior experience in desert hiking and good route-finding skills. Although many of the dangers of specific routes are mentioned in the text, all of them cannot possibly be covered. The information contained in this book should not be considered a substitute for common sense. The author declines all responsibilities for any injuries, physical or otherwise, anyone might sustain while hiking any of the routes suggested herein.

ACKNOWLEDGMENTS

Many people have contributed to the making of this book, directly and indirectly, whom I wish to acknowledge and thank.

First of all, I would like to thank my wife Susan for giving me the freedom to carry out this long enterprise, although it meant countless evenings and weekends apart, and for going through the painstaking task of editing the final manuscript. I would like to thank some of my dearest friends—Janet Ader, Ralph Bergh, Michael Closson, Marc Fermigier, and Bruno Marchon—as well as my wife and my mother, for accompanying me on some of the hikes I took in and around Death Valley, enduring along the way not only the heat and uncooperative rocks and plants, but also the numerous stops I took to write my endless notes. You have made this experience so much more rewarding. A special thanks to Jan and Cliff Lawson also, for sharing with me some of their secrets of Death Valley. My thanks also go to my friend Stewart Kipp for letting me borrow on several occasions his Land Cruiser, an indestructible cross between tank and mastodon that surely saved me a lot of walking.

I am indebted to the staff of Death Valley National Park for their encouragement, support, and advice, especially Esy Fields, former managing director of the Death Valley Natural History Association, and Ed Rothfuss, former superintendent of the monument. I would particularly like to thank Park Naturalist Charlie Callagan, and Cultural Resource Specialist Linda Greene. Their extensive knowledge of the park have been invaluable.

Several people have generously contributed their time to review the book manuscript at various stages. Superintendent Richard Martin and Chief of Interpretation Coralee Hays coordinated the Park Service reviews, which were carried out by Charlie Callagan, Museum Curator Blair Davenport, Park Ranger Dan Dellinges, Mining Engineer Mel Essington, and Linda Greene. I would also like to thank my friend Michael Closson for editing portions of the manuscript, and Lauren Wright, long-time expert of the geology of the Death Valley region, for clarifying several points of geology.

I am indebted to Blair Davenport for her help in the selection and production of the historic photographs included in this book.

I would like to acknowledge Shirley J. Phillips, grand-daughter of Edgar M. Titus, and her husband William L. Phillips, for kindly sharing with me the information they collected concerning the fate of Edgar

Titus in the canyon that now bears his name; park interpreter Kari Coughlin for putting me in contact with them; and David Rogers for allowing me to publish the history of Saline Valley's talc mines, which have been in his family for several decades.

Finally, I want to thank John Evarts, of Cachuma Press, graphic designer Sue Irwin, and Sylvia Vane, of Ballena Press, who provided precious advice and recommendations concerning the formatting and printing of this book.

TABLE OF CONTENTS

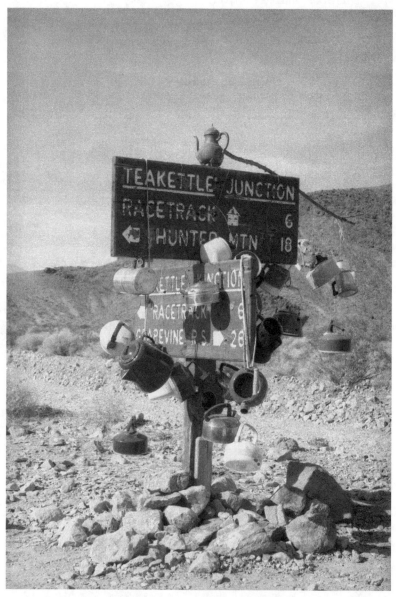

Teakettle Junction, on the edge of the Racetrack Valley. This colorful sign is usually decorated with kettles, a tradition perpetuated by visitors since historic days when this road junction was marked only by a teakettle.

FOREWORD

This book is about Death Valley, about canyons, mountains and open valleys, and about hiking the desert. It is about a vast desert of unique and unspoiled beauty, not as widely known and travelled as other places, perhaps duplicated nowhere else on Earth. This is also, in several ways, a love story. The limitless and uncrowded spaces, the vibrant blue light of spring mornings, the austere beauty of the desert ranges, the ancient rocks distorted behind shimmering heat waves, all conspire to form a primordial, irresistible landscape. I, like many others before me, fell in love with it.

I first approached this desert a little bit at a time, tentatively, overwhelmed by its magnificence and proportions. It took several visits before I dared to venture deeper into its formidable landscape. Here as in other deserts, I found that canyons are natural destinations. They reach into the heart of the most rugged mountains and yet always provide a safe path along which to return. At places, they collapse into mysterious corridors of sheer, naked walls, so deep and narrow that they are rarely probed by the sun. At other places they branch out into intricate labyrinths of side canyons and gulches, offering endless possibilities for exploration. Canyons hold many wonders, from rock formations hundreds of millions of years old to abandoned mines and camps, delicate petroglyphs, bubbly springs of cool water and green oases. Yet the strongest magic of desert canyons may well reside in their meanders, in this random tortuosity that keeps these treasures hidden from view until the long-awaited moment of discovery. The mystery is constantly renewed, pushed back beyond that one ultimate bend that never seems to end.

This book recounts, to a large extent, what I have discovered in Death Valley over the years. The most important message it contains is that behind the apparent austerity and lifelessness of the desert lie incredible beauty and variety, and that Death Valley is a tremendous resource for hiking. A good part of the year the dry weather is surprisingly comfortable, and ideal for hiking—a far cry from the relentless inferno that has been repeatedly depicted in popular literature. The park's mountains and valleys offer a little bit of everything for everyone. Many places can be explored in a single day. Just as many, because of their remoteness or difficult terrain, are best discovered with a backpack and a more generous allotment of time. The contents of this book were selected to reflect this wide variety and to benefit a mixed audience of hikers, from novices to desert rats. Although not as wild, several areas traversed by a primitive road were also included. They give access to spectacular regions and offer a different kind of experience.

My main objective in writing this book was to enhance the visitors' appreciation of this wonderful country. To this end, I have gathered information about the geology, natural history, and natural features of some of the most representative places in and around Death Valley. The emphasis was also placed on the interpretation of historic sites, because this information was not readily available to the general public in a comprehensive yet fairly concise form. The suggested hikes cover a broad spectrum of difficulty and require a wide range of physical skills. In the presentation of the easiest hiking areas, likely to be visited mostly by novices, I have tried to provide a fair amount of detail. On the other hand, for the more remote places—cherished by desert rats, individuals who often thrive on seeking adventure in the wild without knowing too much about their destination beforehand—I purposely omitted many natural features. And for every place I talk about, dozens of equally interesting areas were left out. I have also held out the location of archaeological and most rock art sites, as well as many isolated mining areas, which have been the target of increasing vandalism and theft.

I have often been asked by friends who know me well why I would want to popularize a place I love largely for its solitude. The answer is that my primary goal was not to popularize Death Valley. In the last decade, many of our national parks have been loved to death and profoundly altered by over-visitation. Of all places, Death Valley is the last one I would want to see succumb to the same fate—although its more popular destinations are showing obvious signs of overuse. For one thing, I am planning to spend many more happy days here, preferably with a good friend or alone, certainly without too many other people around to share the scenery with us. Although encounters with fellow hikers are still rare, sooner or later crowds will come to Death Valley, as they have just about everywhere else, with or without this book around. My second, equally important objective in writing this book was to help hikers discover this desert in a responsible way by emphasizing low-impact hiking. I have tried throughout to stress that this is not a free-for-all playground but a fragile landscape that every visitor needs to treat with respect and care, for the sake of the land, for their own sake, and for the benefit of the visitors who will come after them.

My other goal, however dimly realistic, is that this book will reach and influence the lawmakers who set aside our parks and wilderness areas. I hope it will sensitize them to the importance of continuing to set aside more of the eastern California desert and the Basin and

Range. Most of our parks and preserves are too small and fragmented to preserve viable wildlife populations and complete ecosystems. Perhaps more importantly, unless we match their size to the wilderness appetite of the ever-increasing world population, in the long run they will almost certainly not withstand the rising pressure from increasing visitation. This is particularly true of our desert parks, more vulnerable than most environments. It is my most sincere hope that this book will act as an eye opener and help protect what has not yet been ruined.

This is a long book. It covers one of North America's largest national parks, a region extremely rich in natural and human history, and doing justice to it took space. Also, it was my objective to provide descriptions detailed enough so the reader can decide which areas to hike. So, this book is a little heavy. Most hikers don't bother to take a trail guide with them on a hike anyway; photocopies of the few relevant pages suffice. If you do carry it along, a few additional ounces compared to a thinner volume will probably not affect your comfort too much—especially if you are already carrying two gallons of water.

So come on in. This is our largest chunk of unspoiled, unsettled and undivided desert, a land of freedom, stunning light, and eerie landscapes for all to enjoy. If it is the right place for you, its powers will overwhelm you. You will be exhilarated by the heat, dazed by the light, lulled by the serenity, drawn by the smell of danger. As you trudge up that long, hot, desiccated, ankle-twisting alluvial fan on the threshold to some great unknown, you may feel the urge to turn on some music to celebrate the grandeur of the land. Something powerful, dramatic, gut-wrenching, and tear-jerking, as awesome as a slow, giant heart beat—Pink Floyd's "Comfortably Numb," *Carmen*, the Ninth, Led Zeppelin's "Stairway to Heaven," whatever makes you soar. So put on your pack and crank up the volume. Treat the rocks, the flowers, the world around you, with your deepest respect. May you never run out of water. May the coyotes serenade you back to consciousness at dawn. May you find that lovely, lonely, forgotten petroglyph high up on the far cusp of the ridge beyond the canyon head.

Palo Alto, California
April 8, 1997

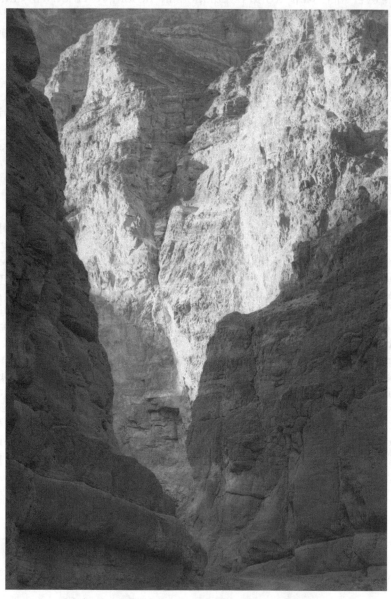

*Majestic walls along the narrows of Titus Canyon,
in the Grapevine Mountains*

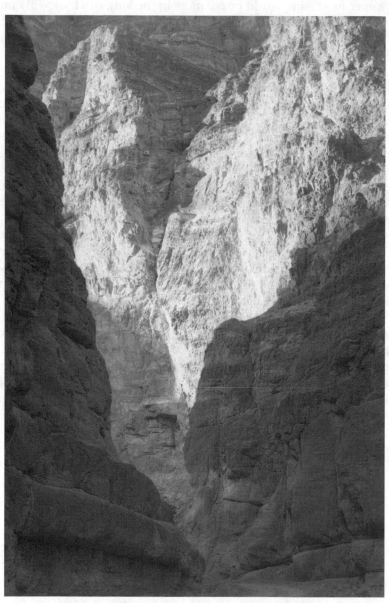

Majestic walls along the narrows of Titus Canyon,
in the Grapevine Mountains

ABOUT THIS BOOK

General Organization of this Book

This book is divided into nine parts. Part I provides general information about Death Valley National Park: natural and human history, hiking tips, and local facilities. Each of the remaining eight parts (II through IX) is devoted to a specific geographic area. They are arranged from north to south and east to west: the Grapevine, Funeral, and Black mountains, the floor and fans of Death Valley, the Last Chance Range, the Cottonwood and Panamint mountains, and the Eureka, Saline, and Panamint valleys. Each part begins with an introductory section including a description of the general area's main features (general location, access roads, geology, vegetation, hydrology, and hiking), a summary table of individual hikes, and a general shaded-relief map. The rest of it contains selected hiking destinations, organized in the same cardinal order.

Organization of Individual Hiking Area Description

Each individual hiking area description contains six common sections, namely a summary of the highlights, three sections entitled "General Information," "Location and Access," and "Route Description," a Distance and Elevation Chart, and a map. When warranted, additional sections are included, such as "Geology," "History," or "Hiking and Driving Suggestions." This information is provided in separate sections for easy reference, and because it may not be of interest to all readers. This chapter summarizes the general purpose of these sections, stressing in particular the definitions that were used and the assumptions that were made in order to avoid potential ambiguities.

About "General Information." This section, together with the summary of the highlights preceding it, provides a synopsis of the most important facts about the hiking area. It is meant as a convenient reference for the reader to decide whether to read on. It includes road access, hiking information (distance, elevation change, and difficulty), main attractions, relevant United States Geological Survey (USGS) topographic maps, and the page(s) where the relevant map(s) are located.

Road access. It mentions whether the hiking area is roadless, or what part of it has a road. For roadless areas, it indicates whether hiking starts from a paved, graded, or primitive road. The type of vehicle

5

required is also shown in parentheses: HC means high clearance, 4WD means 4-wheel drive, and no indication means a standard-clearance car can make it (in dry weather conditions).

Shortest hike/Longest hike. The "Shortest hike" entry lists the distance, elevation change, and difficulty of the shortest hike one might want to take in the area, to get to what I felt was the nearest major point of interest. The "Longest hike" entry gives the same information for the longest hike, in general to get to all the features appearing in the Distance and Elevation Chart. These entries are meant to provide at a glance the extent of hiking required. Distances and elevations are usually one-way figures, measured from the starting point defined by mile 0 in the chart. The elevation change is the total change, ups and downs, and, unless otherwise specified, is one way. These figures do not differentiate between uphill and downhill (which will depend on your starting point). They take into account elevation changes that may not appear in the chart. For example, if two consecutive points are listed in the chart as having the same elevation but are separated by a 200-foot hill, hiking from one point to the other requires a 400-foot elevation change (one way) which is included in the elevation change figure.

Difficulty. Although particular hiking difficulties are mentioned in the text, in many cases the "General Information" section is the only place where the overall hiking difficulty is rated. These ratings are based on distance, ruggedness, and steepness of the terrain, total elevation change, and the number and difficulty of falls and other obstacles. Importantly, they assume that the entire hike, usually round-trip, is to be done in one day (breaking up a long hike into a two-day backpacking trip may well make it less difficult). They also assume cool to warm weather conditions. In very hot weather, bear in mind that the difficulty of hiking *anywhere* worsens considerably, and that these ratings underestimate the difficulty. The following scale was used:

• Very easy: in my book, and therefore in this book, it means a stroll. About as strenuous as a walk around your typical, level, paved and well-groomed city block—a fairly rare occurrence in Death Valley.

• Easy: involves relatively short distances, easy walking on gentle grades, and no obstacles that cannot be dealt with by easily walking around them. Accessible to most people.

• Moderate: fairly demanding, usually with steeper grades and an occasional fall to bypass. Anyone in reasonably good shape should pass this level without feeling they are going through a marathon.

● Difficult: involves steep grades (500-1,000 feet/mile) over moderate distances (6 miles one way), rough and uneven terrains, uneasy footing and/or several falls to bypass or climb.

● Strenuous: implies a large fraction of the way a combination of several of the following: steep grades (1,000 feet/mile or more) over long distances (6 miles one way or more), large rocks in washes, high falls to climb or circumvent on steep talus. This level requires excellent physical condition and recent practice at this kind of activity.

● Grueling: much the same as above but over longer distances (15-20 miles round trip), steeper terrain and unstable footing a good part of the way. It only applies to the one or two most tormented canyons and ridges.

Like any such rating, this scale is subjective. Some of you will find it adequate, while others will curse me the whole way. However, throughout the book I did my best to keep this scale consistent with itself. So even if you disagree with it, you should still be able to use it effectively as a relative scale: just calibrate it against your own scale and adjust it accordingly. For example, you may decide after trying a few hikes that you really cannot hike anything that I have rated strenuous or worse. Or you may feel that what I call moderate is usually easy for you.

Main attractions. The main attractions are listed in decreasing order of importance—again a subjective value.

USGS topographic maps. This entry lists both the older USGS 15' maps (discontinued) and the USGS 7.5' maps required to cover the entire hiking area, as well as the ground between the starting points of the hike and the closest decent road. When several maps are required, the most useful maps are identified with an asterisk.

Maps. This entry lists, in this order, the page location of:
(1) the main map(s) of the hiking area, identified by an asterisk;
(2) in some cases, other maps showing the hiking area in relation to adjacent areas;
(3) the general area map(s) identifying the hiking area's general location, shown in italics.

About "Location and Access." This section gives driving directions to the various points of entry into the hiking area. With only a few stated exceptions, these instructions are meant to be clear enough that readers familiar with the park's main roads should be able to get there without consulting a map. The type of road (paved, graded, primitive) is also mentioned, as well as the vehicle requirement for all unpaved roads (in dry weather only). This last entry distinguishes between passenger cars, high-clearance vehicles (in particular 2-wheel drive pick-up trucks), 4-wheel-drive vehicles (including urban 4WD sedans), and high-clearance 4-wheel-drive vehicles. The distinction between 4WD vehicles is important because very often clearance is more critical than power.

A word of caution about vehicle requirements. This is an *extremely subjective* topic, and in this book it reflects *only* my own experience. I tend to be tolerant of rocks and bushes occasionally scraping the undercarriage or side of my car, and consider that to get there, a few bumps here and there are worth it. As a result, on the park's primitive roads I almost always drive a run-of-the-mill subcompact car, and have recourse to sturdier vehicles only for the roughest roads. I understand and respect that not everyone feels this way. So be aware that on most of the park's primitive roads I claim can be driven with a standard-clearance passenger car, the Park Service recommends a high-clearance and/or 4-wheel-drive vehicle. In fact, several people have come back to me after field testing portions of my book with a variation of "there is no way I could get my car on the Racetrack Valley Road" (a road I have driven numerous times, and many others drive every weekend, with a subcompact car). So if you have little experience driving desert roads with a passenger car, or you do not want to push your car too hard, you should follow the park service recommendations, *not mine.*

About "Route Description." This is the main section. It describes the area's natural features, mines and mining camps, as well as the main attractions and challenges of the hike.

When necessary, route finding and specific difficulties encountered along the route are discussed. For route finding, unless otherwise specified all cardinal directions (such as NNE) are referenced to the true north (North Star). Only in a few stated instances does it refer to the magnetic north. In the park, the magnetic declination is 14.5°-15.5° east.

The location and height of most, but not all, falls requiring either climbing or circumventing are mentioned. Exceptions include fall-riddled places like Grotto Canyon. Fall heights are estimated figures. They are usually not worse than 20% off, which is sufficient to give a reasonable idea of what to expect. When available, the climbing difficulty is also mentioned, using either a simplified scale for non-climbers (such as easy, difficult, or unscalable) or the Yosemite Decimal System favored by rock climbers in the United States. The latter ratings are again personal evaluations and should be considered as estimates. "Unscalable" means a fall so difficult and exposed that even excellent climbers will refrain from attempting it in the middle of Death Valley.

About "History." This section provides basic information about the history of the area you will cross on this hike. Sorting out truth from fiction in the abundant literature on the local history was a major hurdle in putting this book together. To remain as close to reality as possible, I only used information taken from the most reliable sources. There is no doubt in my mind that despite these precautions, many erroneous facts managed to slip in.

About "Archaeology." Native American archaeological sites are relatively abundant in the park. To avoid exposing new sites to vandalism, I have elected to mention only the sites that have been previously described in the popular literature. The only exceptions are a couple of largely unknown and remote rock art sites that I did mention as an incentive for rock art buffs. It is unfortunate for the majority of well-intended hikers, but they will surely appreciate my concerns.

About the Distance and Elevation Charts. Each hiking area description contains a chart, usually on the page facing the map. The chart lists key features along the route, their elevations, and the cumulative one-way distance to each feature measured from the starting point defined in the chart. The only exceptions are features reached by a side trip, away from the main line of travel. In this case, the distance (still one-way) is measured from the last entry along the main direction of travel, and it is indicated in parentheses. For example, in the chart for Golden Canyon, from the Zabriskie Point trailhead at the wash to Manly Beacon, the distance is indicated as (0.4), i.e. 0.4 miles from the wash. In the same direction, the distance to Zabriskie Point, shown as (1.7), is 1.7 miles from the wash. The distances to the next two entries (Fork and Red Cathedral) are again measured from the starting point of the hike, assuming you did not take the side trip to Zabriskie Point.

The hiking distances indicated in these charts and in the text were evaluated by a combination of measurements on 7.5' maps and measurements during actual hikes using a calibrated pedometer. Most of these distances are accurate to ±10%. However, since most hiking areas have no trail, some figures are necessarily approximate, especially on wide washes and fans or around major obstacles. Don't blame me if you find your mileage at odds with mine: this is one of the surprises and pleasures of cross-country hiking.

About the Maps. Each individual hiking area is provided with a map of either the entire area or the most important portion of it. In a few cases, the map is shared with another nearby hiking area; it is then located at the end of the section on one of the two areas. These maps were hand drawn on a computer by the author from USGS topographic maps. Most of them have a scale of around 1:31,800, and an elevation contour interval of 80, 100, or 200 feet. North (North Star) is parallel to one of the edges of the map to within 1°. In some cases, the map had to be split in two sub-maps. When the two sub-maps are separated by a double line, it means that they have no common margin (as in the case of Sheep Canyon). When they are separated by a single line, this line indicates their common margin (as in the case of Echo Canyon). Although not as densely contoured as the 7.5' maps, these maps are accurate enough for most hikes. Furthermore, they show many features (narrows, falls, springs, trails, local names, etc.) that do not appear on USGS maps. Note that not all obstacles are shown, in particular in canyons with many falls, in side canyons away from the main line of travel, in the less traveled portions of the main canyons, and in areas made unreachable by unscalable falls. Given that the hiking areas described in this book involve over sixty 7.5' maps, these maps also represent a serious saving in money and storage space. However, on more extensive exploratory trips, especially those requiring orienteering, they should clearly not be used as a substitute for USGS topographic maps.

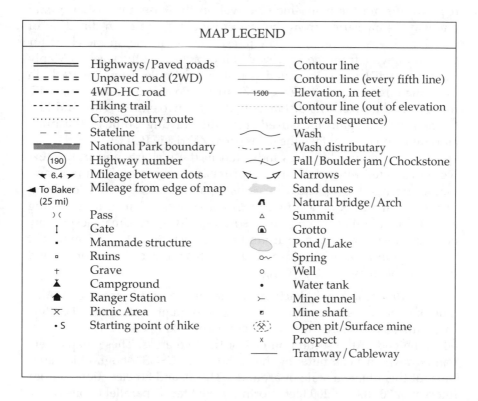

MAP LEGEND		
═══════	Highways/Paved roads	──── Contour line
= = = = =	Unpaved road (2WD)	──── Contour line (every fifth line)
‒ ‒ ‒ ‒	4WD-HC road	──1500── Elevation, in feet
- - - - - - -	Hiking trail	.... Contour line (out of elevation
....	Cross-country route	interval sequence)
– – – –	Stateline	⌒⌒ Wash
▬▬▬▬	National Park boundary	‒·‒·‒· Wash distributary
(190)	Highway number	⌒┬⌒ Fall/Boulder jam/Chockstone
◄ 6.4 ►	Mileage between dots	↘ ↗ Narrows
◄ To Baker	Mileage from edge of map	Sand dunes
(25 mi)		∩ Natural bridge/Arch
) (	Pass	△ Summit
I	Gate	⌂ Grotto
•	Manmade structure	⬭ Pond/Lake
▫	Ruins	o∿ Spring
†	Grave	o Well
⊼	Campground	• Water tank
▲	Ranger Station	⊁ Mine tunnel
⊼	Picnic Area	▫ Mine shaft
• S	Starting point of hike	⟨⊗⟩ Open pit/Surface mine
		x Prospect
		──── Tramway/Cableway

PART I

A FEW BASIC FACTS

NATURAL AND HUMAN HISTORY

The Region

Death Valley and the desert ranges surrounding it were set aside as Death Valley National Monument by President Herbert Hoover on February 11, 1933. Some 60 years later, on October 31, 1994, after a quarter of a century of visionary grassroots efforts to save the California desert, the monument was given national park status and enlarged to 5,264 square miles, an increase of about 63% over its former size. Nearly 93% of its huge land area is officially designated as wilderness. The majority of the park lies in eastern California, along the Nevada border, with a smaller portion wedged in Nevada (the "Nevada Triangle"). By far the largest national park in the lower 48 states, it is surrounded almost entirely by wild lands, including several large wilderness areas.

The Death Valley region forms the northern arm of the Mojave Desert. It is also part of the Great Basin, a vast desert region that contains most of the state of Nevada, the western half of Utah, and parts of southern Oregon and southern Idaho. The Great Basin is primarily one huge sink. Nowhere in this 250,000 square mile chunk of land is there a single river or creek that flows out to the sea. Like most basins in the region, Death Valley is a northwest trending sink. About 140 miles long by 4 to 15 miles wide, it is framed by major mountain ranges. To the east it is limited from north to south by Gold Mountain and the Amargosa Range, the latter being subdivided into the Grapevine, Funeral, and Black mountains. On the west side are the Last Chance Range, the Panamint Range, subdivided into the Cottonwood and Panamint mountains, and the Owlshead Mountains. The eastern ranges are generally lower by several thousand feet. The high point in the Amargosa Range is Grapevine Peak (8,738'). In the Panamint Range it is Telescope Peak (11,049'), the highest summit in the park. The park also includes several

11

of the surrounding valleys—Greenwater and Saline valleys, parts of Eureka and Panamint valleys—and portions of the ranges around them.

Death Valley is hydrologically divided in two parts. The northern part is mostly a dry, sandy, bush-covered plain encroached on both sides by alluvial fans derived from erosion of the ranges. Northward, it gradually tapers down and gains elevation, from just below sea level to about 4,000 feet. The southern valley is very different. A sizeable portion of it, about 500 square miles, lies below sea level. This sink is covered by a 200-square mile salt pan, one of the largest in the Great Basin. Its lowest point is at -282 feet, which is the lowest land elevation in the western hemisphere, and the fifth lowest on Earth (the Dead Sea in Israel (-1,299') holds the record). Telescope Peak, less than 12 air miles away, towers nearly 2.2 miles above the salt pan, which makes Death Valley the deepest depression in the lower 48 states.

Several good two-lane roads traverse the park. The main one is Highway 190, which travels mostly east from Olancha at the foot of the Sierra Nevada to Death Valley Junction near the Nevada state line. It crosses successively Owens Valley, the southern edge of the Inyo Mountains, Panamint Valley, and the Panamint Range, before dropping into Death Valley. From here it cuts across the valley to the foot of the Amargosa Range, continues south to Furnace Creek, and comes out of the park along the southern edge of the Funeral Mountains. Paved roads also run along most of the length of Death Valley. From Highway 190 east of Stovepipe Wells, the Scotty's Castle Road provides access north along the Grapevine Mountains. The Badwater Road travels from near Furnace Creek Ranch south along the Black Mountains, where it joins Highway 178 to Shoshone. East of Stovepipe Wells, the Daylight Pass Road connects Highway 190 to Nevada across the central Amargosa Range. Several graded roads also lead to the surrounding desert valleys—Saline, Eureka, and Greenwater valleys. Hundreds of miles of primitive roads provide access to the park's mountain ranges.

Weather

Temperature. Death Valley is one of the hottest and driest deserts on Earth. The maximum summer temperatures consistently exceed those of any other place. This is largely the result of the unusually low elevation of the valley floor, combined with the trapping of hot air between the high mountains surrounding it. The aridity also fails to provide cooling through evaporation.

The highest temperature in Death Valley was recorded at Furnace Creek on July 10, 1913, with an official reading of 134°F in the shade five feet above the ground. This is the second highest air temperature recorded on Earth, after a reading of 136°F in Al 'Azïzïyah, Libya. It

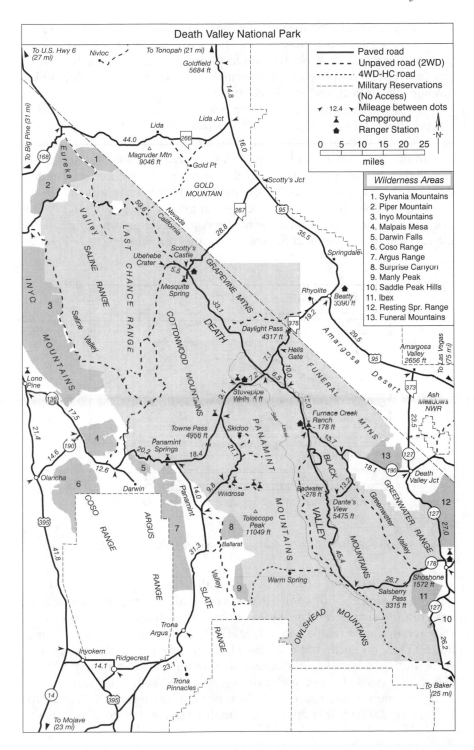

Death Valley National Park

———	Paved road
– – –	Unpaved road (2WD)
- - - -	4WD-HC road
– · – · –	Military Reservations (No Access)
◄ 12.4 ►	Mileage between dots
⚑	Campground
⌂	Ranger Station

0 5 10 15 20 25
miles

Wilderness Areas

1. Sylvania Mountains
2. Piper Mountain
3. Inyo Mountains
4. Malpais Mesa
5. Darwin Falls
6. Coso Range
7. Argus Range
8. Surprise Canyon
9. Manly Peak
10. Saddle Peak Hills
11. Ibex
12. Resting Spr. Range
13. Funeral Mountains

To U.S. Hwy 6 (27 mi)
Nivloc
To Tonopah (21 mi)
Goldfield 5684 ft
To Big Pine (31 mi)
Lida
Lida Jct
Magruder Mtn 9046 ft
Gold Pt
GOLD MOUNTAIN
Scotty's Jct
Eureka Valley
SALINE RANGE
LAST CHANCE RANGE
Nevada California
Scotty's Castle
Ubehebe Crater
Mesquite Spring
GRAPEVINE MTNS
Springdale
INYO MOUNTAINS
Saline Valley
COTTONWOOD MOUNTAINS
DEATH
Rhyolite
Beatty 3390 ft
Daylight Pass 4317 ft
Amargosa Desert
Amargosa Valley 2656 ft
To Las Vegas (75 mi)
Lone Pine
Hells Gate
Stovepipe Wells 5 ft
Furnace Creek Ranch -178 ft
Ash Meadows NWR
Towne Pass 4956 ft
Skidoo
Sea Level
PANAMINT
FUNERAL MTNS
Panamint Springs
Olancha
Darwin
Wildrose
Badwater -278 ft
BLACK
Death Valley Jct
COSO RANGE
ARGUS RANGE
Panamint Valley
Telescope Peak 11049 ft
Ballarat
Dante's View 5475 ft
GREENWATER RANGE
Greenwater Valley
MOUNTAINS
VALLEY
MOUNTAINS
Warm Spring
Salsberry Pass 3315 ft
Shoshone 1572 ft
SLATE RANGE
Trona Argus
OWLSHEAD MOUNTAINS
Inyokern
Ridgecrest
Trona Pinnacles
To Baker (25 mi)
To Mojave (23 mi)

has been argued that because the temperature is generally 4°F higher at Badwater, on the record day of 1913 the temperature at Badwater was probably around 138°F, which would give the record to Death Valley. But for all practical purposes, this issue is academic: Death Valley ranks amongst the hottest, and this is plenty hot.

The temperature chart shown below was computed from official temperature statistics measured at Furnace Creek and averaged over seven decades ending in the mid-1980s. It displays the average mean, minimum, and maximum temperatures, as well as absolute minimum and maximum, for every month of the year. In July, the hottest month, the average maximum is 116°F; the average minimum is still 88.3°F. In January, the coldest month, the average temperature is a balmy 52°F, the average minimum 39.2°F, and the next record-breaking January day will hit above 87°F. The mean annual temperature is an impressive 76.7°F.

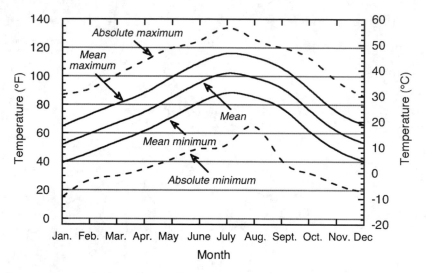

Temperature variations during the year at Furnace Creek Ranch, Death Valley

The first step I took in Death Valley was at 4,956-foot Towne Pass, in three inches of snow. It was very early spring, and instead of entering the searing and waterless desert I had foolishly envisioned, I engaged in a memorable snow fight. Death Valley is quite possibly the hottest place on Earth, but it is also a land of extremes. In the mountains surrounding the valley, the mean air temperature drops at a rate of about 4.2°F per 1,000 feet of elevation gain up to about 5,000 feet, and at a slightly higher rate above 5,000 feet. Because the mountains reach up to over 11,000 feet, this apparently small gradient can go a long way.

When it is 100°F in Furnace Creek, the temperature probably does not exceed a cozy 75°F at 6,000 feet, and it may be less than comfortable on Telescope Peak. And it gets downright freezing up there in the winter.

Precipitation. In the winter, Death Valley receives moisture from the Pacific Ocean, driven in by westerly winds and captured by the surrounding ranges. The main factor contributing to the extreme aridity of Death Valley is the Sierra Nevada. Although 100 miles away, this formidable barrier blocks most of this moisture, and the Panamint Range, the Inyo Mountains, and the White Mountains divert much of what little is left. At the valley floor, the average annual precipitation is only 1.86 inches. Barely enough to fill a cup. This figure does not quite reflect reality, as it varies greatly from year to year—between zero, which occurred in 1929 and 1953, and 4.54 inches, in 1923 and 1983. The rainiest month is February, averaging about a third of an inch. In the wettest spots on Earth it can rain many times as much in a single day, many days in a row. Summer months also receive occasional thundershowers, which originate from the Gulf of Mexico.

In the Death Valley region, precipitation increases with elevation by about 0.7 inches per 1,000 feet up to elevations of about 5,000 feet, and 2 inches per 1,000 feet above 5,000 feet. The mean annual precipitation on the park's highest summits probably does not exceed 15 inches. A significant fraction of it occurs in the form of snow. Every winter, Telescope Peak is a snow-capped beacon visible from miles around.

Winds. Strong winds and sand storms are common on the valley floors, especially in the spring. They arise from strong temperature gradients between the below-sea-level valley and the higher and cooler surrounding ranges. Near Stovepipe Wells, sand storms occur many times a year, especially in the spring. They last anywhere from a few hours to a few days, sending thick clouds of dust up to hundreds of feet in the air and greatly reducing visibility.

Geology

For anyone interested in geology, Death Valley is a fascinating playground. With little vegetation and soil, there is nothing in the way to see the rocks, and geologic events proceed in full view. Looking at a hillside from a distance, one can peer directly into five, fifty, five hundred million years of Earth's history. Often a simple visual inspection will uncover exciting details of the geological past.

Here as everywhere, geologists have divided the thick pile of rocks that form the landscape into a succession of stratigraphic units called formations. A formation is generally made up of a sequence of strata. It is characterized by a thickness (typically tens to thousands of feet), an age, and a duration of formation (a few to tens of millions of years). Formations are often named after an existing name attached to the geographic area where they were first identified. A formation is often, although not always, associated with a specific set of deposition, geographic, and climatic conditions. It may be, for example, the accumulation of limestone at the bottom of a warm sea, or the alternating deposition of mud and volcanic ash in a perennial lake. These conditions generally vary substantially from one formation to the next. The transition between two formations is often the result of a significant change in the local or global environment. In the Death Valley region, which covers a comparatively small land area, many of the same formations recur in most of the mountain ranges. However, because of the lack of uniformity in deposition, as well as subsequent local alterations by erosion, faulting, and metamorphism, the sequence of formations varies greatly between ranges; some formations are even missing at places.

The sequence of formations in a given geographic area is conventionally tabulated in what is called a stratigraphic column. The stratigraphic column of the Death Valley region is shown on pp. 18-21. Each page represents one of the four main geological eras—Cenozoic, Mesozoic, Paleozoic, and Proterozoic—each of which is subdivided into epochs (E=Early, M=Middle, and L=Late). The vertical axis is time. A linear time scale was used, but because of the vast disparity in the time span covered by each era, each page has its own scale. The formations are listed in the order they were deposited, younger towards the top. With the exception of a few formations occurring over limited areas, they represent all the formations encountered in Death Valley.

When two formations were deposited one after the other without any hiatus, they are said to be conformable. In the charts, the horizontal line separating them is then solid (as for example between most Proterozoic formations). When there was a significant time lag between the deposition of two consecutive formations, the boundary between them is unconformable. Such a break in the record indicates, for example, a period of erosion or discontinued deposition. This is represented by a dashed line (as for example between most Tertiary formations). In some cases, it is not known whether the contact between two formations is conformable or unconformable, for example when the contact is buried, or when one of the formations has been removed by erosion. The line is then dotted (as for example between most Cambrian formations).

When out on a hike, the stratigraphic column is useful to identify the age of a formation, the main rocks it is made of (which are listed within each formation in chronological order, younger towards the top), and its average thickness. The age of most formations has not yet been determined accurately. For the very few exceptions, e.g., the Furnace

Creek Formation, the boundary line is drawn all the way across to the "Age" column, and the age is indicated in that column. Otherwise the boundary line stops short of the "Age" column and no age is shown. Particularly ill-defined ages (e.g. the Titus Canyon Formation) are indicated by a question mark. Most of the ages listed are approximate, and generally speaking the older the formation the larger the uncertainty of its age. Whereas the ages of a few late Tertiary formations have been pinned down to just a few hundred thousand years, the error for early Paleozoic formations is around a few million years. The age of the Proterozoic formations is still the subject of considerable debate, and the error for these formations is at least a few tens of million years.

   The Proterozoic: Warm seas and ice ages. Most of the rocks exposed in the ranges of the park are considerably older than the valleys. The oldest rocks, the crystalline basement, date from about 1.7 billion years ago, about a third the age of the Earth. These ancient rocks, mostly gneiss and schist, are remnants of an extensive volcanic belt that became part of the continental shelf, perhaps on the edge of an early version of the Pacific Ocean. The crystalline basement was later buried under miles of younger rocks and strongly metamorphosed by the resulting pressure and heat. Today, this basement is still deeply buried under much of the Southwest. In Death Valley, however, thinning of the crust by tectonic movements and subsequent faulting have brought it back to the surface. The most extensive basement exposures are along the abrupt western side of the Black Mountains and in the Panamints.

   The sedimentary record in the Death Valley region began in the Middle Proterozoic, about 1,400 million years ago—give or take a few. Since then, a thickness of rocks totalling more than 11 miles was deposited on top of the crystalline basement. The oldest rocks of this enormous pile belong to the Crystal Spring Formation, Beck Spring Dolomite, and Kingston Peak Formation, collectively known as the Pahrump Group. The west coast of North America then passed through what is now eastern California. The Pahrump Group was deposited in a large embayment called the Amargosa aulacogen, which extended inland for about 150 miles to the approximate location of Las Vegas. The first two formations are mostly limestone and dolomite deposited in the warm sea that filled this basin. The Kingston Peak Formation is very different. It is mostly diamictite, a conglomerate made of a highly heterogeneous mixture of rocks of all sizes, from grains of sand to boulders several feet across. Geologists speculate that, much like today along the coast of Alaska, this wild assortment was formed during a series of ice ages as glaciers dumped sediments into the aulacogen. Climatic conditions then changed again: the next formation is the Noonday Dolomite. The thickness of these formations varies greatly from place to place, even over

EPOCH		AGE Million years	FORMATION	LITHOLOGY
		1.6	?	•Mostly conglomerate, with basalt flows
Pliocene	L		Funeral Formation	
	E	3.4	Greenwater Volcanics	•Mudstone & sandstone
		5.3	Furnace Creek Form.	☐ 1,500-2,000 feet
		6.3	Artist Drive Form.	
	L	8.0		•Vitrophyre flows layered w/ tuff breccia & conglomerate
		11.2		
Miocene	M			•Mudstone, shale, sandstone •Conglomerate •Mudstone •Basaltic flows & tuff breccia •Basalt conglomerate
		16.6		
	E		?	
		23.7		•Lake mudstone & sandstone, some volcanic conglomerate and tuff breccia
	L			
Oligocene		30.0		
	E		Titus Canyon Form.	•Sandstone •Calcareous mudstone layered with conglomerate •Sandstone & conglom. beds •Limestone & conglomerate ☐ 2,300 feet
		36.6	?	
	L			
		43.6		
Eocene	M			
		52.0	Missing formation(s)	
	E			
		57.8		
Paleocene	L			
		63.6		
	E	66.4		

CENOZOIC

	EPOCH	AGE Million years	FORMATION	LITHOLOGY

		▽ 66.4	?	
		L	↑	
			Granite intrusion	
		97.5		
	Cretaceous			
		E		
		144	?	
		L	↑	
		163	Granite intrusion	
M E S O Z O I C	Jurassic	M		
		187	↓ ?	
		E		
		208		
		L		• Limestone breccia (10-100 ft)
	Triassic		Warm Spring F.	• Andesite flows □ >4,000 ft
		230	Butte Valley F.	
		M 240	? ↓	• Very fine grained laminae of dark gray hornfels
		E ▽ 245	?	□ >4,000 ft

EPOCH		AGE Million years	FORMATION	LITHOLOGY
P A L E O Z O I C	Permian	▷245 258	Anvil Spr. Form.	•Limestone, light gray-white with thinner dark gray beds ❐ 3,600-4,100 ft
			Owens Valley Formation	•Interlayered limestone, shale, sandstone & conglomerate ❐ 1,800-3,100 ft
	Pennsyl.	286	Tihvipah Form.	•Mostly light-gray, platy limestone with beds of calcareous shale and shaly limestone ❐ 200 ft
		320	Rest Spring Shale	•Siltstone, shale (olive gray) •Shale (olive gray) with concretions ❐ 300-750 ft
	Mississip.		Perdido Formation	•Siltstone, shale, limestone, chert conglomerate (*Spirifers, Goniatite*) ❐ 600 ft
		360	Tin Mtn Limestone	•Limestone (med. gray) w/ thin beds of shale and chert nodules (*Spirifers, Corals, Brachiopods*) ❐ 500 ft
	Devonian	374 387	Lost Burro Form.	•Sandstone, quartzite, dolomite (*Cyrtospirifer*) •Dolomite (light gray) •Layered dolom. & limestone (*Corals*) ❐ 1,500 ft
	Silurian	408 421	Hidden Valley Dolomite	•Dolomite (dark gray) •Dolomite (light gray) •Dolomite (med. gray) with chert ❐ 1,400 ft
		438		•Massive dolomite (black) ❐ 400-900 ft
	Ordovician	458	Ely Springs Dolomite	•Massive quartzite (white) ❐ 350 ft
				•Dolomite with some limestone (*Gastropods*)
			Eureka Quartzite	•Shale (thin beds) •Dolomite (*Gastropods*) ❐ 1,500 ft
		478	Pogonip Group	•Shale (*Gastropods*) •Mostly black/light 100-ft bands of dolomite ❐ 1,200-1,500 ft
	Cambrian	505	Nopah Form.	•Mostly thick beds of dark dolomite ❐ 2,000-3,000 ft
		523	Bonanza King F.	•Limestone, shale, silt beds •*Trilobite trash beds* ❐ 1,200 ft
		540	Carrara Formation	•Quartzite, mostly massive and granulated ❐ 150 ft
			Zabriskie Quartzite	•Dolomite
		▷570	Wood Cyn Form.	•Quartzite, shale, quartzite beds ❐ 2,600 ft

EPOCH		AGE Million years	FORMATION	LITHOLOGY
P R E C A M B R I A N	Cambrian	E	Wood Canyon F.	
		570 ?	Stirling Quartzite	•Quartzite, shale ❒ 4,900 ft
		L	Johnnie Formation	•Mostly shale ❒ 2,400 ft
		?	Noonday Dolomite	•Dolomite and limestone ❒ 500-2,000 ft
		900 ?	Kingston Peak F.	•Sandstone and siltstone •Limestone •Diamictite ❒ 1,600-9,000 ft
		? ?	Beck Spr. Dolom.	•Dolomite ❒ 1,000-1,600 ft
	Proterozoic	M 1,300 ?	Crystal Spring Formation	•Thick-bedded dolomite and diabase •Thin-bedded dolomite •Shale (purple) •Quartzite •Conglomerate ❒ 2,300-3,900 ft
		1,600	Missing	
		1,700		
		E 2,500 ▷	Gneiss and Schist	

short distances. Such variations suggest that the aulacogen was sinking, probably as a result of tectonic activity, like in a rift valley.

In the Late Proterozoic the region was part of a coastal delta, with probably no major ranges around. For over 100 million years, rivers relentlessly deposited loads of mud and sand over the ocean shelf, eventually accumulating between 1 and 3 miles of sediments. The muds were later metamorphosed into the colorful shales of the Johnnie Formation, and the sands into the dazzling white Stirling Quartzite and dark quartzites of the Wood Canyon Formation. All three formations are now exposed half way up the eastern slope of the Panamints.

The Paleozoic: A sea of algae, shellfish, and corals. The Paleozoic era started around 570 million years ago, and lasted for some 325 million years. A long spell, represented around Death Valley by some 16 formations with an aggregate thickness in excess of 4 miles. During most, and probably all, of this period the region was immersed under the Pacific Ocean—a warm ocean, as Death Valley was then much closer to the equator than it is today. Over time, the ocean's shoreline fluctuated from just east of Death Valley to much further east. This fluctuation is at the origin of the varying compositions of the Paleozoic formations. When the shoreline was close by, both the sand and silt sediments brought in by rivers were carried out to and settled over the Death Valley region. The silt eventually turned to shale; the sand became the hard white Zabriskie and Eureka Quartzites. When the shoreline was too far east for the heavier sand particles to reach, the sediments were made up primarily of silt. When the shoreline was even further east—hundreds of miles—only the shells of newly-evolved sea animals contributed to sedimentation, forming thick limestone and dolomite beds.

Paleozoic rocks are by far the most common in the Death Valley region. They make up most of the eastern slopes of the Panamints, the majority of the Grapevines, Cottonwoods, and Last Chance Range, as well as the southern Funerals. The Paleozoic formations are also among the most interesting for their fossils. The Cambrian, at the very start of the Paleozoic, was marked by the emergence of the first complex life forms. The warm, shallow ocean covering Death Valley was teeming with countless species of algae, shellfish, and coral reefs, some of which are fairly similar in appearance to the species found in today's tropical oceans. Today their fossils recount several hundred million years of evolution, from the simple-minded Cambrian organisms to the complex animals that had developed by the time the Permian extinction struck—and literally blew them all out of the water. Although fossils of more highly developed sea animals have been identified at a few sites in the park, more primitive fossils are fairly common. The most frequent ones are corals, crinoids (animals that looked like a flower at the end of a tall stalk), trilobites (a distant relative of today's crabs and lobsters), and shellfish, in particular brachiopods and other bivalves.

The Mesozoic: Granitic intrusions. The beginning of the Triassic saw the deposition of the Butte Valley and Warm Spring formations, now exposed almost exclusively in the southern Panamints. This was to be the last sedimentation for about 200 million years. Towards the end of that era, about 100 miles to the west, the Pacific plate started to push under the continental plate. It forced a long range of volcanoes to emerge along the coast, which brought major transformations to the western edge of the continent. As the volcanoes spewed out thick lava flows, the ocean that had been covering Death Valley for the best part of one billion years withdrew. Death Valley had finally dried up.

Through the Jurassic and Cretaceous, while the dinosaur empire rose and fell a few hundred miles to the east, Death Valley was scoured by alternating waves of volcanism, metamorphism, and plutonism. To the west, extreme underground heat and pressure forced the intrusion of an enormous batholith of granite, later uplifted to form the Sierra Nevada. Probably as a side effect, Death Valley saw much thrust faulting activity and the intrusion of several granitic plutons. Large swells of granite-like rocks called quartz monzonite and granodiorite pushed their way up through the native sedimentary rocks to just a few miles below the surface. These plutons are now exposed at Hunter Mountain in the Cottonwoods, in upper Hanaupah and upper Warm Spring canyons in the Panamints, and around Skidoo. This is also the time the large bodies of schist and gneiss found in the Funerals were metamorphosed. The Hunter Mountain Pluton, one of the largest in the region, has been dated at around 165 million years. The Skidoo granite was formed later, sometime in the last 20 million years of the Cretaceous. These intrusions contained the gold and silver that sparked the famous strikes of Skidoo and Harrisburg.

The Cenozoic: The opening of Death Valley. The earliest known records of Cenozoic rocks around Death Valley are the lake and stream deposits of the Titus Canyon Formation. Death Valley was then probably a region of broad valleys, rolling grasslands, and woodlands dotted with lakes, with a warm and wet climate. The hodgepodge of sandstone, mudstone, and conglomerates of this formation is exposed mostly in a narrow strip along the crest of the southern Grapevines and northern Funerals. Its claim to fame is that it has yielded the fossilized remains of several Oligocene mammals, including rodents, tapirs and horses, and the well-preserved skull of a titanothere.

The slow pulling apart that produced the Basin and Range began in the Middle Miocene, long after the last breath of the last titanothere. Over a land area of more than 100,000 square miles, tectonic movements produced a gradual thinning of the crust, which locally collapsed into long, northwest-trending basins. In Death Valley these forces first developed around 14 million years ago, along the two long faults that frame the valley. The Northern Death Valley-Furnace Creek Fault Zone, which runs down the western foot of the Amargosa Range and up Furnace Creek Wash, started first. The Southern Death Valley Fault Zone, along the western foot of the Black Mountains, became active a couple of million years later. Combined, they are still today one of the longest active fault systems in California.

Movements along the Furnace Creek Fault opened a long, narrow, southeast-trending basin from today's Mesquite Flat down across the northern Black Mountains, clear across the future site of Death Valley. For a few million years this trough gradually filled up with sediments washed down from the emerging ranges around it, early incarnations of the Black, Funeral and Panamint mountains. Combined with volcanic ashes, these sediments produced the 4,000-foot thick Artist Drive Formation, one of the most colorful in all of Death Valley. From 6.3 to 5.3 million years ago, and probably for quite some time earlier, the basin was at least episodically submerged under Furnace Creek Lake. Ancestors of today's mammals, reptiles, and birds lived along the lakeshore—mastodons, camels, one-toed horses, wading birds, lizards, and rodents. Their fossil tracks grace a similar lake playa exposed in the Black Mountains. Vast quantities of sediments and periodic blankets of ashes and lava accumulated at the bottom of the lake, resulting in the thick beds of the Furnace Creek Formation. Boron-rich minerals were leached out of the mountains into the lake, occasionally precipitating to form rich borate deposits. This soft formation was later uplifted and eroded into the eerie badlands near Zabriskie Point. From the 1880s until recently, it is this formation that produced most of the local borax—Death Valley's "white gold."

The final touch in the creation of Death Valley—the sinking of the Badwater Basin—is relatively recent, beginning around four million years ago. The two ranges that now frame Death Valley were then partially in place, although on average perhaps only half as high as they stand today. Geologists generally agree that the valley was formed when these two land masses were pulled apart by the enormous tensions that developed along the Southern Death Valley Fault Zone. As the Panamints were uplifted on their west side, they dipped eastward, deepening Death Valley in the process. Erosion steadily brought down huge amounts of alluvia from the rising mountains, which filled the bottom of this giant graben as it was forming. Today, after a few million years of simultaneous rising, sinking, and filling, the Panamints loom two miles above Death Valley. The valley fill is equally impressive: the alternating layers of clay, gravel, and rocks under the valley floor reach down more than 9,000 feet. And the tilting and filling are still on-going.

During the Pleistocene Ice Age, glaciers did not reach this far south but Death Valley did change significantly. Increased precipitation and meltwater from the Sierra Nevada filled most of the region's closed basins with lakes interconnected by rivers. Death Valley was flooded by a succession of lakes. The last one was Lake Manly, a 100-mile long, 600-foot deep body of water that stretched from the mid-Grapevine Mountains to around Saratoga Spring. Today's desert lakes, like Pyramid Lake in northern Nevada, are probably good examples of what Death Valley looked like then. The salt pan that coats the valley floor today is made mostly of the carbonates, sulfates, and chlorides that precipitated when Lake Manly began to evaporate for good, about 11,000 years ago. Smaller lakes have periodically flooded the valley since then, but the largest flood, about 2,000 years ago, was only 30 feet deep.

Flora

Discovering the flora is one of the great pleasures of desert exploring. Each plant has a unique story to tell, about its habitat, survival skills and growth habits, or simply its fragrance or the beauty of its flowers. Being able to identify and name just a few plants and knowing a little about them can greatly enhance one's appreciation of the desert. This section is meant as a short introduction. For more information, get a copy of Roxana Ferris' *Death Valley Wildflowers*. It is the most specific field guide to get started. At a later stage you can consult more exhaustive references, in particular Edmund Jaeger's classic *Desert Wild Flowers*. Experts may want to check the bibliography references on the flora of specific park areas and Mary DeDecker's *Flora of the Northern Mojave Desert, California*.

Though Death Valley is one of Earth's driest deserts, probably more than 1,000 plant species call it home. This surprising diversity is largely the result of the wide altitudinal range and the variety of soils prevailing in the park. Each species has inherent characteristics and tolerance ranges that enable it to inhabit specific regions, defined primarily by their elevation, water availability, soil chemistry, drainage, and exposure to sun. In and around Death Valley, these parameters cover a broad spectrum and the pattern of vegetation is fairly complex. Botanists divide the flora of a given biogeographic region into zones. A zone is a subdivision that exhibits similar altitudinal and broad climatic influence, and contains species with related compositions and physiognomy. It is generally subdivided into associations, smaller ecological units characterized by essential uniformity and a few dominant species. Several of the park's biogeographic regions (mountain ranges and valleys) have been studied by botanists. Not unexpectedly, the corresponding zones of different regions contain many of the same dominant species, although they may differ in the details of their plant associations.

Based on these similarities, and although this is not strictly correct from a botany point of view, I have tabulated the main plant zones encountered in the park on the following page. For each zone the table lists the habitat usually associated with it, the approximate range for the lower and upper elevation where this zone occurs, and its dominant and most common species (which are all perennials), in decreasing order of importance. These are the plants you are most likely to encounter and should learn to identify first. Remember that many more species are present (though not as abundantly as the plants listed), that some of the plants listed may not be present in some mountains, and that not all zones are present in all ranges (even if the elevation is right).

Another important plant community, not represented in the table because it transgresses all other zones in climatic and altitudinal conditions, is found near springs and perennial streams. It includes riparian plants like willows, cottonwoods, common cane, reeds, and even plants one would never expect in a desert, like ferns, mosses, and orchids. Phreatophytes—plants that must have their roots near water—are also found around springs (see *Mesquite Flat*).

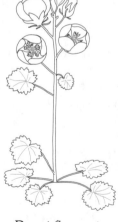

Desert five-spot

Contrary to popular belief, cacti are not generally abundant in deserts, especially in Death Valley. They need a good seasonal water supply, as well as good drainage. In the park, this happens only at higher elevations. Cacti are found up to 9,500 feet, but not usually on low valleys or fans below about 600 feet. The park supports about 15 species of cacti. The cottontop, beavertail, pricklypear, and calico cacti are the most common. Even so, they occur infrequently, although they are common where found. All other species are uncommon to rare. The rarest are the pencil, Mojave fishhook, and pincushion cacti—you'll have to do a lot of walking before running into one of these.

The wild flower displays in the springtime are without a doubt one of the desert's greatest treasures. In a good year vast areas are carpeted with extravagant arrangements of annuals, including primroses, sand verbena, desert gold poppy, desert gold, and phacelias. More rarely you will see desert five-spot, one of the most popular flowers, or

PLANT ZONES OF DEATH VALLEY			
Zone	**Elevation range**	**Habitat**	**Dominant and common plants**
Alkaline Sink	-250' to ~100'	Valley floors	Mesquite, arrowweed, inkweed, alkali sacaton grass, salt grass, rush, pickleweed
Creosote Bush	-240'/800' to 4,600'/6,000'	Fans, lower washes and slopes	Creosote bush, desert holly, cattle spinach, sprucebush, ephedra, shadscale, beavertail cactus, cholla, thornbush, brittlebush, ragweed
Mixed Shrub	3,200'/4,500' to 6,200'/7,200'	Mid/upper canyons and slopes	Shadscale, blackbrush, bitterbrush, thornbush, ephedra, hopsage, cliff rose, beavertail cactus, cholla, calico cactus
Sagebrush	2,000'/4,600' to 6,000'/9,000'	Upper canyons and slopes	Low sagebrush, big sagebrush, rabbitbrush, Mojave rubberbrush, bitterbrush, ephedra, cliff rose, Joshua trees
Pinyon Pine	~6,000' to ~8,000'	Upper canyons and slopes	Pinyon pine, Utah juniper, low sagebrush, mahogany, big sagebrush, Mormon tea
Limber-Bristlecone Pine	~8,000' to ~11,000'	Highest summits	Limber pine, bristlecone pine, big sagebrush, tansybush

Mojave desert-star. Gravelghost is one of my favorites. Perched at the tip of a long, slender stem that merges into the background, its white flower seems to float above the ground, stirred by the slightest breeze. Many perennials are also quite showy. One perennial that is hard to miss is the indigo bush. In the spring, this large shrub is dotted with innumerable tiny flowers the deepest purple you'll find in the desert. At higher elevations, the canyon washes are adorned with prince's plume, globemallow, and the amazingly profuse pale yellow flowers of the stingbush. When in bloom, the often dense cover of brittlebush can turn entire washes into a sea of sunflowers. Another favorite of mine is the desert prickle poppy, a handsome and fairly infrequent flower. The high mountains, where moisture is greater, support many more pretty flowering species, including desert mariposa, Mojave aster, penstemons, larkspur, and lupines. If you are lucky you may run into such endemics as Panamint daisies (some years they put on ephemeral shows in lower Wildrose Canyon), bear poppy, or rocklady maurandia, which ranks amongst the rarest in the park. Perhaps the most striking flowering plants of all are the cacti. In the late spring and early summer many of the park's species sport clusters of the most brilliant flowers, from pale yellow to bright magenta, a treat easy to spot against the grayish-green desert flora.

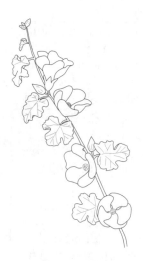

Desert globemallow

The bulk of the blooming season usually occurs on the alluvial fans and lower canyon washes between the second week of March and the first week of April. The best years are when the rainfall is above average and evenly distrib-uted throughout the winter and early spring. The first floral displays occur on the valley floors, which are the first ones to get warm enough for germination. After a few weeks these flowers wither and die, but as the season march-es on higher elevations warm up and the flower belt migrates higher up the fans, then into the mountains. By May the upper canyons are awash with blossoms. A local saying claims that there is always a plant in bloom somewhere in Death Valley. I have come here every month of the year, and I do not recall a single visit when I did not see a few wild flowers.

The topography of the Death Valley region—high, insular mountain ranges isolated by deep basins—provides habitats for a partic-ularly large number of endemic plants—species that grow here and nowhere else on Earth. Endemics in the Black Mountains, for example, account for about 8% of the total flora in that range. Some endemics are common in several areas of the park and surrounding region. Death Valley sage (*Salvia funerea*), for example, originally discovered in the Funeral Mountains, occurs in several neighboring ranges. Others are limited to one or a few small areas. For example, a systematic study of the Cottonwood Mountains turned up only one specimen of a rare mal-low. Some of the plants endemic to Death Valley National Park and its vicinity are listed in the table on p. 30. Many other species, though not endemic, are fairly rare in the park. Experts will enjoy looking for these unique plants. Check the bibliography for references on the flora of specific mountain ranges, which provide complete lists of rare, threatened, and endangered plants in these areas.

Here as in other deserts, the flora has devised clever strategies to cope with the fundamental challenge of desert living—the scarcity of water. The objectives are dealing with the heat, acquiring water, and minimizing water loss. As far as the heat is concerned, many plants have evolved cells that are resistant to the stress associated with expansion during extreme water loss. This applies in particular to the widespread creosote bush and desert holly, two of the desert's heat-resistant champions. Other plants, like cacti, slow down their metabolism during droughts and live off stored energy and water. Others simply avoid the heat. A good example is the stingbush: it manages to extend its range to low-elevation fans by growing at the foot of arroyo banks, which offer a little more shade. Competition for water is fierce, and here again different strategies have evolved. Mesquite trees send roots as much as 100 feet underground to reach the water table. Many shrubs have a shallow root system spread over a large area to collect as much water as possible during short bursts of rain. Several tricks are also used to minimize water loss through evaporation. Most desert plants have evolved small leaves. Some plants drop their leaves during extremely dry periods. Others, like cacti, have replaced leaves with spines and developed thick skins. The cleverest trick of all may be that used by annuals. They survive as seeds for extended periods, sometimes years, waiting for the right conditions to come out of dormancy; then they quickly grow, flower, produce more seeds, and die.

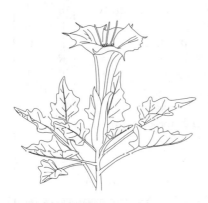

Sacred datura

By pointing out such wonderful minutia, modern biology teaches us a great deal about survival. But the most powerful lesson perhaps comes from the western Shoshone, who have lived here far longer than us and acquired a highly practical knowledge of desert plants. The number of applications they used them for is as amazing as the number of plants they used. You may walk the desert for years and never even suspect the wealth its scrawny-looking plants hold in store. For food the Shoshone used pinyon pine nuts, the beans of mesquite trees, prickly-pear cactus joints, yucca buds, evening primrose seeds, and many other seeds, grasses, and greens. Strands of willows and the roots of bulrush and yucca were used for basketry. Hunting bows were made of juniper,

SELECTED REGIONAL ENDEMIC PLANTS			
Species	**Common name**	**Status**	
Astragalus funereus	Death Valley locoweed	R	U
Boerhaavia annulata	Wet-leaf	R	W
Camissonia cardiophylla robusta	Heart-leaved primrose	R	U
Camissonia claviformis funerea	Brown-eyed eve. primrose	R	A
Eriogonum hoffmannii robustius	Robust Hoffman buckwheat	E	I-R
Eriogonum intrafractum	Napkin-ring eriogonum	E	I
Eriogonum rixfordii	Pagoda buckwheat	R	W
Galium hilendiae carneum	Panamint Mtns bedstraw	E	
Gilmania luteola	Golden carpet	E	I-R
Lupinus magnificus magnificus	Magnificent lupine	E	I
Nama demissum covillei	Coville's purple mat	R	U
Petalonyx thurberi gilmanii	Gilman sandpaper plant	E	U
Perityle villosa	Hanaupah rock daisy	E	I
Salvia funerea	Death Valley sage	R	C
Sclerocactus polyancistrus	Mojave fishhook cactus	R	I
Tetracoccus ilicifolius	Holly spurge	E	I

Key: *Endemism:*   R=regional endemic E=Death Valley endemic
        Abundance: W=widespread A=abundant C=common
                U=uncommon   I=Infrequent R=rare

the string from wild hemp, and the arrows from willow, common reed, or arrowweed. The straight stems of the arrowweed also went into the construction of dwellings, windbreaks, and sweat houses. Medicinal uses were also numerous. The creosote bush was used to induce vomiting, big sagebrush for stomach aches, brittlebush for toothaches, juniper bark for fever, and yerba mansa for open sores—to name a few. Sacred datura was a favorite to induce visions in shamanic activities, and Mormon tea was brewed into a fine tea. One can only marvel at the inquisitive nature of the minds who learned, by trial and error, over countless generations, to make such clever usage of the desert's scant resources, not only to survive but to lead a better and richer life.

Fauna

In spite of its extreme temperatures and aridity, the Death Valley region supports a surprisingly varied wildlife. This is in fact one of the largest desert sanctuaries, and a wonderful place to observe desert critters in their natural habitat. Keep wildlife in mind while out on a hike: a chance encounter with a rare desert dweller, be it a bighorn sheep or a collared lizard, is one of the best rewards of desert hiking. Much of the fauna does not have a strong geographic habitat specificity and can be encountered over large areas.

Desert bighorn. Of all large desert mammals the bighorn sheep is one of the rarest and most beautiful. For several decades it was threatened by the diversion of water from springs for mining operations, then by increasing competition with wild burros. In 1955-1960, the monument's bighorn sheep population was estimated at between 600 and 1,400. Today, following the nearly complete discontinuation of mining activities and the dramatic reduction in the burro population, the bighorn is faring better. Its population is even believed to be on the rebound, in contrast with the rest of its North American desert range where its numbers are generally decreasing.

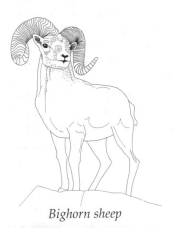

Bighorn sheep

Although bighorn sheep are commonly sighted at low elevations near the major springs at the foot of the Funeral Mountains, they are mostly confined to the more remote and seldom traveled higher elevations, and therefore they are rarely encountered. The numerous canyons draining the desert ranges provide the most direct access to their mountainous territory. The sheep's majesty and scarcity make an encounter with this elusive animal one of the great rewards of desert hiking.

Coyotes. Omnipresent in Native American traditions and myths, the coyote has long been a symbol of the North American desert. A visit here would not be complete without sighting this beautiful canine, or at least a treat to a few howls at night from this talented vocalist. Chances of encounter are fairly good in the low desert, especially around the lower fans of the Funeral Mountains, Furnace Creek Ranch, and Stovepipe Wells. Even the salt pan receives an occasional visit. Unfortunately, with increasing park visitation, in the more populous areas coyotes have turned to begging for food from passing cars—a bad habit they have contracted from misinformed visitors who just can't resist feeding them. Do not feed coyotes. Scare them away instead. For their own survival, they must learn that humans are their worst enemy. If you see people feeding wildlife in general, scare *them* away too.

Wild burros. Originally native to northeastern Africa, burros were introduced to the Mojave Desert by prospectors beginning in the late 1800s. They proved to be so well adapted to the arid climate that they multiplied to large populations. Too much for their own good. In the mid-1930s, the monument's burro population was estimated at more than 2,000, a figure as frightening as the burro's reproduction rate of 20-25% per year. The main problem is that burros compete directly with the native bighorn sheep. On a hot day, a burro will drink and eat at least three times as much as a bighorn. As burros tend to congregate around springs and contaminate the water, they also probably affect how much other animals are able to use these springs. In their widespread forage, burros create extensive networks of trails and damage vast areas, often uprooting the plants they eat and thus increasing soil erosion. The competition became so unbalanced that by the 1940s, and probably earlier, the survival of bighorn sheep in Death Valley was threatened.

In an attempt to solve the problem, between 1939 and 1969 periodic programs removed a total of about 3,600 burros. But by 1983 they were back in full force, and the National Park Service (NPS), in collaboration with the Bureau of Land Management (BLM) and various animal protection groups, carried out a master plan to remove all wild burros from the monument. This was, to say the least, a major undertaking. Over a five year period around 5,700 animals were removed, bringing the population close to zero.

Years have passed, the land has healed, and the bighorn sheep population is on the rebound. The burro population is still doing quite well in adjacent areas, in particular BLM and US Forest Service desert lands, where they are protected. In Death Valley, in spite of periodic population control, the burros are making a slow and limited comeback. You may well run into small groups of burros in the Cottonwoods, Funerals, and eastern Panamints. They are certainly common in and around Saline Valley. Chances of encounter are good year-round: even in the middle of a hot day, burros don't seem to mind standing motionless in the heat. If they feel their territory is threatened by your presence, they may try to scare you away with one of their alarming calls. In the middle of nowhere, after hours of deep desert silence, it can be a jarring experience!

Other mammals. Other mammals are represented by numerous species, with habitats covering all elevations. Lower elevation dwellers include the kit fox, badger, ringtail cat, bobcat, antelope and roundtail ground squirrels, and several species of rabbits, woodrats, kangaroo rats, mice (including pocket and deer mice), and bats. Kit foxes are spotted on occasion near campgrounds, especially at night. Higher elevations support some of the same species as well as scattered populations of pocket gophers, porcupine, mule deer, and gray fox. Mountain lions have also been spotted, although extremely rarely (see *Hazards* in *Desert Hiking Tips*).

Reptiles. On a typical day in the wild, even if you do not see any other wildlife you are likely to catch a glimpse of a few lizards scurrying to shelter. Lizards are common at all elevations. They include the banded gecko, the desert iguana, the western whiptail, side-blotched, zebra-tail, horned, collared, and leopard lizards. The chuckwalla is the largest of them all. Confined to rocky areas, it is rarely seen.

The park is home to at least 18 species of snakes. The most common ones include the gopher snake, king snake, red racer, and the beautifully banded shovel-nosed snake. There are also several species of rattlesnakes, including the Mojave and Panamint rattlesnakes, and the sidewinder. Because snakes are cold-blooded and do not fare well in high temperatures, they are not nearly as common at lower elevations (see *Hazards* in *Desert Hiking Tips*), although at least one species (the western blind snake) has been sighted below sea level.

Desert tortoises are another reptile perfectly adapted to the harsh local conditions. In the summer they can go for months without eating or drinking. They endure the cold months by hibernating. Desert tortoises are not commonly encountered in the park, although small populations do exist, mostly at elevations higher than 3,000 feet. The Owlshead Mountains are one of their best sanctuaries in the park. The desert tortoise is listed as a threatened species. If you see one, remember to approach it slowly, to enjoy it from a reasonable distance, and to not touch it (you may pass on fatal diseases).

Birds. Several hundred species of birds have been identified in Death Valley, and at just about any elevation. Although most of them are migratory, this number includes many resident birds. One certainly would not recommend Death Valley as a mecca for bird watching, but birders should not rule it out while exploring the park. The most commonly encountered species are ravens, turkey vultures, wrens, hummingbirds, hawks, and Gambel quail. The list goes on with sparrows, owls, ducks, finches, larks, thrashers, and many others. The largest populations are found at the well-watered and shaded artificial oasis around Furnace Creek Ranch, around natural springs, and at higher elevations, especially in the pinyon pine-juniper forests.

Native American History

Archaeologists have identified several prehistoric cultures in the Death Valley region, some of them thousands of years old. Archaeologists Alice Hunt and William Wallace have divided the chronology of this long period of occupation into four stages, referred to as Death Valley I through IV. These stages of human activity were separated by long time periods showing little to no record of human occupancy. The exact social, cultural, and ethnic connections between them are not known, but much has been inferred about each of these cultures from evidence found throughout the park.

The earliest sites (Death Valley I stage, or the Nevares Spring Culture) may be as old as 12,000 years. This was the end of the Pleistocene ice age, a time when the last vestige of Lake Manly was still present in Death Valley. During this relatively wetter period, game was probably more plentiful. These early inhabitants subsisted by hunting, as suggested by the abundance of scrapers, believed to have been used to skin kills, found at Death Valley I sites. This period was followed by a hotter and drier one, during which the lake was completely dry and the area probably received only sporadic visits.

The second stage of human occupation, Death Valley II (the Mesquite Flat Culture), lasted from about 3,000 B.C. to A.D. 1. In the early part of this period, the climate was wetter than it is today. A shallow lake filled the valley at least part of the time, and hunting was still the basis of subsistence. This period is characterized by a proliferation of stone knives and scrapers. Towards the late Death Valley II stage, the area became warmer again, and the lake dried up. The springs that supported the aboriginal population progressively dried up, game presumably became more scarce, forcing the valley's inhabitants to migrate or, for those who stayed behind, to gradually shift their subsistence practices from hunting to gathering.

The Death Valley III stage (the Saratoga Spring Culture) started around the beginning of the Christian era and lasted between 500 and 1,000 years. The climate was generally the same as it is today, large game was scarce, and subsistence was based on gathering and small game hunting using the bow and arrow. The large number of grinding tools, including metates and manos, mortars and pestles, recovered from Death Valley III sites shows an increasing dependence on plant gathering, while the introduction of smaller, lighter arrowheads suggests the pursuit of smaller game.

The Death Valley IV stage (the Death Valley Shoshonean Culture) occurred during the second millennia A.D. This fourth wave of occupation is characterized by frequent exchanges with neighboring cultures, in particular the Pueblo cultures of the Colorado Plateau and the Yuman cultures that existed along the Colorado River. Pottery was introduced then, at first imported from eastern Native American cultures, and later locally made.

Up until the late 1800s, Death Valley was occupied by Shoshone-speaking tribes. They were part of a much larger Shoshone Nation that inhabited a vast region stretching from western Wyoming to eastern Oregon, eastern California, and central Nevada. The Shoshone

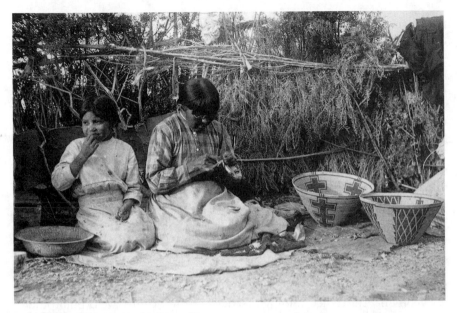

Timbisha girl and woman, circa 1925 (Photo courtesy of U.S. Borax Inc.)

who lived in the Great Basin, including the Death Valley region, are known as the Western Shoshone. They were divided into small extended family groups, each one confined to a particular geographic area. Those who lived in Death Valley called themselves Timbisha. This name derives from *Tumpisa* (red rock), the name they gave to Furnace Creek. They made the mouth of Furnace Creek their home because of the proximity of abundant and reliable water at Travertine, Nevares, and Texas springs. Another group was based around Warm Spring, in Panamint Valley. Several other villages were scattered throughout the region, invariably near the best springs. Areas to the south of Death Valley were occupied by Kawaiisu Indians, and to the west and south by Paiute Indians, in particular around Owens Lake and Owens Valley.

Over the centuries, these indigenous peoples adapted amazingly well to an environment that gradually became one of the harshest on Earth. To meet their scant subsistence needs, they learned to make use of just about every available resource, and to keep their numbers low. Even at its apogee, the Death Valley area was inhabited by relatively few individuals, estimated around 100. They moved frequently, following the rhythm of the seasons. In the winter they lived at lower elevations, in roofless brush shelters or conical dwellings made of logs. Much of their meat supply was provided by rabbits and other rodents, birds, reptiles, and bighorn sheep. They ranged far to harvest wild plants, grasses, and mesquite beans. One of their main food sources, the beans were eaten raw or made into flour. In the summer, they moved to the cooler high mountains. Their main summer staple, pinyon pine nuts, is what primarily attracted them to the higher elevations. In the late summer, the pine cones were knocked off with a hooked pole, and their nuts were roasted in coals overnight. They ate the nuts either whole, boiled, or ground into a flour and used in soups. Pine nuts are high in fat and calories and constituted a definite improvement over the meager food supply of the lower desert. In the winter they returned to the warmer, more comfortable valley floors. This age-old migration pattern is what enabled them to survive for untold centuries in this hostile desert. As much as can be ascertained, most of their time was dedicated to food gathering. Little time was left for other activities such as art, although they had mastered pottery making and were deft basket makers.

The arrival of the first immigrants in the mid-1850s, and the gradual influx of miners over the following decades, completely destroyed this self-sufficient society. By the 1870s Death Valley's native population had already been significantly reduced by displacement. Newcomers established mining districts, erected camps, and manipulated water sources without regard for prior Native American uses of the land. With their traditional hunting and foraging grounds gradually taken over, they became slowly acculturated. During the mining rush they often carried out manual labor for road building, construction, ranching, and mining. The beginning of tourism in the late 1920s further accelerated this disruption. A few families continued to visit the Death Valley area annually until the late 1930s, but eventually they also left or died, and with them part of their unique culture and the precious knowledge and wisdom they had accumulated. Today, a few Timbisha Shoshone families live on a 40-acre village next to Furnace Creek Ranch. Tribal members from neighboring towns still pay periodic visits to their ancestral land at Panamint Valley's Indian Ranch. Other Shoshone and Paiute families share a few small reservations in Owens Valley. Altogether, they cover under 2,000 acres—a tiny fraction of their original territory. The Death Valley Shoshone did not even receive official recognition as a tribe by the Bureau of Indian Affairs until the end of 1982.

Signs of ancient cultures have been found throughout the park—rock shelters, house circles, bone and stone tools, pottery sherds, storage pits, and rock alignments. Many of the canyons used as travel routes across the mountains and as residences in the summer still display vestiges of their occupancy, including petroglyphs, cave shelters, ceremonial sites, and burial grounds. On the alluvial fans leading up to them are old campsites, the hunting blinds they used to hide from bighorn sheep, and the slender traps they made to catch small rodents. With a little imagination, they will help you reconstruct the story of the vanished cultures that, for centuries, called this place home. If you come upon some of these remains, do not disturb them. They are sacred to the Shoshone people, and should be treated with respect.

Mining History

Death Valley has always fascinated fortune seekers. Its isolation and roughness, its dreadful name and unbearable summer heat, all conveyed images of hidden riches no one had the courage or strength to unearth. Although the payoff hardly ever matched expectations, this overwhelming attraction sparked innumerable mining ventures, well into the second half of the twentieth century.

The earliest prospecting took place on the heel of the historical passage of the forty-niners through Death Valley. On his way through the area in 1849, one of the immigrants picked up a piece of rich silver ore. When he reached the coast, he had a gunsight made with it, and before long rumor had it that he had left behind a mountain of silver. The search for the Lost Gunsight Lode was on. The following year, two of the forty-niners returned to search for the lost lode. In the fall, Dr. Darwin French lead the first full expedition, then gave it another try 10 years later. Dr. Samuel George also led a party to Death Valley at the end of 1860. Instead of silver he discovered antimony in Wildrose Canyon, and he opened one of Death Valley's very first mines. Other enticing tales of "lost mines" grew over the years, instigated by prospectors who wandered back from the desert with a handful of gold-specked rocks but no exact recollection of where they came from. The lost lodes of Charles Alvord in 1860, and Charles Breyfogle in 1864, were the most famous. For decades, in spite of repeated failures, these elusive treasures lured party after party of lost-ledge hunters back to Death Valley.

Real mining emerged slowly. In 1871, a civil engineer and land surveyor named August Franklin discovered a silver-lead deposit at what became Chloride Cliff in the Funeral Mountains, and started the first mine on the east side of the valley. A decade later borax was in the limelight. The Eagle Borax Works, on the west side of Badwater Basin, operated less than two years, but the Harmony Borax Works near the mouth of Furnace Creek was Death Valley's first mining success. Until the late 1880s, it publicized Death Valley with enduring images of its 20-mule teams painstakingly hauling wagons full of boron ore across the barren Mojave Desert. There were other isolated enterprises—Jean Lemoigne's lead mine in the Cottonwoods, and copper mining around the Racetrack Valley—but they were limited in scope.

Most of Death Valley's historic mines started between 1904 and 1906, and they had climaxed and died by 1930. The three main players were gold mines—the Bullfrog Hills mines in the eastern Grapevines,

Skidoo in the Panamint Mountains, and the Keane Wonder Mine in the Funerals. Unlike most, they had plenty of good ore. They were also led by experienced managers, who early on developed the right mining and processing infrastructure. At Skidoo, it was the famous pipeline that brought water from below Telescope Peak some 20 miles away. The water allowed the Skidoo quartz mill to run inexpensively, thus reducing the weight of the ore and shipping costs, and making operations profitable. At the Keane Wonder Mine it was the aerial tramway used to transport the ore down from the hard-to-reach lode, and the mill and processing plant that again reduced shipping costs and squeezed out leftover gold from mill tailings. In spite of its isolated location, it eventually ranked third, behind legendary Skidoo. With a production exceeding 1.5 million dollars, the Bullfrog district was the richest. It gave birth to Rhyolite, for several years an important mining center and the largest town around. The area is still exploited today. There were scores of smaller mines, including the Cashier, Inyo, and Leadfield mines. A few of them had plenty of good ore and were fairly successful. The Carbonate/Queen of Sheba Mine, Death Valley's largest lead producer, brought in over $300,000. The Eureka Mine had enough gold to support its owner and sole operator, Pete Aguereberry, for most of his life. But many mines were just not rich enough, and they rose and fell several times, following the hopes and disappointment of successive owners.

Single-blanket jackass prospectors—the hardy souls who searched the desert for mineral wealths, with a burro as their only companion—made many of the original strikes. Their names are forever celebrated all over the land they loved—at Harris Hill and Aguereberry Point, at Lemoigne Canyon, Ashford Peak, and Bradbury Well, and of course at Scotty's Canyon, named after legendary Death Valley Scotty, who never discovered much but through his fantasy tales had everyone convinced he had.

Throughout this time period, most enterprises suffered greatly from the difficulties inherent to desert mining. Of all of them, isolation was the most severe. The closest railroads, in Nevada and in Owens Valley, were far away, and roads were few and rough. As a result, transportation of the ore to market was generally expensive, and only the highest grade ore could be economically hauled out. Another serious problem was the lack of water. It made living conditions difficult, but it also precluded the use of water-powered equipment, a common and economical practice in the gold fields of northern California. The rough terrain did its share to impede development, and so did the heat—operations were often forced to close down in the summer months.

There were other, unforeseeable difficulties. One of them was the San Francisco earthquake and fire of 1906, which all but destroyed

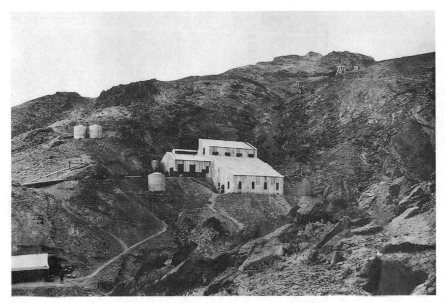

The Keane Wonder Mill in its heyday
(Courtesy of the National Park Service, Death Valley National Park)

northern California's financial center and profoundly disrupted the state's economy. Soon after, the United States Panic of 1907, a financial crisis brought about by reckless speculation and improper management of financial institutions, reduced available funding even further. These two crises occurred at the worst possible time, when many mining enterprises were just starting and needed financial support the most. Many claims and prospects died still unexplored. Many camps never had a chance to develop into real mining towns.

Perhaps the biggest problem of all stemmed from the blind faith Death Valley inspired in investors. From the Ubehebe Mining District down to the Amargosa River, many mining companies were started with only minimal evidence of valuable ore in the ground. Their history followed a similar pattern—a small strike, a mad rush, the creation of a few companies, the influx of a little cash, then a quick collapse upon realization of the low ore quality and the enormous difficulties and high cost of desert mining. More often than not, the only people who came out ahead were the prospectors who made the strike, when they were wise enough to sell their claims for cash—often at a price wildly disproportionate to the magnitude of the discovery.

The most spectacular example is undoubtedly Greenwater Valley's 1905 copper rush. It was the largest and most spectacular boom in the history of Death Valley, and one of its most notorious failures. Over the course of four years, it involved more than 2,000 people, four

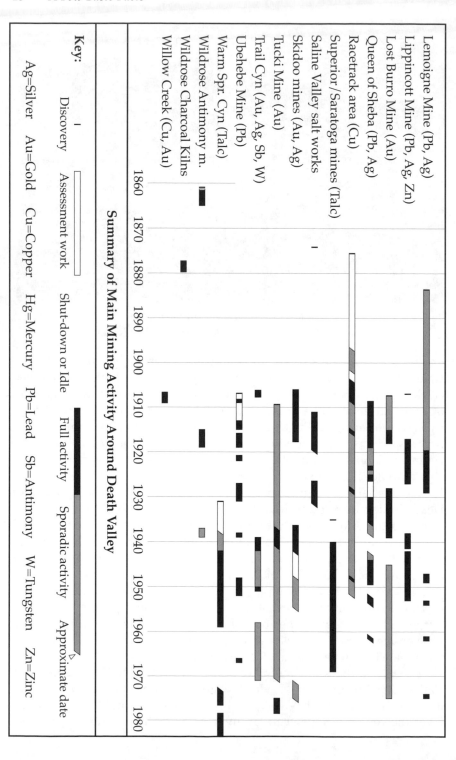

Summary of Main Mining Activity Around Death Valley

Key:

| Discovery | Assessment work | Shut-down or Idle | Full activity | Sporadic activity | Approximate date |

Ag=Silver   Au=Gold   Cu=Copper   Hg=Mercury   Pb=Lead   Sb=Antimony   W=Tungsten   Zn=Zinc

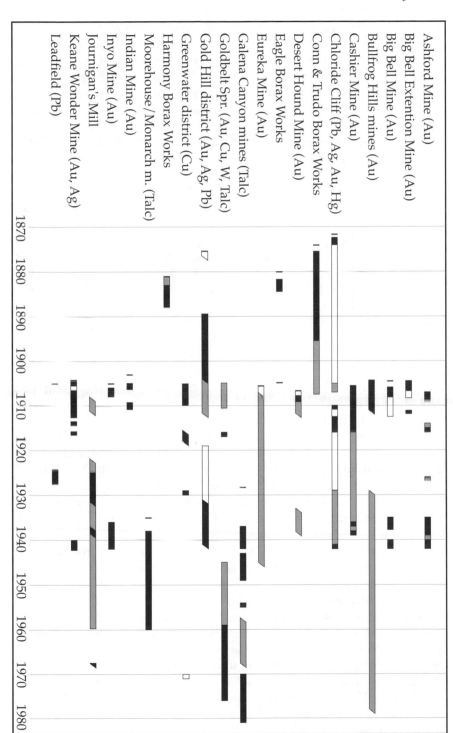

towns, 73 incorporated mining companies, over 140 million dollars in capitalization, and extensive exploratory work including a 1,400 foot shaft. But the copper ore was not as rich and plentiful as speculators had hoped, and the new-born district was dead by the end of 1909.

In the 1930s, with improved roads and means of transportation, new exploitations were started throughout the region, though by then the area's national monument status restricted mining to existing claims. Several mines, in particular at Skidoo, were also reopened after passage of the Gold Reserve Act in 1934 and the ensuing increase in the price of gold. Lead and silver mining, which had been slow going, also underwent a revival, in particular at the Lippincott Mine, up in the Last Chance Range. By the early 1950s most of the heavy-metal mining had peaked and died.

Gold, silver, and lead made the glory days of Death Valley, but it is less noble materials—borax and talc—that produced the biggest bonanzas. Though they were both largely ignored for decades as too cheap a commodity, the value of the talc and borax eventually recovered from Death Valley exceeds all the heavy metal productions combined. The main talc mining efforts took place in Warm Spring and Galena canyons in the southern Panamints, starting in the mid-1930s. Smaller operations also flourished in the Ibex Hills after the 1940s. The Warm Spring Canyon mines were by far the most productive in the region and, for many years, in the country. Operated until the 1980s, they produced over 700,000 tons. After decades of dormancy, borax mining came back to life in the 1970s, this time backed by the full power of modern technology—strip-mining for the most part. The Boraxo Mine, in upper Furnace Creek Wash, was active until the 1980s and produced several hundred thousand tons. Those were Death Valley's last mining efforts.

A few mines are still operating today on the edge of the park. The Billie Mine is still producing borax. Gold mining is back in full force near Rhyolite and at the south end of Panamint Valley near Manly Fall. But as a visit to these sites will not fail to reveal, contrary to most historical mines, these large-scale operations do a lot of damage to the land.

The main mining ventures of the Death Valley area are tabulated on the previous pages. For further reading, the most detailed source is *A History of Mining in Death Valley National Monument*, a four-volume government-sponsored research study by Linda Greene and John Latschar. Much of the historical data found in this book was compiled from this source. It is out of print as of this writing, but it is available in university libraries around the country. Another very useful reference is *Death Valley and the Amargosa: A Land of Illusion*, by Richard E. Lingenfelter. It is well researched, well written, and highly entertaining.

■

DESERT HIKING TIPS

This chapter provides basic information about the features, hazards, ethics, and regulations of hiking in Death Valley. It also goes over the difficulties most commonly encountered while driving primitive roads, and suggests a few pointers to deal with them. Like the old NPS brochure that depicted travelers reduced to skeletons as they drove through Death Valley in a convertible, this is not meant to alarm you but to make you aware of potential dangers. It is by no means exhaustive. Refer to one of several excellent survival books (see *Bibliography*), which cover these topics to a level of detail beyond the scope of this book.

Best Seasons for Hiking

Temperature versus season and elevation. Death Valley has always had a bad reputation for heat. It ranks amongst the hottest deserts on Earth, and this fact tends to linger, rightly so, on the mind of anyone planning a visit here. However, it's a popular misconception that Death Valley is *always* hot. The first key feature to bear in mind is that temperature variations from winter to summer are very large. In the winter on the valley floor, days are balmy but at night the thermometer can dip below 40°F. On the other hand in the summer the temperature at Furnace Creek may not drop much below 100°F for days on end. Between these two extremes, there is a long time period during which the temperature is quite comfortable. Because the air is so dry, for most people the comfort zone for lower lying areas extends approximately from mid-October to mid-May. Obviously this window is subjective and depends on your personal tolerance for heat. Consult the temperature chart in the previous section to assess when you can safely come here.

The second, equally important key feature about the weather is that because the elevation in the park covers such a huge range (from below sea level to above 11,000 feet), at any given time the temperature varies substantially with location. In the dead of winter the highest peaks are often snowbound, while the valleys usually remain comfortable. In the summer the lowest elevations can be unbearably hot, while the temperature is reasonable at elevations above 4,000 or 5,000 feet. Year-round there are pleasant places somewhere in the park.

Peak seasons. As expected, the three peak tourist seasons of Death Valley National Park fall during the comfort zone defined above: Easter, Thanksgiving, and Christmas/New Year. From mid-December through January, it may not be very warm during the day, and it will freeze at night above a few thousand feet. The days are also quite short, which reduces hiking and sightseeing time. October and March are probably the ideal months, as they offer a fairly balanced diurnal and nocturnal temperature, and longer days. Early spring is probably the best of the two. The days are longer, the higher mountains are often still graced with snow, and the desert blooming season is at its peak.

Summer hiking. In the summer, when temperatures exceed 110°F in the valley, most people are reluctant to stray too long from air conditioning, let alone hike anywhere. The resolution of all but the most determined desert rat may falter. Unless you know from previous experience that you can tolerate long exposures to sun and heat, hike first at higher elevations, where the air temperature usually doesn't exceed 90°F (remember that the temperature drops by ~4.2°F per 1,000 feet of elevation gain). Hike at lower elevations later on, in small doses at first to assess your tolerance to sun and heat. You may kill a myth and discover that it can be a pleasant, even exhilarating experience. Allow a couple of days to become adjusted before doing any extensive hiking.

Sand storms are common year-round. In the summer they can be unpleasant and dangerous. They can also cause sleepless nights. Try to escape to slightly higher elevations until the storm dies out.

Winter hiking. Winter days can be cold and windy. Below a few thousand feet you will not need arctic wear, but a sweater and a warm jacket are in order for the evening and early morning, as well as a decently warm sleeping bag. It has also been known to rain, and although it is often just a drizzle, a few hours of it will get you wet. Bring along rain gear and a tent. If you are planning to spend time at higher elevations, keep in mind that it is just like any other mountain up there. Expect snow, ice, and frigid nights.

Winter days in Death Valley are deceptively short. In December sunset occurs around 4 p.m. This significantly reduces how far you can hike in a day. If you are planning a long hike, get an early start. Bring a flashlight, just in case you get caught out there after dark.

Water: Needs and Availability

One of the most fundamental characteristics of Death Valley is that it is essentially waterless. Unlike in more temperate mountainous terrains where one encounters some form of water every day, be it a lake, stream, spring, or rain puddle, in Death Valley fresh water is exceedingly rare. When planning a desert hike in the hot season, from mid-May to mid-October, the most critical concern is obviously water. Here more than anywhere else you will need to carry your own.

Water needs. How much water is enough? The answer depends on several factors, starting with the time of year. On a sunny day in February I drank only one quart in a five-hour, 14-mile hike down Titanothere Canyon. But early morning one hot day in July I took one gallon of water with me up Mosaic Canyon, had gone through half of it after three miles, and had to turn around. During the six to eight cooler months, your water needs will be comparable to what they are when hiking in temperate regions. Count on one to two quarts a day for any reasonable amount of ground you cover. But in the summer the sun means business. With rocks too hot to touch, air pushing three-digit temperatures in the shade, and no shade, you'll need a lot more.

Your water needs also depend on humidity, the amount of shade and wind, your metabolism, clothing, level of physical activity, and the terrain difficulty. As a good rule of thumb, if you are walking on level ground in 100°F weather, allow a minimum of one quart per hour. You'll need less while resting, about one or two cups per hour. Walking up steeper terrain, you may need as much as two quarts per hour. This may seem like a lot of liquid to ingest but don't underestimate this most vital of your body's needs. A common mistake is to think you can personally get by with drinking less and to become dehydrated. If you have not done so before, keep track of your personal water needs on your next trip here to better plan future trips. To monitor your water consumption safely, start with short, easy walks. Slowly work up towards longer hikes, increasing the water you take with you accordingly.

In hot weather, you don't lose only water through perspiration, but also minerals and salts. To make up for this loss, take multi-vitamin/mineral tablets, or drink a mineralized drink, like Gatorade, instead of straight water. This is important. The salts and minerals prevent your muscles from cramping, in particular your stomach, and after a tiring hike it helps keep the water down.

Water is dense. To complete a 10-hour hike in the summer you may need to start with 10 to 20 pounds of the stuff on your back. The only redeeming feature is that your load will lighten up as you drink it and sweat it off, so that on the average you will be carrying only half what you start with. But this is still heavy, and it may adversely affect your enjoyment of the desert. It will also impact how far you can hike.

Spring water. There are several hundred seeps and springs within the park, so that the probability of encounter is not all that low. However, many of them carry no surface water. Most of the ones that do have never been tested, and in general they should be used only as a last resource. Always treat the water, either by boiling, filtering, or chemical treatment, as it is likely to be used by wildlife and biologically contaminated, in particular with giardia. I always carry with me a vial of iodine pills for such emergency. Before drinking the iodine-treated water, make sure to splash some of the water around the bottle opening, and let it do its job for at least 10 minutes (longer in cool weather). A touch of Kool Aid or equivalent helps disguise the bad taste of iodine. This treatment obviously does not get rid of minerals. If the water is heavily mineralized, it may upset your stomach (which still beats heat exhaustion).

Water caching. A good way to handle the water weight problem is to cache water ahead of time along your anticipated hiking route by a combination of driving and walking. This is a common strategy in multiple-day desert treks. It can also make day hikes more enjoyable. On a day hike that requires returning along the same route as going in, stash some water on your way in and pick it up on your way back. An optimum arrangement is to drop off one third of your water after traveling one third of the total distance. Plan ahead and keep your water in appropriately sized containers. When caching water for longer than a few hours, bury the containers to avoid unpleasant surprises. Animals have been known to chew through plastic jugs to get a free drink. Make sure to retrieve your containers, even if you don't need the water.

Always keep at least a couple of gallons of water in your car, for both human and machine emergency needs. This may be the best water caching tactic yet: these thoughtfully stored jugs may some day give you the most priceless, lukewarm and plastic-tasting swigs you've ever had.

Handling the Terrain

Desert hiking. Most hiking in Death Valley is cross-country. It means walking on alkali flats, sand, alluvial fans, gravel washes, canyon bedrock, and mountain slopes, most of which have very uneven surfaces. This is not very different from typical cross-country hiking, except for a few points. When applicable, the heat is one. Another one is that canyons are interrupted, more often than not, often more than once, by falls that must be climbed or bypassed. Also, when traveling up canyon, chances of wandering off into the wrong fork are amazingly good. When hiking down canyon, it takes special effort to get lost. Gravity is a foolproof guide: follow the path of least resistance and, barring major obstacles, you will eventually get to the canyon mouth. But when hiking up canyon in unfamiliar terrain without directions, at the first fork where the two branches look alike you'll have a 50% chance of taking the wrong branch. It is frustrating if you are trying to get to a good spot, a lot more serious if you are trying to get back to your car. The easiest remedy is to use a good map and keep track of where you are. Another one, if you have to go down canyon first and then return up the same canyon, is to pay attention to the turns you make on your way down.

Cross-country hiking provides a greater sense of freedom than hiking on trails, but it is more strenuous, and slower. If you are not familiar with it, start with easy places and slowly graduate to more challenging places. Travel with a friend. Other than the pleasure of sharing a great place with someone you like, it makes traveling safer and easier.

The park also offers a few maintained trails and hundreds of miles of abandoned mining roads and trails to hike on. The condition of these roads is variable, although because of the slow rate of erosion it is often surprisingly good.

To cope with the rough terrain, use lightweight hiking boots, especially if you are prone to twisting your ankles. I prefer running shoes padded with air or a gel. Though not as sturdy, they are lighter, more comfortable, and on long hikes the padding greatly reduces wear and tear on knees, ankles and hips.

Hiking time. In the text I seldom mention hiking time, a variable that depends too strongly on individual performance and traveling conditions to be meaningful. To fill this gap, here is a guideline specific to desert hiking. On fairly level cross-country terrain, count on hiking at about 80% of your normal hiking speed on established trails—from a typical 3 mph to 2.5 mph. With a light daypack you can expect to cover 12 to 14 miles in an eight hour-day, including breaks. Allow for additional time when traveling uphill, about 10 minutes per 1,000 feet, and for handling difficult falls and other obstructions. If you are carrying a backpack, count on 1.5 to 2 mph, including breaks, a little less in very hot weather, when you might need to rest 10 minutes or so every hour.

USGS maps. On any serious hike, take a topographic map with you. If hiking is old hat to you, this is an obvious statement. Otherwise, you may need to learn how to read topo maps to be able to venture out there without wandering aimlessly. Topos also come in handy to figure out what this small side canyon you are passing by may have in store, how far a potential goal is, or to plan a trip from your home.

USGS topographic maps of the Death Valley region are available from many USGS outlets and sporting goods stores throughout the country, and from the Visitor Center. The most useful maps for hiking are the 7.5' maps, which provide the greatest level of detail. The 15' maps (which are being discontinued) are helpful to zero in on distant features for orientation. Unless you intend to cover a good fraction of a map, you may want to take with you only photocopies of the targeted areas. They are easier to carry and consult in the field than original maps, and they can be mistreated.

As essential as they are, the USGS topographic maps are not free of errors, especially the 7.5' maps. The most common errors range from mildly annoying to confusing, and should not cause you much trouble. They include occasional mislabelled contours, and missing or misplaced features. The location of Desolation Canyon, for example, was wrong on the 15' map, and it is still wrong on the 7.5' map. On the 7.5' map the Grotto Canyon and Twenty Mule Team Canyon roads are incomplete. Unfortunately, the 7.5' Death Valley maps also contain worse errors that may put hikers in trouble by making them think something exists that is actually not there (or vice versa). This includes a few imaginary roads (as in Sheep Canyon), missing springs (as in Marble Canyon), and the omission of most impassable falls. In many cases, these falls are high and wide enough that, according to the 7.5' map accuracy claimed by the USGS, they should show as contour lines running into each other. Such errors are potentially dangerous. If you blindly trust the map and find yourself stopped by a fall just when you thought you were home, you may face a much longer return trip than anticipated. One way to avoid a nasty surprise is to look on the map for particularly steep, narrow, and deep places. They are usually potential fall areas. Also check the book maps and text, which mention most high falls.

Backcountry Regulations

To protect the park's environment, its resources, and its visitors, the NPS imposes a number of regulations for backcountry use, reproduced below. Since they are likely to change over time, make sure to also obtain a current list of regulations before heading out.

Backcountry camping. Backcountry camping is permitted 2 miles beyond any developed area, paved road, and "day use only" dirt road. The latter include:
- Racetrack Valley Road from Teakettle Jct to Homestake Dry Camp
- Titus Canyon Road
- Keane Wonder Mine Road
- Cottonwood Canyon Road (first 8 miles)
- Mosaic Canyon Road
- Grotto Canyon Road
- Skidoo Road
- Aguereberry Point Road
- Wildrose Canyon Road
- West Side Road

Camping is *not* allowed
- at the Lost Burro Mine
- at the Ubehebe Mine
- at the Inyo Mine

- on the valley floor from 2 miles north of Stovepipe Wells down
  to Ashford Mill
- within 200 yards of all water sources to protect them for
  wildlife use

Camping should also be avoided near all mining areas both for personal safety and to protect these fragile resources. Overnight group size is limited to 15 people and no more than six vehicles. Larger groups should contact the Chief Ranger for a Special Use Permit.

Off-road driving. Driving off roads is prohibited. Stay on established roadways to prevent vehicle damage.

Mountain bikes. Bicycles are allowed on all paved and open dirt roads and on the bike path near the Visitor Center. They are *not* allowed off roads, on trails, or in the wilderness areas of the park.

Horseback riding. Horse use is allowed except in developed campgrounds and on paved roads. Because water and forage is scarce, grazing animals are discouraged.

Fires. To prevent wildfires and conserve the scant supply of desert wood, ground fires are not allowed in the backcountry, even in portable fire pits. For the same reasons, the gathering of native wood, dead or alive, as well as lumber from historical structures, is unlawful. If you intend to cook, bring a stove and your own fossil fuel.

Garbage. Pack out all garbage; do not bury any of it, biodegradable or not. Bury human waste at least six inches deep.

Wildlife. Feeding wildlife, including coyotes, ravens, and roadrunners, is prohibited. When wild animals are fed by humans they tend to depend on this food source rather than forage for their natural diet. Some wild animals also carry communicable diseases, like rabies.

Pets. Pets are permitted in developed areas and on roads. They must be leashed and restrained at all times. Pets are not allowed off roads, on trails, and in the wilderness areas of the park.

Weapons. Weapons are strictly prohibited. This applies to firearms, air guns, bows and arrows, slingshots, and similar weapons.

Private properties. Please respect all private properties, including the many patented claims located within the park boundaries.

Natural environment. The removal of rocks, historical and prehistorical artifacts, plants, or animals is strictly prohibited. Leave the park undisturbed for others to enjoy. The use of metal detectors is prohibited.

Backcountry permits. At the time of writing no permit is required for overnight backcountry use. However, this policy may change in the future, so check with park rangers. Also, for safety reasons the NPS advises backpackers to get a permit. A sound idea. If you get in trouble in an isolated spot, it could be weeks before anyone happens to come along, and this simple measure could save your life. Permits are available at the Visitor Center, in person or over the phone. All you need to do is indicate where you intend to travel, for how long, and basic information about your party to facilitate a search. You can optionally request the NPS to initiate a search if you fail to check in within 24 hours of the time of your planned return. In this case, after your return you must check in at one of the ranger stations, either in person or by phone ((760) 786-3244 from 8 a.m. to 7 p.m. in winter, 6 p.m. in summer) to let them know you are back and they are off the hook. A permit can be used for a multiple-day overnight trip or just for a day hike. Try to take advantage of this unique option. Most parks don't offer to come and get you if you don't show up!

The other reason for wanting a permit is that in the state of California a vehicle left parked on the side of the road for more than 48 hours may legally be considered as abandoned by the highway patrol. On one occasion, returning from a day hike to my car parked on Highway 190 I found a sticker on the windshield politely pointing out that "Section 22669 Vehicle Code provides for removal of a vehicle when an officer has reasonable grounds to believe it is abandoned." Given that in Death Valley, removal of a vehicle (and the water and food thoughtfully stashed in it) could create a life-threatening situation for an exhausted hiker, it is doubtful that an officer will have it towed, even after a few days. But to be on the safe side, register, especially if you are planning to leave your car unattended for several days. If there is a question about your vehicle, the highway patrol will contact the Park Service, realize you are out there hiking, and leave your car alone.

Rock Climbing

One of the pleasures and greatest challenges of canyon hiking is climbing the dry falls that often block the way. Falls are near vertical discontinuities in the floor of a canyon, ranging from a few to tens of feet in height. Sooner or later, when hiking around Death Valley, you'll come upon a fall you can't circumvent and must climb. Although many falls can be easily and safely climbed, others are extremely difficult to scale, even for experienced climbers.

If you have never done serious rock climbing, be aware that climbing can be dangerous and should not be attempted carelessly, especially far from well-travelled areas. The best advice I can give to novices is not to climb alone, or at least to let someone know where you are. In case of an accident, having a partner can save your life. Also, where one person finds it impossible to climb, two or more people can sometimes make it by helping each other. To this end, bring a short length of rope or webbing. A crucial point to remember is that climbing down is often much more difficult than climbing up. To avoid getting stuck, before climbing up make sure that you can come back down. Finally, don't push your luck. If a fall looks too difficult, look for a safer way around it. Alternative routes often exist, and they can be more fun. If none is available, turn around. There is plenty more to see elsewhere.

Rock climbers will find throughout the park hundreds of good climbing areas, most of them for bouldering, others for wall climbing, with difficulties covering the full spectrum. For obvious reasons, I mention only a fraction of the climbing possibilities in this book. Narrows and high falls, which are generally indicated in the text, often offer good climbing surfaces. Most high climbing walls are in the range of tens of feet high, rarely higher than 100 feet. However, many of the high falls have been polished to a glass finish, and they can be a great challenge even for the best climbers. When hiking in canyons likely to contain falls, bring your climbing shoes.

Top-roping is often not possible because of the lack of natural anchors or bolts. Death Valley National Park does not have a set policy on rock climbing, largely because it is so infrequently practiced. However, should some climbing areas become cluttered with bolts, chalk marks, bits of webbing and other beautifying artifacts, chances are that stricter policies will be adopted. To keep this park hassle free as long as possible, inquire before establishing an artificial route. In the limited confines of a canyon, bolts are much too conspicuous, and they will destroy the unspoiled character of the wildest place. Also, refrain from using chalk. Rain will not clean up after you, and chalk marks in the wild are an eye-sore. Unless you are tackling difficult moves (5.11 or higher) in humid weather, there is little reason to use it.

Carefulness is the motto of climbers. Because of the remoteness of the Death Valley region, be more careful than ever.

Hazards

Dehydration and strokes. For about three months of the year and at low elevations the combination of heat and low humidity creates a serious potential for dehydration. It is important to be able to recognize the symptoms of dehydration to take timely measures. The first symptom is thirst, which is not simply a physical discomfort but a signal that your body has lost water and needs to be hydrated. Most people will feel thirsty after a water loss of less than 0.5% of their body weight, or about 0.5 to 1 quart. Look for signs of dehydration, such as persistent thirst or dark urine, and immediately increase your water intake.

Prolonged exposure to heat without sufficient intake of water produces further body water loss and may lead to heat exhaustion. Blood is then directed away from the brain to irrigate and cool the skin, resulting in excessive sweating, dizziness, tiredness, and vomiting. Take these warning signs seriously: they are telling you that you may be in trouble. Find a place sheltered from the sun and breeze, and rest. Drink plenty of mineralized water, at least a couple of quarts. Often this will restore sufficient strength to travel again.

If water loss and exertion are allowed to persist, a heat stroke may occur next. Blood becomes too thick to be pumped fast enough through the body and glands stop producing sweat. The main body cooling mechanisms essentially shut down. The symptoms are red, dry skin, headache, fever, dizziness, delirium, and nausea. This serious condition requires prompt medical attention. In the meantime keep the victim cool, in the shade, covered with wet clothes, if possible.

By using simple preventative measures based largely on common sense, these heat-related problems can be easily avoided. First and foremost, drink often. Don't save your water for later: stockpiling it in your canteen doesn't do you any good. Thirst lags behind your body's need for water, so *don't wait until you are thirsty to drink*. In hot weather, drink every 15 to 30 minutes, even if you think you don't need it. Always take plenty of water with you. *Do not wander into the desert without water, even for an intended short walk.* You never know how long you'll be out there.

Your clothing can help your body handle the heat better. Wear a wide brimmed hat. Granted, a hat can be a silly looking thing, and it does tend to mess up your hair, but the benefits greatly outweigh these minor inconveniences. Wearing a hat reduces water loss through your head and exposure to harmful ultraviolet radiation. Dress lightly, but do wear a light-colored long-sleeved shirt and long pants. Covering your skin reduces water loss by insulating your body from the heat source. As your sweat-soaked clothes cool down through evaporation, they will also bring some measure of comfort. Use high-potency sunblock lotion and chapstick, liberally and often.

Avoid hiking around midday. Get an early start, preferably before day break for long hikes, and benefit from the most enjoyable morning hours. By mid-morning, when the temperature has soared to uncomfortable levels, find the deepest available shade and relax for a while. Resume hiking in the late afternoon when the sun is lower, there is a little more shade, and the temperature has started to drop.

Windy conditions are fairly common in Death Valley. A good breeze makes you feel better by cooling your body, but it does so at the cost of accelerated water loss. In hot weather, stay away from the wind.

If this is not possible, keep your clothes on, even just a thin layer, to cut down the drying power of the wind.

If you run out of water, and you are too far from potable water to reach it without getting in more trouble, check your map for less than reliable water. If your situation is not so desperate as to warrant taking a chance at drinking questionable water, use it to soak your clothes and a cloth to wrap around your head, which will cool you down. I have used this natural form of refrigeration in deserts around the world, sometimes with dubious well water, and it has gotten me out of trouble several times. If there is no water around, rest in the shade, and do not resume walking until the temperature has dropped.

Mine hazards. Old mining areas are prime hiking goals in the desert. Entering mines, like tunnels and caves, somehow holds a special fascination that some people, including myself, just can't seem to resist. Many of the mine tunnels out there are old, unsupported, and very dangerous. Existing supporting structures have not been checked in decades and are generally shaky and equally dangerous. Other potential dangers include concealed pits, sharp rusted tools, collapsing ground, pockets of odorless and deadly carbon monoxide, etc.

To avoid trouble, the first basic rule is quite simple: don't enter any mine tunnel. If you decide to break this first rule, at least follow the second rule: do not go in without a flashlight. For example, rattlesnakes are known to hole up in old tunnels, and you certainly don't want to make one of these little buggers feel cornered. If you decide to break both of the first two rules, do follow the third one: don't venture beyond where you can see. Sometimes a tunnel will lead into a hidden slanted drift or vertical shaft. If you decide to break all three rules, chances are pretty good nothing will go wrong. But then again, it may be years before someone finds out exactly what happened to you.

In the vicinity of a few particularly dangerous mining areas, the NPS has posted warning signs. It's a good idea to read them. For your protection, in some popular areas the most treacherous openings have been covered with wiring, boarded up, or fenced off. Take the hint seriously and stay away. Consider all mines as hazardous.

Snakes. If you are new to the desert, it may well conjure up images of empty spaces infested with temperamental and very deadly snakes. To alleviate your concerns, bear in mind these few facts. Snakes are nowhere numerous, especially in Death Valley. They are largely nocturnal. Of the numerous species residing here, only three are venomous. The desert night snake and California lyre snake have mildly toxic venom. Rattlesnakes are the only ones with strong venom, and they are rarely encountered. In the last 15 years, I have seen only three rattlers in the park. A snake's body temperature is the same as the ambient temperature. When the air temperature exceeds 90°F, which implies ground temperatures well above 100°F, rattlers do not survive very long in full sun. Being smarter than your typical hiker, at such times they generally hole up in shaded areas and wait it out. So in hot weather it's relatively safe to walk on ground fully exposed to the sun. Like other snakes, rattlers are not vicious; they don't strike for the hell of it. Unless molested or cornered, upon detecting your presence they are much more likely to escape than fight. Just give them a chance and move out of their way; remember *you* are the intruder.

That's the good news. But the danger is still real. Of all the potential natural hazards that are largely out of your control—such as being hit by falling rocks, lightning, or flash floods—I would rank a nasty encounter with a rattler as the most probable. A rattlesnake bite is a major accident that requires prompt medical assistance. It can be painful, quite harmful, sometimes fatal, certainly at least temporarily disabling, and if it happens in the middle of nowhere you are not going to be able to walk very far to get help.

Here are a few precautions you should take while hiking. Stay alert. Do not jump onto a shaded area or an area you can't see well. Be particularly careful when climbing up. Learn to tell a rattler from harmless snakes. Carry a snake bite kit with you, and be familiar with its contents and how to use it properly (read what Dave Gancy has to say about it in his desert survival book). Be familiar with the physiological effects of a bite, and learn what you should do to take care of it.

Mountain lions. These rare predators don't exactly abound in the park, but they have been sighted and should be mentioned as a potential hazard. Should you encounter a lion showing hostile behavior, here is the current wisdom. Do not approach it, and don't run from it either, or you may trigger a chase. Do all you can to appear as large as possible. Spread out your arms, open your jacket if you have one. Do not crouch or bend over. Speak firmly in a low voice. If attacked, fight back. On several reported occasions, throwing stones worked. All this being said, one should add that the probability of an encounter with a lion is extremely low. I have seen in the wild about two dozen lions, all of them in East Africa. Don't let the thought of lions spoil your day. It would be like staying indoors to avoid getting hit by a meteor.

Flash floods. Although Death Valley's climate is extremely dry, it does rain a little, and a little rainfall over a large area can go a long way. Precipitation, especially in the summer, can occur in violent cloud bursts. These downpours are so sudden that much of the water runs off the nonabsorbent and sparsely vegetated desert soil to the nearest drainage, where it can collect into a forceful stream with devastating power. For a short time, usually no more than a few hours, normally dry washes are alive with raging torrents of slurry, powerful enough to transport anything from gravel to boulders over several miles.

Numerous accounts of such violent rainstorms have been recorded in the 150-year history of Death Valley. In 1901 a flash flood swept away much of Panamint City, a mile-long silver-mining town of more than 200 stone buildings in Surprise Canyon. In July 1950, a huge cloudburst over the Funeral Mountains sent boisterous mud torrents down Furnace Creek Wash. In a few hours it gauged six-foot deep channels in the highway that runs along the wash and buried it under as much as four feet of gravel. In the summer of 1990 the road above Scotty's Castle was closed for four weeks after a violent storm covered miles of asphalt with alluvia. Just about every year, somewhere in the park a main canyon gets vigorously scoured.

If you do any extensive hiking in the summer, keep floods in mind. The simplest precautionary measure is to consult the weather forecast. The Visitor Center and the main ranger stations receive weather report updates every day around 10 a.m. Inquire about the forecast by phone or in person. If a major storm is expected, either postpone your trip or be particularly careful. The second preventative measure is to stay alert. Periodically inspect the sky up canyon. Listen for what has been described as the roar of an approaching freight train, perhaps the best advance warning you'll ever get. If a storm is threatening while you are in a canyon, walk on higher ground as often as possible. In narrows, keep an eye out for escape routes to higher places. By climbing 10 feet above the wash you'll be above the water level of most flash floods. Twenty feet should take care of the worst situations, except in the tightest narrows, where far higher floods can occur. Always camp at least 20 feet above the wash, and never in narrows.

Perhaps the best protective measure against flash floods and all other hazards is to let someone know where you are going and when you are planning to return (see *Backcountry permits*).

Backcountry Driving

Road conditions and vehicle requirements. To reach some of the most remote areas in the park requires driving on its extensive network of primitive roads. The one thing that should be said at the outset about the condition of these roads is that it can change dramatically with time—temporarily or irreversibly. After a good rain, unpaved roads can become impracticable for a few days until the ground dries out. The obvious corollary is that if you are several miles out on a primitive road with a passenger car and it starts pouring, don't hang around too long or you may not be able to drive back for some time. Over longer periods of time, storms and wear take their toll and perfectly good roads become impassable, even for the most sturdy vehicles. The reverse also happens when the Park Service grades an old beat-up road. So bear in mind that the road conditions mentioned in the text may have become partially or completely incorrect.

In general, though, maintained roads are in good shape and passable with standard 2-wheel-drive vehicles. Unmaintained roads often require high clearance, more rarely 4-wheel drive as well. This is an important point to remember: clearance is often more critical than power. "Urban" 4-wheel-drive sedans often don't fair better than a normal vehicle because their clearance is only marginally higher.

Your determination to get there is also an important factor. It depends on how daring you are, and how willing you are to take your car—or your favorite rental agency's car—on a "bad" road. A friend and I once drove my Honda Accord down the Gold Valley Road towards Willow Spring, a good archetype of a "bad" road. At the worst spots one of us walked ahead of the car to move the largest rocks out of the way. We gave up before the spring, but we had driven far enough to backpack the rest of the way in the limited time we had left. Driving a rough road with a lightweight vehicle can be an adventure—in fact, more so than with a rugged vehicle. If you do it right (meaning if you bring enough food and water, let someone know where you are, and don't have an important meeting on Monday morning) it can be a lot of fun.

If you like this kind of experience, one thing you should know is that park rangers are asked to advocate caution—a sound policy, which undoubtedly prevents a lot of people from getting in trouble. The down side is a general tendency to cry wolf. Even if you know how to drive backcountry roads with a less-than-optimum vehicle, I still advise you to inquire about road conditions beforehand. Just be aware that the information you'll get may need interpretation. Rangers will tell you if the road is closed to motor vehicles, washed out, or snowed in, and suggest alternate routes, possibly saving you a lot of needless driving.

Seasonal road closure. In the winter some of the roads may be closed for a few days due to snowstorms, especially Highway 190 at Towne Pass. Highway 190 to Death Valley Junction and Highway 178 to Shoshone go over lower passes and are hardly ever closed.

It has been a park policy in the past to close a few backcountry roads to motorized traffic during the summer. The main reason is that cars get stranded in the middle of nowhere, usually from overheating, and the limited staff cannot afford to patrol every single backcountry road every day to rescue unfortunate travelers. The roads subject to closure are the Titus Canyon Road, the West Side Road north from the Warm Spring Canyon Road, and the two short roads into Desolation and Natural Bridge canyons. The exact closure period varies from year to year, but it is generally from May through mid-October. During this period these roads remained open to hiking. Also, the Titus Canyon Road and the West Side Road can still be driven by obtaining the key to the gates at the Visitor Center. You will have to tell a ranger where you are going and for how long. If you prefer to be alone, you can also check whether another party is going to be in the same area. If you get in trouble and fail to return the key at the prearranged time, the Park Service will send out a rescue patrol. This policy may or may not remain in effect in the future. Inquire at the Visitor Center.

Getting unstuck. If you put in enough unpaved miles with a standard passenger car, sooner or later you will get stuck. The usual scenario goes something like this: the car stops going forward, the rear wheels loose traction, spin into the ground, and bury themselves part way to the axles. Bad news. The first thing to do is to stop feeding gas as soon as your car is stuck. If you are on a slope, it is usually easy to push your vehicle out of the bad spot and try again. On level ground, pushing or driving the car forward and backward repeatedly and slowly acquiring momentum is often effective. Otherwise, try to dig the wheels out. For such emergencies, always keep in your trunk a shovel, a few sturdy boards, and a jack. Dig a trench in the front of the buried tires deep enough to jam a board underneath both of them for better traction, or jack up the car to slip a board or rocks underneath the tires, and slowly drive out of the ruts. At high noon in July it can be a painful process, but the alternatives are usually worse, so give it a serious try.

Looking for help. If you can't get unstuck, or if your vehicle breaks down and you can't fix the problem, stay with your vehicle and wait for help to come to you. It's a lot easier for rescuers to spot a stranded vehicle than a wandering human being. Open all doors to make your vehicle more visible and to provide some shade. Use the horn and headlights for signals. Be prepared for such emergencies. Always keep in your vehicle plenty of water and food, a flashlight, matches, a rope, jumper cables, a tool box, at least one spare tire, and a good book. Leave your vehicle only if you are certain you can walk to help safely.

Wilderness Ethics

Some day others will visit this place after you, and they probably would prefer not to be reminded that you were here. So please practice minimum impact hiking. When other hikers are nearby, be as quiet as possible. Minimize the traces you leave behind: walk softly, on gravel rather than on the plants, on bedrock rather than gravel. Most perennial desert plants are slow growers. The scrawny-looking bushes you walk by on fans and washes have been giving it their best for usually much more than a decade. Even plants looking half dead are half alive, therefore alive. Avoid stepping near or on them, as they heal very slowly. Pack out what you pack in. Practice low impact camping. Do not discard organic matter, which may take months to decompose in the dry climate. Build cairns only when absolutely necessary, and make sure to destroy them on your way back. They will otherwise mislead other hikers, and will often be resented as an intrusion.

One of my strongest recommendations is to avoid hiking in large groups. Besides violating the wilderness spirit, this form of hiking can have a strongly negative impact on the desert. Where a few hikers will often fan out and scatter their tracks over some area, large groups tend to walk in a single line and leave a more pronounced trail. In the desert the soft soil gets marred easily, rain does not clean up anything fast, and such tracks take years to disappear. Groups are also almost always noisy and highly visible. This is quite unfair for lone hikers who have the misfortune to run into one of them miles from nowhere.

Leave everything where you find it for others to enjoy. The bits and pieces of metal scattered around old mines and camps have great historical value and are irreplaceable. If every visitor was to take away one item, one of Death Valley's greatest treasures would be forever gone in just a few years.

Archaeological sites, in Death Valley as elsewhere, are protected by law. In 1980, the Bureau of Land Management estimated that as many as 35% of the desert archaeological sites in the United States showed signs of degradation by vandalism, and that despite public education, wilderness designation, and enforcement, about one percent continue to be damaged or stolen every year. In Death Valley National Park, some rock art sites are being increasingly damaged by graffiti, and artifacts have been stolen. Here again, common sense spells out what should be avoided. The best rule is not to touch anything. It applies to rock art (which tarnishes and wears under repeated contact), rock alignments (which lose their significance when disturbed), and ruins and artifacts (which should remain intact for others to enjoy and study).

The prehistoric and historic archaeological sites found in the park, including the few sites mentioned in this book, are strongly tied to the heritage of the contemporary Native Americans of the Death Valley region. As such, they are very important to their traditions, and many of them are sacred. They are also protected by the law. Treat them with respect, and leave them the way they are for others to enjoy.

■

SERVICES

This chapter lists the main services available in the park, including restaurants, stores, service stations, campgrounds, and accommodations. Also check the free NPS visitor guide, available at the Visitor Center and check-in points, which also provides the current operating hours of these and other services.

Food

After a tiring day hike or few days in the wild, you may want to eat out and relax rather than do your own cooking. Furnace Creek Ranch offers several restaurants, including a steak house and a cafeteria. Hours are flexible, and not all of them are opened year-round. The buffet breakfast at the steak house is actually quite all right. Furnace Creek Inn serves food that might even tease a French palate, although their prices are just on this side of extortionate. If you are looking for a hearty breakfast prior to hitting the trail, or a good, down-to-earth American dinner, try the dining room at Stovepipe Wells. It serves some of the best food in the valley in a homey atmosphere, quieter than at the ranch. It is open all year, although it is buffet style in the low season. There is also a small snack bar at Scotty's Castle. While visiting the west side of the park, you can also eat at Panamint Springs, a privately-owned resort opened year-round where locals like to hang out. It has a rustic dining room, a small patio, and a pleasantly shaded veranda.

Two general stores, at Furnace Creek and Stovepipe Wells, carry groceries and basic supplies. Costs run high and selections are understandably limited, so stock up before coming here. Greater selections are available from some of the surrounding towns, in particular Beatty, Lone Pine, Trona, and Ridgecrest.

Public Showers

Public showers are available at Panamint Springs and Stovepipe Wells (inquire at the motel office). The public showers at Furnace Creek Ranch, closed some time ago, may be re-opened in the future. Inquire at the motel desk for possible use of the swimming pool showers.

Campgrounds

Death Valley National Park offers 11 campgrounds to choose from, widely distributed throughout the central portion of the park and ranging in elevation from -196 to 8,200 feet. Nine of them are operated by the NPS. The other two, namely the small resort at Panamint Springs and the small Fred Harvey RV Park at Stovepipe Wells (which does not allow tenting), are privately owned. All campgrounds have flush toilets, except for the three campgrounds in Wildrose Canyon, which have pit toilets only. Refer to the general map of the park for the location of these campgrounds, and to the table below for more information.

During the peak season and on long weekends, the Furnace Creek campgrounds are generally full by mid-afternoon, if not sooner. Advance reservations can be made from October through April at the Furnace Creek (all sites) and Texas Spring (group sites) campgrounds. Reservations can also be made at Panamint Springs, but they are only needed on long weekends, holidays, and in the summer. All other campgrounds are available on a first come, first serve basis. The Stovepipe Wells Campground is hardly ever full for trailers, but it quickly runs out of tent-only sites. If you don't want to have to pitch your tent between two trailers, secure a tent site in the morning. Remember that these sites are coveted. Before taking off for the day, put up your tent or leave an "occupied" sign (preferably bolted to the table), or chances are amazingly good you'll find your site occupied when you return.

Quiet hours are 10:00 p.m. to 7:00 a.m. Generators may be operated only between 7:00 a.m. and 7:00 p.m., except at Texas Spring where generators are not permitted. In spite of these rules the campgrounds are often quite noisy well into the quiet hours. If this is likely to bother you,

Campground	Elev.	Season	Sites	Water	Firepits	Sanitary Station
Furnace Creek	-196'	All year	136	✓	✓	✓
Texas Spring	0'	Oct.-Apr.	92	✓	✓	✓
Sunset	-190'	Oct.-Apr.	1,000	✓		✓
Stovepipe Wells	0'	Oct.-Apr.	200	✓	✓	✓
Fred Harvey RV Park	0'	All year	14	✓		✓
Panamint Springs	1,930'	All year	84	✓		✓
Emigrant	2,100'	Apr.-Oct.	10	✓		
Mesquite Spring	1,780'	All year	30	✓	✓	✓
Wildrose	4,100'	All year*	30	Apr.-Nov.	✓	
Thorndike[+]	7,500'	Mar.-Nov.*	8		✓	
Mahogany Flat[+]	8,200'	Mar.-Nov.*	10		✓	

* Weather permitting
[+] Dirt road; no trailers, campers, or motor homes; 4WD may be necessary

you may find it worthwhile to sleep at more remote campgrounds or in the wild (see *Backcountry Regulations* in *Desert Hiking Tips*).

Lodging

Panamint Springs, Stovepipe Wells, Furnace Creek Inn, and Furnace Creek Ranch offer motel accommodations. If they are all full, which happens for several weeks during the milder months, the closest alternatives are Beatty, Nevada (which has several motels), the Longstreet Inn 7 miles north of Death Valley Junction, or better yet the Amargosa Hotel at Death Valley Junction.

Service Stations

The service stations in the park are at Furnace Creek, Stovepipe Wells, Scotty's Castle, and Panamint Springs. Diesel fuel is available at Furnace Creek, Beatty, Panamint Springs, Trona, Olancha, and Lone Pine. The only mechanics on duty are at Furnace Creek. If they can't do the job, they usually farm it out to closest services in Beatty. Towing services are available from the Furnace Creek gas station and Beatty, Nevada. If you are in trouble and don't have their number handy, call 911. If you need a 4-wheel-drive vehicle, you can rent one from the Furnace Creek Chevron. If you need it for just one or two days, it may be cheaper than to drive your own guzzler all the way from home.

Visitor Center

The Visitor Center at Furnace Creek is a great source of information about Death Valley and the Mojave Desert. In spite of the size of the area under the NPS jurisdiction, there is almost always someone knowledgeable about your particular interest to give you an answer. You can also browse through an impressive selection of books, pamphlets, and articles about the human and natural history of the region. The Visitor Center offers daily ranger-led hikes, evening programs, and a variety of slide shows on the natural and human history of Death Valley. The complete series of USGS 7.5' topographic maps covering the park area is also available for purchase. The 15' maps are displayed for consultation.

If you are planning an extended trip on some of the primitive roads in the park and vicinity, it is a good idea to first stop by or call the Visitor Center or a ranger station to inquire about road conditions. You can also ask about the weather forecast, the hours of various local services, the condition of the passes in the winter, etc. Given that it can take several hours to drive to your destination, this knowledge can represent a significant time saving.

This information is also available from any of the ranger stations at Stovepipe Wells, Grapevine, Scotty's Castle, Beatty, and Shoshone. These smaller operations have more restricted hours and limited staff, but if need be their staff will contact the Visitor Center to get the information you need.

Death Valley National Park is a fee area. Fees are collected at the Visitor Center in Furnace Creek and at the Grapevine Entrance Station. This will give you a permit valid up to one week, and renewable up to a maximum yearly stay of four weeks. You can also purchase an annual pass (Golden Eagle Passport), valid in all federal recreation fee areas for one year from the date of issue.

Useful Phone Numbers
(Area code 760, unless otherwise specified)

Lodging
Furnace Creek Ranch	786-2345
Furnace Creek Inn	786-2361
Panamint Springs	(775) 482-7680
Stovepipe Wells	786-2387
Amargosa Hotel	(800) 952-4441
	or 852-4441

Campgrounds Reservations
Furnace Creek & Texas Spring	(800) 365-2267
Panamint Springs	(775) 482-7680
Emergency (24 hours)	786-2330
	or 911
Fire Department	786-2444
Furnace Creek Auto Repair	786-2232
Furnace Creek Visitor Center / Information	786-2331
Hiker's check-in	786-3244

Ranger Stations
Furnace Creek	786-2331
Scotty's Castle	786-2342
Stovepipe Wells	786-2387
Ashford-Shoshone	852-4308
Towing (Furnace Creek Ranch)	786-2232

■

PART II

GRAPEVINE MOUNTAINS

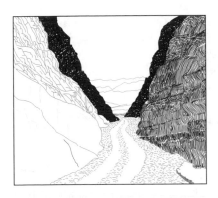

THE GRAPEVINE MOUNTAINS form the eastern boundary of northern Death Valley. The northern section, north from Grapevine Canyon, is a sprawling range lower than 8,000 feet, about 25 miles wide, and surrounded on all sides by valleys at least 3,000 feet high. The southern section, wider, higher and more rugged, rises almost 9,000 feet above the much lower floor of Death Valley. The highest summits there are Grapevine Peak (8,738') and Wahguyhe Peak (8,628'). As elsewhere in the Amargosa Range, the Grapevine Mountains are more steeply sloped on their western side, particularly near their southern end, between Red Wall and Titanothere canyons. In contrast, on their eastern side they drop only a few thousand feet to high desert country—Sarcobatus Flat and the Amargosa Desert.

Access

The southern Grapevine Mountains are surrounded by paved roads and generally fairly accessible. The easiest access to the greatest number of canyons is provided by the Scotty's Castle Road, which parallels the mountains fairly closely along Death Valley. From this road it is generally no more than a two-mile hike to the foot of the range. The eastern side of the Grapevine Mountains can be reached from the Daylight Pass Road and its Nevada extension, Highway 374. From around Beatty, Nevada, several unpaved roads cross the Bullfrog Hills and the Bullfrog Mining District westward. These high-clearance roads lead close to several east-side canyons, often reaching within a couple of miles of the crest. Titus Canyon is the only canyon in the southern Grapevines that is traversed by a road. This scenic backcountry road crosses the mountains from near Beatty all the way to Death Valley, and accesses some of the most rugged areas in the Grapevines. The portion of the northern Grapevine Mountains that belongs to the park, just north of Scotty's Castle, is best reached from the Big Pine Road.

Geology

The type of rocks you are most likely to see in the Grapevine Mountains are Paleozoic sedimentary rocks of marine origin. They make up most of the steep western front of the range. From Grapevine Peak to Boundary Canyon, the southern crest of the Grapevines is capped with Miocene volcanic rocks, mostly rhyolite. These rocks are fringed on their west side by small, fault-bound exposures of Oligocene volcanic rocks from the Titus Canyon Formation. The foot of the range is paralleled by the Furnace Creek Fault Zone, which more or less coincides with the Scotty's Castle Road. The scattered hills between the fault and the western foot of the range, in particular the Kit Fox Hills and the foothills stretching 10 miles south from the Grapevine Ranger Station, are made of younger deposits, mostly fanglomerates from the Funeral Formation.

Vegetation and Hydrology

Like the other ranges on the east side of Death Valley, the Grapevines lie in the rain shadow of the higher Panamint Range to the west. Thus they are fairly dry, and springs are generally scarce. The largest springs are Grapevine Springs, west of Scotty's Castle. Marked by conspicuously lush vegetation, they rise along a horizontal fault at the base of the western foothills. Their water has long been appropriated for human use at Scotty's Castle. Other springs on the west side include the luxuriant oasis in Grapevine Canyon around Scotty's Castle, Surprise Springs just south of Grapevine Canyon, Klare Spring in Titus Canyon, Lostman Spring in Titanothere Canyon, and Daylight Spring at the head of Boundary Canyon. The main springs on the Nevada side are Brier Spring near Strozzi Ranch, McDonald Spring, and Willow Spring. Despite their general dryness, the Grapevine Mountains are high enough to support a relatively extensive pinyon pine-juniper woodland, in the vicinity of the two highest peaks.

History

Although the portion of the Grapevine Mountains within the park has been left largely untouched by mining, it witnessed three major historical events. The first one is, of course, associated with Scotty's Castle. Located in the midst of lush springs in Grapevine Canyon, the site was first developed as a ranch in the 1880s by Jacob Staininger.

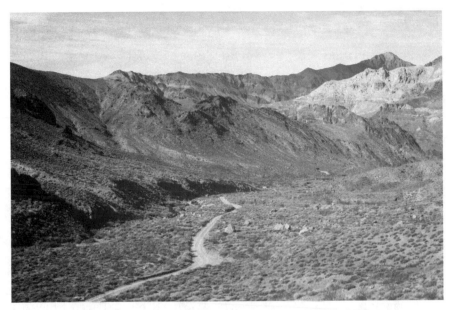

Grapevine Mountains from the Titus Canyon Road near Red Pass

Originally a farm boy from Pennsylvania, Staininger stayed here the rest of his life, raising mustangs and quails, and tending a small vineyard. Long after his death, Albert Johnson, a wealthy insurance executive from Chicago with a life-long involvement in the area, acquired Staininger Ranch. He and his wife used it as a base camp on their frequent visits to Death Valley, and their long-time friend Walter Scott, better known as Death Valley Scotty, occupied it between their visits. In the mid-1920s, Johnson used his personal fortune to build a mansion on the property, which was eventually named Scotty's Castle. Today, the alluring castle, in its contrasting setting of greenery and stark mountains, is the most visited site in the park.

The second significant historical area in the Grapevines is the Bullfrog Mining District, which was centered around the Bullfrog Hills, in the southeastern foothills of the mountains. Between 1904 and 1908, this was the site of one of the most feverish gold rushes in the history of Death Valley. The area eventually produced more gold than any other mine around, and it is still exploited today. The other notorious site is Leadfield, in a fork of Titus Canyon. In 1925 and 1926, prospectors and miners swarmed the area to investigate what was being hailed as the biggest lead-silver mine in the West. Although the venture quickly turned out to be unprofitable, the massive advertising campaign conducted by mining promoter Julian raised a lot of interest in the property for a while, and left a lasting imprint on the local lore.

Suggested Hikes in the Grapevine Mountains					
Route/Destination	Dist. (mi)	Elev. change	Mean elev.	Access road	Page
Short hikes (under 5 miles round trip)					
Fall Canyon to confluence	2.3	830'	1,355'	Graded	76
Leadfield	<1.0	<100'	4,040'	Graded	85
Titus Canyon first narrows	1.8	660'	1,270'	Graded	92
Titus Canyon (upper canyon)	2.1	950'	4,200'	P/16.5 mi	85-86
Intermediate hikes (5-12 miles round trip)					
Fall Canyon					
through tightest narrows	3.7	1,470'	1,670'	Graded	76-78
through lower narrows	4.3	1,660'	1,770'	Graded	76-78
Klare Spring	5.9	2,180'	2,030'	Graded	86, 92
Lostman Spring	4.3	1,900'	4,060'	Graded	95-98
Red Wall Canyon					
to first fall	3.2	1,520'	1,160'	Paved	69-70
through third narrows	5.7	3,000'	1,900'	Paved	69-74
Titus Canyon second narrows	4.0	1,480'	1,680'	Graded	92
Long hikes (over 12 miles round trip)					
Fall Canyon					
to third side canyon	6.9	2,640'	2,260'	Graded	76-78
Titus Canyon up to Leadfield	8.5	3,100'	2,490'	Graded	85, 92
Suggested overnight hikes (over 2 days)					
Fall Cyn-Red Wall Cyn loop*	29.8	12,800'	3,560'	Graded	76-80
Red Wall Canyon					
from highway	10.6	7,010'	3,900'	Paved	69-74
from mouth of Titus Cyn	14.7	7,950'	3,090'	Graded	70-74
Titanothere Canyon (rd to rd)	12.0	4,090'	2,560'	Graded	95-98
Titus Canyon Road	26.9	6,910'	3,950'	Paved	84, 92
Titus-Fall canyons loop*	18.3	7,560'	2,700'	Graded	85-86
Wahguyhe Peak (via Fall Cyn)	14.5	7,690'	4,780'	Graded	76-80

Key: P=Primitive (2WD)
* =Total distance and elevation change (ups + downs) for all loops

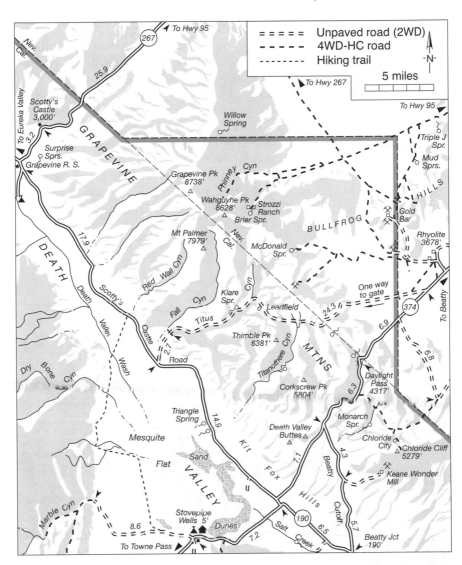

Hiking

The western slopes of the Grapevine Mountains are drained by several major canyons, most of them unnamed. Although not the most popular hiking destinations in the park, they can be the grounds for beautiful treks in totally wild country. Most of these canyons, especially north of Fall Canyon, are about a one-hour walk from the Scotty's Castle Road—a jaunt by Death Valley standards—yet long enough that seclusion is guaranteed. Since all but one of them are roadless, you will not be bothered by motor vehicles. Where the canyons cut through the steeper western scarp, they form deep, narrow, and spectacular swaths offering a combination of grand sceneries and narrow passages. The southern Grapevines contain, in fact, some of the longest consistently deep and narrow canyons in the park, especially Titus and Fall canyons.

The eastern Grapevines go through a smaller elevation change and are generally less spectacular, although equally wild. In the mid range, Phinney Canyon and Strozzi Ranch are the most interesting for their springs. They are both accessible via high-clearance roads and a little walking. These roads can also be the starting point of longer hikes, in particular to the wooded crest of the Grapevines. The crest can be reached by foot fairly easily from this side, and constitutes one of the attractions of hiking here. The extensive Bullfrog Mining District is also an exciting area to explore old gold mines.

■

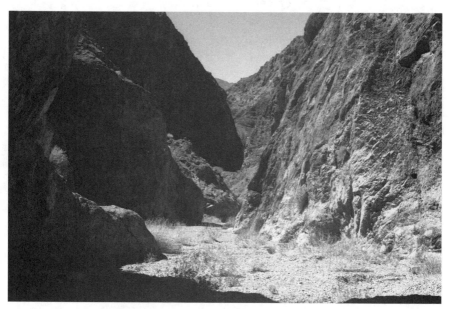

In the first narrows of Red Wall Canyon

RED WALL CANYON

Red Wall Canyon has some of the finest narrows in the park, a succession of tight corridors that wind deep beneath soaring red walls. The impressive first narrows have a 25-foot fall most people will find a challenge to climb. The second narrows also have a fall, much easier, nicely polished brecciated walls, and startling displays of slickensides illustrating the area's turbulent tectonic history. The challenge of the falls, the scenic beauty, and the unusual geology of this colorful outdoors museum combine to make a particularly delightful day hike.

General Information

Road status: Roadless; hiking from paved road
Shortest hike: 3.2 mi, 1,500 ft one way / moderate
Longest hike: 10.6 mi, 7,000 ft one way / difficult
Main attractions: Good narrows, geology, falls, rock climbing
USGS 15' topo map: Grapevine Peak
USGS 7.5' topo maps: Fall Canyon, Grapevine Peak
Maps: pp. 73*, 67

Location and Access

Red Wall Canyon is in the central Grapevine Mountains, north of Fall Canyon. It can be reached from either the Scotty's Castle Road or the end of the two-way dirt road at the mouth of Titus Canyon. For the first route, park anywhere around mile marker 19, 19 miles north of Highway 190 (13.8 miles south of the Grapevine Ranger Station). The mouth of Red Wall Canyon is the red gap at the apex of the alluvial fan a couple of miles away. For the second route, the starting point is the same as for Fall Canyon.

Route Description

The approach. The route from the Scotty's Castle Road is the shortest, requiring an easy, 45-minute walk up a moderately steep fan. An interesting feature to look for here is the varied fan vegetation and its distribution. Many plants grow only in specific niches defined by their heat tolerance and moisture requirement. The fairly uncommon strawtop cholla is found mostly at lower elevations, while the beavertail cactus occurs higher up, closer to the canyon mouth. Creosotes are larger and healthier near the toe of the fan, and the stingbush is often wedged along the cooler and moister banks of the washes. Desert-trumpet eriogonum and the hardy desert holly thrive all over. Look for large logs stranded on the gravel. These peeling, water-worn trunks were once trees growing more than eight meandering canyon miles away and 7,000 feet higher, in the sparse woodland visible near the crest of the Grapevines. The views of northern Death Valley get increasingly finer. The faint track cutting across the valley westward from the Scotty's Castle Road is the west side trail to the Niter Beds and Stovepipe Wells, which has been closed off to motor vehicles for decades. It is a good landmark to locate your car on the way back.

The second route, from the mouth of Titus Canyon, follows the base of the mountains for about 4.5 miles to the mouth of Red Wall Canyon, which is the fifth main canyon past Titus Canyon. It requires walking over or around several hills, and it is quite time consuming. However, it's a good backpacking route, passing by four narrow canyons, including Fall Canyon, all of which make exciting side trips.

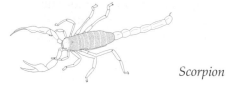

Scorpion

The first narrows. The first narrows start 0.5 mile in, at a conspicuous gateway where the wash squeezes between two high rock pillars. The next half a mile is an unevenly narrow corridor winding beneath high walls, rising sheer and flat like sandstone cliffs. These walls of dolomite and limestone stained by oxides are the namesake of this canyon. Their rich red prevails throughout the first two narrows, producing one of the most colorful canyons in Death Valley.

This tight stretch gradually deepens, passes by a nice alcove up on the north side, and is then blocked by the first fall, a 25-foot obstruction topped by a giant chockstone. The fall is climbed in three phases, first up a 10-foot polished chute to a small recess under the chockstone, then around the chockstone to a wide ledge, and finally over a 7-foot boulder jam. The only potentially dangerous part is the second step, which calls for an awkward move around the bulging chockstone on a slanted polished wall devoid of good holds. Rock climbers can also climb from directly underneath the boulder jam. Both routes are moderate (maybe only 5.6) but exposed, and the dolomite can be dusty and slippery. Climbing shoes help. If you are not a rock climber, it definitely helps to come here with a friend, who can provide that one missing foothold or handhold. The climb down is more difficult, and some people may find a rope handy, if only to lower heavy packs. At the top of the fall there is a gap between boulders to set a temporary 60-foot rope.

The remaining part of these narrows, above the falls, is the nicest in this canyon. In the afternoon this barren passage glows with the rich red light reflecting down from the narrow opening overhead. Most of these narrows are in dolomite, wildly shattered, brecciated, and folded, bearing witness to the tumultuous geological past of the Grapevine Mountains. This stretch contains striking examples of these intense deformations. Brecciated rock walls have been worn by water into colorful pastel mosaics. There are also some amazing displays of folded rocks. On the north wall just above the fall, severely deformed strata form an entangled pattern of folds bending as much as 180° over only a couple of feet.

The second narrows. The second narrows, 0.9 mile long, start just a little further. They boast colorful red walls, deeply undercut and hollowed at places, but their most unusual feature is slickensides. Red Wall

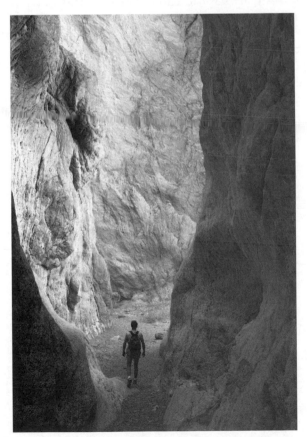

The author in the first narrows just above the 25-foot fall

Canyon was formed along a minor fault. As the two facing rock surfaces along such a fault grind past each other during tectonic activity, they gouge into each other parallel grooves called slickensides. The most conspicuous slickenside is on the south wall just above the wash, in a left bend about 0.3 mile into the second narrows. This bright red, smooth wall is covered with fine horizontal grooves and dark, glazed and polished streaks, created when it ground against the huge block leaning against it on the right. The sheer size of this block bears witness to the tremendous energy involved. In the mountains of Death Valley, motion along fault lines is usually vertical, but here it is horizontal. This type of fault is called a strike-slip. There are many other slickensides in these narrows; periodically look back and higher up on the walls.

The narrows gradually taper down and deepen to a tortuous core, then open up slowly. Near the neck there is a second high fall. Twelve feet high and well polished, it has good footholds and handholds and is relatively easy to climb, both up and down. Above it the narrows boast numerous undercuts and a few alcoves.

Just beyond the second narrows is the first significant side canyon, on the north side. In 0.15 mile this narrow passage is blocked by a towering drop-off, impressive high walls, and beautiful polished cascades banded in gray and orange.

The third narrows. The third narrows, starting shortly past the side canyon, are somewhat similar to the first two, although shallower and not as colorful. They narrow gradually to a 12-foot wide passage

	Red Wall Canyon	
	Dist.(mi)	Elev.(ft)
Scotty's Castle Road	0.0	400
Mouth	2.3	1,460
1st narrows (start)	2.8	1,710
25-ft fall	3.2	1,920
1st narrows (end)	3.3	2,005
2nd narrows (start)	3.7	2,230
12-ft fall	4.2	2,600
2nd narrows (end)	4.6	2,820
Side canyon	4.7	2,860
3rd narrows (start)	5.0	3,020
3rd narrows (end)	5.7	3,400
4th narrows	6.9	4,150
Head	10.6	7,410

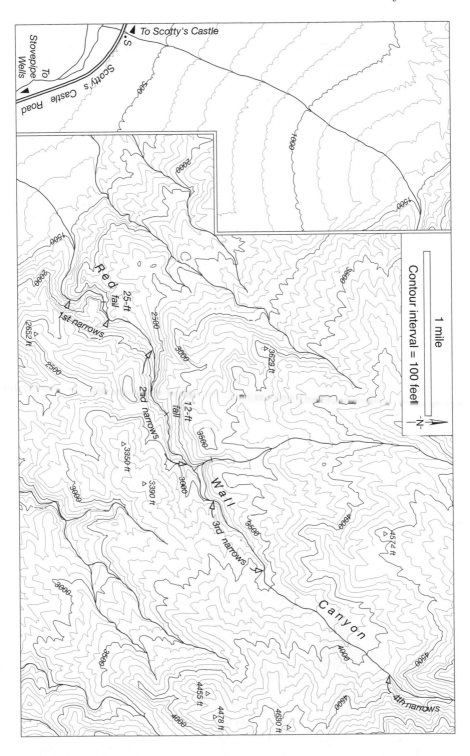

with a few tight curves between walls of gray dolomite. Look along the way for a small arch against the skyline, for cacti and the entangled vines of coyote melon, and for a deep cave with a strange upside-down plant hanging from its ceiling.

   The upper canyon. Although the end of the third narrows is the likely turning point for most day hikers, this canyon continues much further and offers the potential for longer overnight trips (see *Fall Canyon*). At the end of the third narrows the canyon opens onto a broad valley. At the head of this valley, a little over a mile away, there is a massive 1,500-foot escarpment through which the canyon has cut a fourth set of narrows. From there it is 3.7 miles to the head of Red Wall Canyon, with the last mile or so above timberline—a rare treat in the largely barren Grapevine Mountains.

■

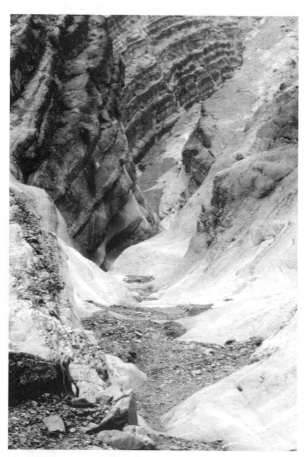

Fall Canyon narrows from the top of the 18-foot fall

FALL CANYON

You can't go wrong with Fall Canyon. It is easily accessed, easy to walk, and one of the two or three most consistently deep and narrow canyons in the park. Its majestic cliffs and winding corridors are likely to inspire even the most seasoned desert hiker. The high fall that blocks the way 2.5 miles in is the gateway to one of the best narrows around, to a remote upper canyon and wonderful high country in prime bighorn sheep habitat.

General Information

Road status: Roadless; easy hiking access from graded road
Shortest hike: 2.3 mi, 830 ft one way / moderate
Longest hike: 15 mi, 7,700 ft one way / difficult
Main attractions: A long, deep and narrow canyon, excellent narrows, peak climbs, rock climbing
USGS 15' topo map: Grapevine Peak
USGS 7.5' topo maps: Fall Canyon*, Thimble Peak, Wahguyhe Peak, Grapevine Peak
Maps: pp 79*, 87, 67

Location and Access

Fall Canyon is the first major canyon north of Titus Canyon. To get to it, take the Titus Canyon Road, which branches off the Scotty's Castle Road 14.9 miles north of Highway 190 (17.9 miles south of the Grapevine Ranger Station). Drive it 2.6 miles to the mouth of Titus Canyon and park. This road is graded and suitable for passenger cars.

Geology

During a notable storm in 1991, hundreds of thousands of cubic feet of mud were dislodged somewhere in the upper drainage of Fall Canyon and a virgin flow of almost pure, fine-grained silt came pouring down the wash. The stream was so powerful that it did not exhaust its momentum until it was within half a mile of the canyon mouth. For several months thereafter, the wash was covered under a wall-to-wall carpet of cracked dry mud several inches thick for many miles. The mud flow's smooth surface preserved rain drops, bird and coyote tracks, as well as clear traces of the eddies and turbulences of the ephemeral stream. Mud along the base of the canyon walls recorded high-tide marks as deep as a foot. In the tightest narrows above the lower fall,

75

waves had splattered mud as much as six feet up the polished walls.

Although this mud flow was important, it did not last long. During the following year, at least one other flash flood came along, carrying gravel this time, and completely wiped it out. Today, except for traces above the first fall, you would never know it was there. But mud flows are not all that infrequent, and with a little luck you will run into one somewhere—preferably in its dry form! These giant ribbons of mud are reminders that not so long ago, the dry canyon you are passing through was briefly alive, as in the old days, with the rumbling sounds of rushing water.

Route Description

Access. At the mouth of Titus Canyon, look for the small trail to Fall Canyon just left of the "Do Not Enter" sign. It first follows the foot of the range, then veers right and climbs into a small ravine. Turtleback, a pretty gray-green plant that well deserves its name, grows along the fan. After about 0.6 mile the trail reaches a high bank and drops into the wide wash of Fall Canyon, a short distance from the canyon mouth.

The lower canyon. This is one of the most spectacular canyons around. For more than 3 miles starting shortly above its mouth Fall Canyon is a deep gorge, getting deeper and more magnificent further into the mountain. At several places the wash squeezes through good narrows, impressive not so much for their tightness as for their high walls, which soar vertically straight from the wash for hundreds of feet—and they are topped above by even higher walls. The sheer, bare rocks are particularly colorful, ranging from yellow to tan, dark brown, and red, and the color arrangement evolves during the day as the sunlight strikes at varying angles. In the evening, the slanted rays of the sun pick up deeper shades of red as they reflect back and forth between the walls, and they turn this wonderland of rocks into a flaming gorge.

The first obvious landmark is the confluence with the first side canyon. This deep amphitheater, dominated by an imposing tower and large boulders, has the grandeur of a cathedral. The side canyon runs after a short distance into a 13-foot fall with a shaded grotto just above it, closed on its back side by an impassable 20-foot fall.

Fall Canyon follows a minor fault, marked by abundant slickensides. The largest and most conspicuous one is about 0.25 mile before the first side canyon, on the south side, about 20 yards above the wash. Other large ones can be seen within half a mile of this side canyon up and down canyon, high up on either wall.

Along this entire stretch, rock climbers will find plenty of good traverses on the smooth, sturdy dolomitic walls.

The fall and the tightest narrows. About 2.5 miles into the canyon progress is interrupted by a slick 18-foot fall, which presumably gave this canyon its name. It's a difficult climb (perhaps a hard 5.10) but unless you want to challenge it you will not need to, as there is an easier way around it. The bypass, usually marked by a small cairn, starts about 300 feet before the fall, on the south side. The route involves first an easy (class 4) climb up a short chimney. Above it a small trail, steep at places, leads up to a wide inclined ledge that leads down to the wash just above the fall.

This bypass is the crux of this hike and well worth the effort. Above the fall the wash squeezes through the tightest narrows of Fall Canyon. Although only a third of a mile long, they are among the best around and the most exciting part of this hike. Bounded by high vertical

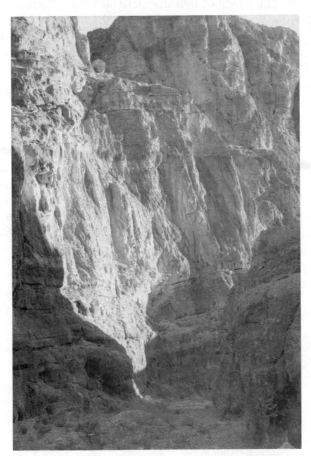

Sheer walls bathed in sunlight await hikers
along the lower part of Fall Canyon

walls polished tens of feet up, this deep, dark, and winding passage is reminiscent of some of the deepest narrows of Grotto Canyon.

The mid-canyon. Further on the canyon remains impressively deep. It goes through a couple of nice narrows, then slowly opens up until it reaches the second and third side canyons, which are next to each other on the east side about 3.5 miles above the fall. The second side canyon is a possible route to upper Titus Canyon, although I have not hiked it. The third side canyon, about 1.5 miles long, is a shallow ravine with a series of easy short falls. This area, which is the beginning of the upper canyon, is about as far as most hikers will go for a day hike.

The upper canyon. Fall Canyon retains the same character for several more miles—fairly deep and narrow, framed by high-rising walls of sedimentary rocks, often distinctly striated. There is a short narrows along the way, a fall not as difficult as the lower one that most people will prefer to bypass, a few side canyons, some tight and challenging, one of them with a little spring. The main canyon gradually changes character, eventually turning into a long and narrow valley, rimmed on all sides by a ridge more than 2,000 feet higher. This is a beautiful, wild area, graced by scattered pinyon pines and junipers, some of them in healthy stands as high as 20 feet—a sharp contrast with the lower canyon. One winter I had the good fortune to encounter a band of six ewes just after they had drunk at a small, rain-filled tinaja.

The rims of the upper canyon are dominated by Mount Palmer (7,958') on the east side, and Wahguyhe Peak (8,628') to the north. These two peaks are natural destinations if you spend a few days here. The easiest, though far from easy, approach to Mount Palmer is up the rough, forested side canyon at elev. 5,220', to where it opens up

Fall Canyon		
	Dist.(mi)	Elev.(ft)
Mouth of Titus Canyon	0.0	940
Mouth of Fall Canyon	0.9	1,235
First side canyon	2.3	1,770
18-ft fall	3.4	~2,270
End of tightest narrows	3.7	2,390
End of narrow section	4.3	2,600
Third side canyon	6.9	3,580
Side canyon to Mt. Palmer	10.7	5,220
Mount Palmer	(3.3)	7,958
Wahguyhe Peak	~15.0	8,628

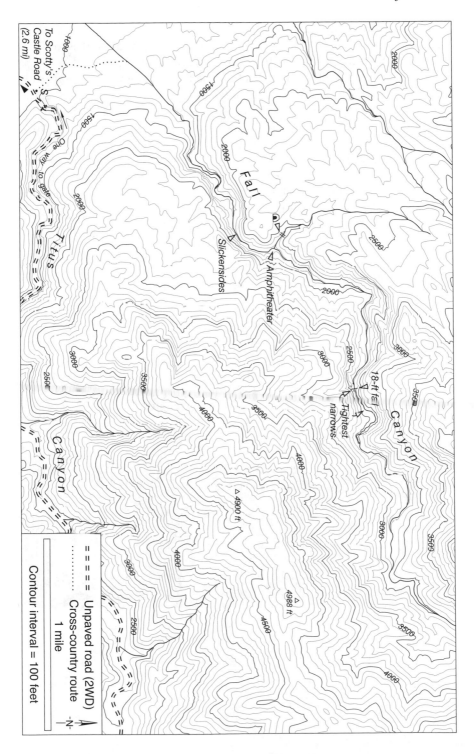

To Scotty's
Castle Road
(2.6 mi)

One way to gate

Titus

Fall

Slickensides

Amphitheater

Canyon

18-ft fall

Tightest
narrows

Canyon

△ 4900 ft

△ 4988 ft

===== Unpaved road (2WD)
·········· Cross-country route

1 mile

Contour interval = 100 feet

-N-

(~6,560'). Then climb southwest to the ridge and follow it to the summit. The views are great all around, from the dizzying depths of Red Wall Canyon to Bare Mountain, Badwater Basin, and Telescope Peak.

Seen from Fall Canyon, Wahguyhe Peak is an even more appealing goal—a striking conical mountain covered with long dark basaltic flows and scattered trees. The route is more straightforward, by way of the saddle west of the peak, but it is tougher, taking some heavy-duty scrambling at the end.

Another great target for a multiple day trip, which is not as difficult and will give you two canyons for the price of one, is to continue up one of the two last western side canyons of Fall Canyon, cross the ridge, and return via beautiful Red Wall Canyon.

■

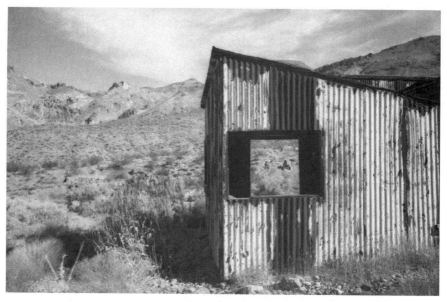

Building at Leadfield

LEADFIELD AND UPPER TITUS CANYON

> *If you are looking for a scenic and adventurous backcountry drive, try the Titus Canyon road, a scenic mountain byway that will take you clear across the Grapevine Mountains. One of its many highlights is the small ghost town of Leadfield; its scattered buildings have an unusual story to tell. There is a small spring and petroglyphs along the way, the geology is interesting, and the spectacular drive through the narrows in the lower canyon is truly unique.*

General Information

Road status: Primitive road in lower canyon; upper canyon roadless
Shortest hike: Short strolls / very easy to easy
Longest hike: 12 mi, 4,350 ft one way (or more) / moderate
Main attractions: Scenic backcountry road, ghost town, petroglyphs,
    spring, lead mines
USGS 15' topo maps: Grapevine Peak*, Bullfrog
USGS 7.5' topo maps: Fall Canyon, Thimble Peak*, Daylight Pass*,
    Wahguyhe Peak
Maps: pp. 87*, 67

Location and Access

Titus Canyon is a major canyon of the southern Grapevine Mountains. A primitive road, originating in Nevada, goes down the lower half of the canyon to the Scotty's Castle Road. Except for the short, two-way stretch below the canyon mouth, this road is one way westward (about 27 miles). To get to it, drive the Daylight Pass Road 6.9 miles east of the pass to the signed Titus Canyon turnoff. Officially, the Park Service recommends a 4WD vehicle to tackle this road. However, people often drive it with standard-clearance vehicles, in spite of a few short stretches of soft gravel in the wash. In the summer, the Titus Canyon Road may be closed to motorized traffic. At such times, you can get the key to the road's gates from the Visitor Center. The road may also be closed in the winter for a few days when it is snowed in.

History: Leadfield's Boom and Bust

Among the few mining towns Death Valley had, Leadfield undeniably gets the prize for the shortest lifetime. It rose to fame in a matter of weeks, soared to promising heights for a few months, then turned to a ghost town almost overnight. What started it all was a group of lead-silver deposits located in a fork of Titus Canyon. Lead was first discovered here in 1905, when a few claims were filed, briefly exploited, and soon abandoned because of their remoteness. The Leadfield rush didn't start until nearly two decades later, in March 1924, when three prospectors staked several claims in what was probably the same location. They worked them for about a year before selling out to Jack Salsberry, a persistent mining promoter who had been involved earlier at Greenwater, in the Ubehebe Mining District, and at the Carbonate Mine. Soon thereafter, Salsberry formed the Western Lead Mines Company. By the end of 1925, the company had accumulated no less than 50 claims, bored a long tunnel into the most promising ledge, and put a large crew to work on a road to Beatty. In January 1926, the construction of a pipeline to Klare Spring, a couple of miles down canyon, was under way. In response to this enthusiastic effort, other companies were filing claims all around Salsberry's property. Twenty-four hours after Western Lead entered the stock market in San Francisco, 40,000 shares had been sold, and shares quickly climbed to $1.50. The scattering of tents and boarding houses that had sprouted near the mines was officially named on January 30. Leadfield was born, and the boom was on.

The general euphoria reached new heights in early February, when a promoter from southern California, Charles C. Julian, bought into the Western Lead Mines Company. Julian had succeeded in the oil business, and all interests saw his arrival as a guarantee of Leadfield's future. He became the company's main stockholder and new president, and Salsberry its manager. Over the next few months, as Julian invested his personal fortune in the enterprise, Leadfield witnessed tremendous activity. In late February trucks rumbled down the newly-completed Leadfield Road, bringing in lumber and mining equipment. The work force exceeded 100. By March, a dozen companies were working just as feverishly on adjacent ground. The second largest outfit, the Leadfield New Roads, had just installed an office and was getting ready to ship its best ore while waiting for additional equipment. Western Lead's main tunnel was now more than 600 feet long. With 8% to 30% in lead and 7 ounces of silver per ton, its ore was rich enough for profit if the vein persisted with depth. The town was keeping up with the boom. It soon had its own newspaper, the *Leadfield Chronicle*, and announced plans for a large hotel to host the many miners coming in from all over the country.

The excitement was generated not so much by the value of the ore, which was good but not phenomenal, but by Julian's sizeable financial investment and the wholehearted support of Inyo and Nye County officials, who saw in Leadfield a much-needed revival in the local economy. The positive response of the market was partly the result of Julian's fundraising talents. When his stock went public, Julian placed advertisements in Los Angeles newpapers advising investors who could not afford to gamble on his company not to buy any stock. He also invited mining engineers from around the country to visit his property, adding the dangerous offer that all travel expenses would be reimbursed to anyone who found the mine showings at odds with Julian's claims.

His offer didn't go unnoticed. On March 15 a specially chartered train pulled into Beatty, carrying Julian's first promotional excursion. Some 340 visitors and potential investors disembarked, joined by an even larger crowd from Tonopah and Goldfield—over 1,000 people drove down to Leadfield that day. The Lieutenant-Governor of Nevada gave the keynote address that touched off a series of speeches praising Julian's determination. Geology experts were taken on a tour of the mines, and dinner was served to everyone. The trip was a resounding success. Two weeks later shares reached $3.30. In anticipation of upcoming growth, in April the town site of Leadfield was officially surveyed on land donated by Western Lead. The plan, which allocated some 1749 lots over 93 sprawling blocks, was approved in May by Inyo County.

Everybody seemed happy, except for the California State Corporation Commission. Early on, the Commission was after Julian for failing to obtain a permit to sell his stock. Around April 1926, it took a brokerage company to court for selling Western Lead stock. The Commission's investigations raised indignation among local officials, who refused to let anyone interfere with Leadfield. It was argued that what was being sold was Julian's personal stock, which didn't require a permit. Several qualified geologists testified that Western Lead was quite legitimate. The Commission remained undeterred. In June it dealt its second blow, ordering Julian's personal stock in Western Lead to be removed from the Los Angeles stock exchange.

While Julian took this decision to court, mining developments continued as strong as ever. Western Lead announced plans to install a 400-ton concentration plant. To reduce the cost of ore transportation by road, the possibility of extending the railroad to Leadfield was investigated. Smelting companies and the Tonopah & Tidewater Railroad sent out representatives to Leadfield. In the meantime a few companies were trucking their best ore out to Beatty. Several new strikes were made, and more machinery installed on various properties. By the end of summer the town had expanded to include a general store, barber shop, a restaurant, the Leadfield Hotel, and a post office.

But these noble efforts weren't meant to last. In late October the Commission put a halt on the sale of stock in the Julian Merger Mines, a holding company Julian had incorporated as his last resort. At the same time, the main Western Lead tunnel reached the vein it had been aiming for all along and only hit low-grade ore. With Julian's financial structure destroyed, Western Lead didn't get a second chance to look for better ore. Leadfield's three main companies, all financially dependent on Julian's estate, went under. Julian appealed the decision but lost again. The boom had run out of steam and the mines folded one by one. The post office closed in January 1927. The mining equipment and pipeline were hauled out early in the summer. By July only a few miners were still working on one of the properties.

In subsequent years, newspapers and writers hastily blamed Julian for Leadfield's boom and bust. In fairness, Julian did not start Leadfield, and his business was never proved to be illegal. There was, and still is, decent ore at Leadfield, and whether it should have been exploited was certainly a judgment call. Without the interference of the state, a couple of the Leadfield companies may well have turned out a small profit. We'll never know. Decades later, Julian's peculiar story still adds a touch of mystery and lore to an empty corner of the desert.

Route Description

Red Pass. The colorful exposures in the foothills on the way up to Red Pass, at the crest of the Grapevines, are lava flows (dark brown), ash beds and tuffs (yellow, green, and pink). The dark pinnacles protruding from the mountain slope on the north side are volcanic plugs, the hardened lava cores of the volcanoes that spewed out these volcanic debris, sometime between 5 and 10 million years ago.

The ride up to the crest of the Grapevines, along switchbacks cut into steep, high-reaching slopes, is quite spectacular. Upon reaching Red Pass, you'll get an eye-filling view of the deep valley you are about to enter. The pass is named after the red calcareous mudstone widely exposed here, which is the same strata that yielded the fossil titanothere bones in Titanothere Canyon. It is part of the Titus Canyon Formation, a thick stack of sedimentary rocks deposited by streams and lakes in the Oligocene. This formation prevails down to the Leadfield area and across the upper reaches of the valley, and it is responsible for the vivid colors that stain this entire area.

From here the road drops 1,100 feet into the canyon along tight switchbacks. At the bottom of the switchbacks, it overlooks a deep gorge on the south side. If time allows, take a stroll back up into it, starting where the road reaches the wash. It is a narrow little canyon, slithering along a high wall of dark gray limestone scoured by hanging falls. The ghost town of Leadfield is about half a mile down the road.

Leadfield. The few structures of rusted corrugated iron on the canyon slopes stand as an epitaph to a small town that once stirred interest throughout the West. The large house close to the wash is the old store building. The large gray tailing above it, next to another large house, bears witness to the sizeable effort expended here. The faint trace of a road that passes in front of the lower house was Salsberry Street, the main street. Much of the ground on both sides of it is covered with tent sites. Follow the main street east, past a large concrete foundation, which may have been laid down for the concentration plant. The street climbs on to another frame building, which was the property of Western Lead. The nearby sealed adit was the company's main tunnel. Several other tunnels, prospects, shafts, and tailings are scattered along the canyon for a couple of miles on either side of town. Most of the town buildings stood on the other side of the wash. Look there for faded streets lined with tent sites, wood floors, retaining walls, and for a couple of dugouts by the road. Imagine this place on March 15, 1926, with a hundred cars parked all over. Was the rusted carcass by the side of the road one of them? Where was Ole's Inn, where some 1,120 meals were served that night?

Upper Titus Canyon. Past Leadfield the canyon narrows. At a posted sign "When Rocks Bend," a syncline of well-stratified rocks is exposed in the wall, striking for its regularity. A little further the road drops into Titus Canyon.

Uphill from here the canyon is roadless. It is fairly narrow at first, with eroded walls of thick folded limestone and dolomite strata dipping sharply. In 0.4 mile the wash branches out. The map suggests that the east fork may be a good place to hike up to the crest of the Grapevine Mountains. The shorter west fork enters a wide open and relatively level area. In 1.7 miles it leads to a spectacular divide overlooking Fall Canyon. The red exposures along the way are again beds of calcareous mudstone from the Titus Canyon Formation, older than at Red Pass. In the 1930s and 1940s Chester Stock and Francis Bode, prominent geologists with the California Institute of Technology, uncovered around here fossils of several Oligocene mammals—the skull remains of a titanothere, bones and teeth from a tapir, a small horse (*mesohippus*), rodents, and rhinoceros. For a good day hike, continue down the facing side canyon to Fall Canyon, then down this canyon to the mouth of Titus Canyon. Be aware of the high fall on this route (see *Fall Canyon*).

Petroglyphs,
Klare Spring

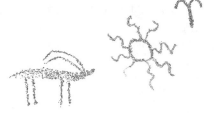
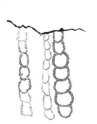

Klare Spring and the mid-canyon. Down canyon from the confluence, the road continues along a narrower passage, then follows the wide wash for several miles. Along this stretch, the formations exposed on the high canyon walls, often strongly folded, are mostly Cambrian, generally younger down canyon. The rocks below the spring are mainly quartzites (Wood Canyon Formation and Zabriskie Quartzite). The orange shales common further down belong to the Carrara Formation. The Bonanza King Formation begins near the narrows.

The main attraction here is Klare Spring, which is right by the road. A small creek, rising along the Titus Canyon Fault, gathers among thickets of arrowweed, rush, cane and rabbitbrush surrounding two young palm trees, and heroically flows for about 150 yards—on a good year—before vanishing in the gravel. In early spring you may be fortunate and find stream orchis blooming by the creek—yes, an orchid, not too uncommon in redwood country but rare in Death Valley. Bighorn sheep frequent this area, as is often evidenced by their tracks and droppings. On a large boulder above the spring there is a fine panel of petroglyphs with uncommon designs, including anthropomorphic figures, a sun, and the rain symbol (short parallel wavy lines dropping from a horizontal line), as well as more frequent subjects, like bighorn sheep.

Titus Canyon is named after Edgar Titus, a mining engineer who perished mysteriously near here in 1905. Titus and his brother-in-law Earl Weller had just moved to Bullfrog, Nevada. They came from Telluride, Colorado, where they were involved in the mining industry until a dispute with union miners forced the Weller's family to close their gold mine and move on. On June 20, Titus, Weller and an assistant named Mullin headed out from Bullfrog to a rich gold ledge Titus had recently discovered in the Panamints. According to Mullin, the party

Leadfield and Upper Titus Canyon		
	Dist.(mi)	Elev.(ft)
Highway 374	0.0	3,505
Red Pass	12.6	5,290
Leadfield	15.8	4,040
Titus Canyon	16.5	3,750
Fall Canyon overlook (hike)	(2.1)	~4,700
Klare Spring	18.4	3,120
Facing side canyons	19.6	~2,700
Narrows	20.3	2,420
Mouth	24.3	940
Scotty's Castle Road	26.9	169

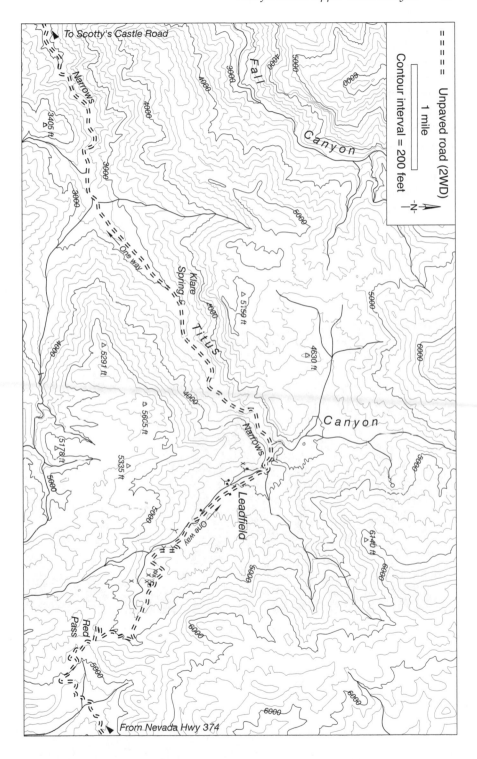

lost its way and set up camp for the night in the Grapevine Mountains. The next day, Titus and Weller went scouting for a route to Death Valley while Mullin stayed at the camp with the burros and supplies, but they never came back. Mullin was rescued from his camp in mid-July, after enduring three weeks of summer heat with little water. Although three men were found dead in the valley on July 1, and Weller's father organized several search parties the following two years, the bodies of Titus and Weller were never identified with certainty. They may have perished from dehydration, or they may have been murdered by miners from Telluride, who had also arrived in Bullfrog that month. To this day their disappearance remains a mystery.

The narrows start a few miles below the spring. Refer to *Titus Canyon Narrows* for a description of what to see there.

■

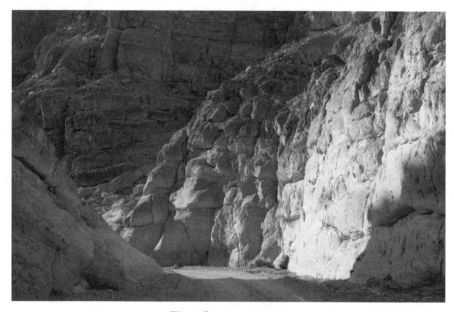

Titus Canyon narrows

TITUS CANYON NARROWS

Four miles long, hundreds of feet deep, and as narrow as 15 feet, the narrows of Titus Canyon rank among the longest and deepest in the park. They are easily accessed, the grade is moderate, and they teach a wonderful lesson about the power of stream erosion in the desert. A must-see if you like narrows.

General Information

Road status: Primitive road through narrows
Shortest hike: A short walk/easy
Longest hike: 4 mi, 1,480 ft one way (or more)/moderate
Main attractions: Long and deep narrows, geology
USGS 15' topo map: Grapevine Peak
USGS 7.5' topo maps: Fall Canyon*, Thimble Peak
Maps: pp. 91*, 67

Location and Access

This section complements the previous one by describing the narrows of lower Titus Canyon. To hike the narrows, start from the canyon mouth, which is reached by driving the lower end of the Titus Canyon Road. The signed turnoff to this good graded road is on the Scotty's Castle Road 14.9 miles north of Highway 190 (17.9 miles south of the Grapevine Ranger Station). After 2.7 miles you'll reach a small parking area at the canyon mouth. Park and hike from here (the road continues into the canyon but it's one way the other way). You can also drive through the narrows by taking this road the other way (see *Leadfield and Upper Titus Canyon*).

Hiking Suggestions

The best hike in Titus Canyon is probably the narrows. It takes about half a day, and it is only moderately difficult. To hike to Klare Spring and back takes a day, and Leadfield a very long day. If you back-pack in, remember that camping is prohibited within 2 miles of the road. The canyon drive being quite popular, hikers should expect an occasional car to drive by, especially in the high season. In the confined narrows, an approaching vehicle can be heard long before it gets anywhere near you. If you like your canyons natural, come here in the summer when vehicle access is limited (see *Seasonal road closure* in *Desert Hiking Tips*).

Parts of the narrows are well shaded, and you may find the heat preferable to sharing them with combustion engines.

Geology: Erosion and Desert Flash Floods

When walking down this or any other bone-dry canyon, it may
be hard to believe that water erosion is still significantly altering the
landscape. However, although local rains are rare, they are often violent
enough to generate raging torrents with tremendous erosional powers.
For example, a single, 1-inch rainfall over the entire 35-square mile
watershed of Titus Canyon can excavate a few hundred thousand cubic
feet of debris–enough to cover tens of fan acres a few inches deep. Such
moderate floods reportedly occur about every 10 years in Titus Canyon.
At this rate, it would take only about 50,000 years to carve out the lower
gorge. This is a reasonable time span: a few percent of the estimated age
of Titus Canyon. This simplistic calculation does not prove that the narrows were formed by flash flood erosion. But it does show that even in
dry weather stream erosion can be a significant agent. This is a good
example of a most powerful principle of geology: a small effect repeated
enough times can produce profound changes.

The Titus Canyon narrows have a typical "wineglass" shape: a
narrow lower gorge topped by high-reaching, more widely flaring
slopes. The lower gorge is the product of stream cutting, while the upper
V-shaped section results from widening by tributary erosion and land-
slides. The shape of a canyon is governed by which of these two processes dominates, and over what period of time. Worldwide, most stream
valleys have a V-shaped section. On the other hand, the deep and narrow canyons of the Colorado Plateau result from prolonged stream
downcutting. In Titus Canyon the narrow gorge shows that stream cutting has been dominant in recent times.

Titus Canyon Narrows		
	Dist.(mi)	Elev.(ft)
Mouth	0.0	940
Tightest spot	0.3	1,040
Brecciated walls	0.7	1,170
First narrows (end)	1.8	1,600
Second narrows (start)	2.2	1,760
Second narrows (end)	4.0	2,420
Klare Spring	5.9	3,120

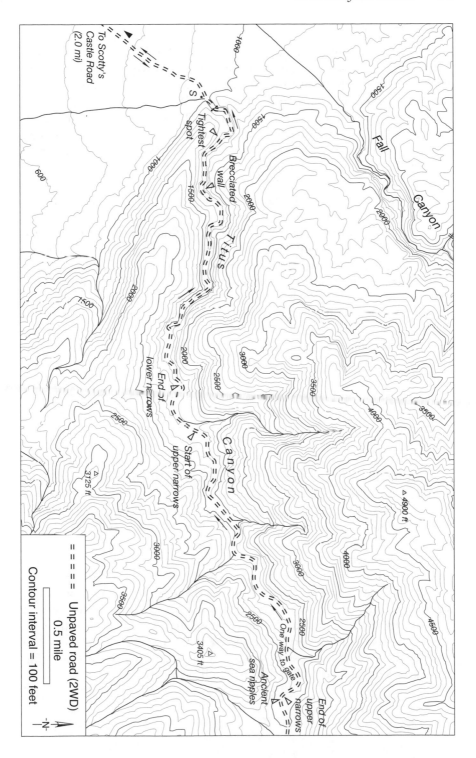

To Scotty's
Castle Road
(2.0 mi)

S

Tightest
spot

Brecciated
wall

Titus

End of
lower narrows

Start of
upper narrows

△ 3125 ft

Canyon

△ 4900 ft

Fall

Canyon

One way to gate

Ancient
sea ripples

△ 3405 ft

End of
upper
narrows

===== Unpaved road (2WD)

0.5 mile

Contour interval = 100 feet

-N-

Route Description

The narrows of Titus Canyon are undoubtedly the crowning glory of this spectacular canyon. They start right away, abruptly. It may take your eyes a moment to adjust, as you walk in seconds from blinding open desert to dim confined spaces. The high vertical walls are banded in light shades of orange and gray. These are the hard interbedded layers of dolomite and limestone of the Bonanza King Formation. The passage is narrowest about a third of a mile above the mouth, where the walls are less than 15 feet apart at their base, which is barely wide enough for the road. With the exception of a 2,000-foot stretch, the canyon remains narrow for the next 4 miles, and along the first mile it is often less than 30 feet wide.

Throughout the narrows look for ominous signs of water erosion, both recent and old. The lower walls have been polished smooth by flowing water. Gravel stranded on ledges 10 feet or more above the wash mark the high tide of past floods. In an abrupt left bend, a deep overhang was cut into the base of the wall by running water.

About 0.7 mile in, the passage is adorned with two spectacular facing walls of giant polished mosaics. These are breccia made of large, dark, and angular blocks of limestone, some several feet across, cemented by white calcite. Shattering of the limestone into blocks probably occurred thousands of feet underground, where hot water dissolved some limestone and redeposited it as calcite in the gaps between them. The blocks were displaced very little with respect to each other after shattering, as shown by the matching orientation of cracks in adjacent blocks.

Another sign of erosion is a rock fall at the foot of the south wall, at the head of the first set of narrows. Its angular blocks, not yet rounded by erosion, indicate that it is recent. It was formed when the wall collapsed after heavy rainstorms in 1976, contributing to the relentless widening of the canyon. The temporary opening in the wash is a good place to see the typical "wineglass" shape of the narrows.

Although not as tight, the second narrows are equally impressive. A good part of the way the walls soar more than 500 feet up. Quite a few neatly stratified walls are exposed throughout this section, some strongly folded. The narrows end after a couple of windy miles, almost as abruptly as they started. At their upper end, look at the south wall, where the road comes very close to it. On the flat, 45° slant above the base of the wall are exposed parallel ripple marks left by a Cambrian sea—an event recorded more than 520 million years ago.

∎

TITANOTHERE CANYON

> *If you appreciate seclusion and grand sceneries, you will enjoy the long solitary trek down this deep, stately swath through the Grapevine Mountains, its wildness and tormented geology, and the sweeping vistas where it opens up on to the valley floor. For unconditional Death Valley lovers.*

General Information

Road status: Roadless; hiking from paved or graded road
Shortest hike: 4.3 mi, 1,800 ft one way / moderate
Longest hike: 12 mi, 4,900 ft one way / difficult
Main attractions: A deep and spacious canyon, spring
USGS 15' topo maps: Grapevine Peak*, Stovepipe Wells
USGS 7.5' topo maps: Thimble Peak*, Stovepipe Wells N.E.
Maps: pp. 97*, 67

Location and Access

Titanothere Canyon is the southernmost major canyon in the Grapevine Mountains. To hike in from the upper canyon, drive the Titus Canyon Road, which intersects the canyon near its head. This one-way, graded road, usually passable with a passenger vehicle, branches off Nevada Highway 374 6.9 miles east of Daylight Pass (or 6.1 miles west of Beatty, Nevada). After 9.6 miles it reaches a first pass and drops gently into the drainage of Titanothere Canyon. Park about 0.6 mile beyond this pass. The wide opening to the south is a side canyon that leads into Titanothere Canyon. You can also park 1.1 miles further, and hike down the ravine to the south, which is in the main drainage. This is 1.2 miles before Red Pass. If you have gone too far you will have to walk back on this one-way road.

To get to the canyon mouth, drive the Scotty's Castle Road 7.5 miles north from Highway 190 (or 25.3 miles south of the Grapevine Ranger Station). Titanothere Canyon is at the apex of the large alluvial fan to the east. Park near the north end of the Kit Fox Hills (the low hills east of the road), to help locate your car from the canyon mouth on your way back.

Geology: 40-Million-Year-Old Titanotheres

The crest of the southern Grapevine Mountains, in particular around the head of Titanothere Canyon, is made of ancient stream and

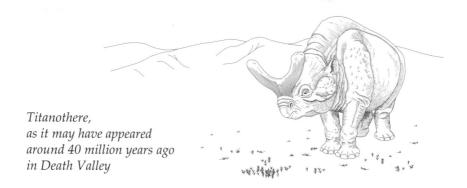

Titanothere,
as it may have appeared
around 40 million years ago
in Death Valley

lake deposits known as the Titus Canyon Formation. They were forming about 40 million years ago, when this area was probably a region of broad valleys, lakes, and a few mountain ranges with volcanoes. The climate, warm and much wetter than today, supported rolling grasslands and woodlands alive with numerous species of mammals. Titanothere Canyon was named after the fossilized remains of a titanothere discovered in the red calcareous mudstone beds of the upper part of this formation. Titanotheres and other, now extinct mammals lived here 35 to 40 million years ago. These browsers resembled modern rhinoceros, with massive bodies and legs. Two broad and blunt horns grew on either side of the nose. They reached North America from Asia in the Middle Eocene. Over time they grew in size, until by the Early Oligocene they were the largest animals around, reaching 12 to 14 feet in length, 7 to 8 feet in height, and 4 to 5 tons in weight, like a good-size white rhinoceros. They became extinct by the end of the Early Oligocene, perhaps incapacitated by their small brain and an inability to adapt to grazing.

The titanothere remains were originally discovered in 1934 by Donald Curry, a paleontologist and then ranger-naturalist at the monument. While traveling along the Titus Canyon Road he found a portion of a titanothere jaw in a road cut near the head of an unnamed canyon then referred to as "the canyon east of Thimble Peak." Although titanothere fossils had already been discovered on the continent, in particular in the famous White River deposits of the western Great Plains, this discovery was the first evidence of early Oligocene land mammals in the Great Basin, and it stimulated much scientific interest. Subsequent excavations unearthed from this general location other mammal fossils, including rhinoceros and artiodactyls (see *Leadfield and Upper Titus Canyon*). They also uncovered a well-preserved titanothere skull nearly 70 centimeters long and jaw bones (a cast of it is displayed at the Visitor

Center Museum). It represented a new species, which was named *Protinatops Curryi* in honor of its discoverer. The "canyon east of Thimble Peak" later became Titanothere Canyon.

Route Description

The upper canyon. From the Titus Canyon Road you can go down into Titanothere along either of the two drainages mentioned above. The east fork is the most interesting, as it goes over an 80-foot drop-off. This sweeping fall is the only obstacle in this canyon. Going around it is straightforward, down the boulder-strewn talus slope on its west side. The canyon continues as a broad V-shaped gully. In about 1 mile, just before the confluence with the west fork, it goes through short narrows with a few polished chutes and whirlpools.

Below the confluence the canyon widens and cuts deeper into the Grapevine Mountains. The openness of the straight wash is compensated by vast panoramas, starting with good views of Thimble Peak to the west, with its vertical curved walls and pyramidal cap. As the elevation drops, more craggy peaks and mesas fill the horizon, reminiscent of sceneries in the inner Grand Canyon.

About 2.7 miles from the road a small side canyon enters from the east. Before reaching it, look for two small arches on the eastern skyline, dwarfed by distance. The confluence is an interesting area, a vast

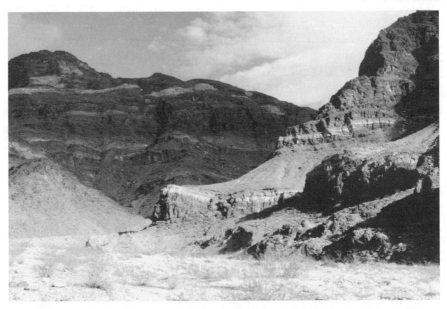

Titanothere Canyon cuts a majestic swath through the Grapevine Mountains

amphitheater bounded by thousand-foot cliffs and littered with huge
boulders shed by the cliffs. A large grove of dark pinnacles stands on its
south side. On the bench just east of the confluence are the remains of an
old rock shelter, a semicircle of stacked rocks against the flat face of a
large boulder. Like others in this windy canyon, it may have been used
as a wind break. Scattered modern artifacts such as railroad ties and
rusted cans suggest contemporary occupancy. A host of cacti—beavertail, calico, and cottontop—thrive nearby, encouraged by the higher elevation.

The Neck. Perhaps the most interesting part of Titanothere
Canyon is what I named the Neck, the area just above the spring where
the walls come together to form a 50-foot wide passage. The area starting about 0.5 mile above the Neck offers an unusual display of standing
strata. The bedrock was deeply folded and subsequently eroded, so that
now the strata exposed in the surrounding hills are vertical. Erosion has
preferentially removed the softer alternating layers, producing acres of
shallow parallel ridges, like the furrows of a ploughed field. In this
strangely serrated landscape, nothing much grows except for alien-looking clusters of cottontop cactus.

In this same area the wash offers a good example of segregation
among desert plant communities. At this intermediate elevation (~3,000
feet) the land supports plants from different zones. The light green bushes in the wash are sagebrush. The darker green, leafless bushes on the
banks are Mormon tea. Both are typical of the Upper Sonoran zone,
while the ubiquitous creosote bush is typical of the Lower Sonoran zone.
The sage grows exclusively in the wash, the Mormon tea and creosote
only on the banks, and the cottontop cactus only on the higher rocky
slopes. These preferential distributions are based on a combination of

	Titanothere Canyon	
	Dist.(mi)	Elev.(ft)
Titus Canyon Road	0.0	5,000
Drop-off	0.25	4,840
Fork	1.1	4,310
First side canyon	2.7	3,690
The Neck	3.9	3,200
Lostman Spring	4.3	3,110
Main side canyon	6.8	~2,040
Mouth	8.9	1,200
Scotty's Castle Road	12.0	110

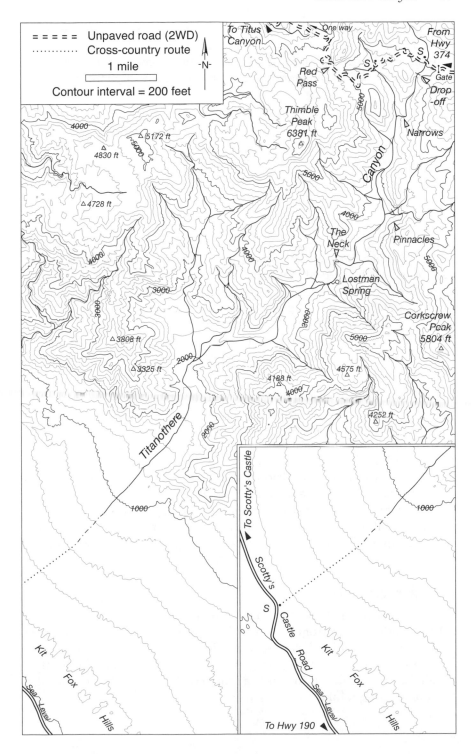

= = = = = Unpaved road (2WD)
.... Cross-country route
1 mile
Contour interval = 200 feet

-N-

To Titus Canyon
One way
From Hwy 374
Red Pass
Gate
Drop-off
Thimble Peak 6381 ft
Narrows
4000
5172 ft
4830 ft
5000
5000
Canyon
4728 ft
4000
The Neck
Pinnacles
4000
5000
Lostman Spring
3000
Corkscrew Peak 5804 ft
3000
5000
3000
3808 ft
2000
3325 ft
2000
4575 ft
4188 ft
4000
4252 ft
Titanothere
2000
1000
To Scotty's Castle
1000
Scotty's
S
Castle Road
Kit Fox
Sea Level
Kit Fox Hills
Sea Level
To Hwy 190

heat tolerance, soil chemistry, water availability, type of water (ground or surface), and resistance to flash floods. In the next few miles down canyon, most of these plants disappear as the creosote gradually takes over the wash, eventually forming a sea of unusually large bushes.

*Coyote tracks
in dried mud*

Lostman Spring. This small, incongruous spring is on the south side of the wash just past the Neck. A few old cottonwood and mesquite trees cling to the steep talus, surrounded by a dense tangle of cane. Surface water is usually non-existent. In the cold season it is a barren place, too thick and thorny to penetrate, rustling with fallen leaves, and somewhat disappointing. In the late spring and summer, when the trees have foliage, it is a welcome oasis and a pleasant spot to rest from the sun.

The lower canyon. Past the spring the wash gradually opens up. A few side canyons enter from the north, most of them as broad as the main canyon. The most interesting one is 2.1 miles below the spring, before the main side canyon. It is choked with boulders, making progress difficult at places, but it quickly turns to a fairly narrow passage between abrupt walls. Below the main side canyon, the wash opens on to a broad alluvial plain over 0.7 mile wide, thickly vegetated with unusually tall creosote bushes. In another 2 miles the canyon opens on to its long alluvial fan. The rest of the walk is somewhat tedious, over braided runoff channels in coarse gravel, but the dramatic views of the golden dunes against dark Tucki Mountain certainly make up for it.

Hiking Suggestions

A great way to see this canyon, if you can arrange a shuttle, is to hike its entire length from the Titus Canyon Road to the Scotty's Castle Road. This downhill trek can be easily done in a day. For a shorter day hike, go only as far as the spring and back. The hike from the Scotty's Castle Road up to the spring takes a long day. You may want to consider it for an overnight hike.

∎

PART III

FUNERAL MOUNTAINS

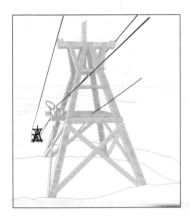

THE FUNERAL MOUNTAINS ARE located on the east side of central Death Valley, from Boundary Canyon to the north (their boundary with the Grapevine Mountains) down to the dry bed of Furnace Creek to the south. They are the smallest (about 220 square miles) and lowest of the mountains bordering Death Valley. Roughly in the center of the Funerals is a low point called Indian Pass (about 3,050'), with high points near Chloride Cliff (5,279') to the north and Pyramid Peak (6,703') to the south. On their west side, the alluvial fans climb for several miles from the floor of Death Valley to the western front of the mountains, which rises abruptly 2,000 to 3,500 feet to the crest. This escarpment is generally less pronounced than elsewhere in the Amargosa Range. On the east side, the Funerals slope down gently to the Amargosa Desert, dropping an average of 2,000 feet over several miles. The southern tip of the mountains is protected as the Funeral Mountains Wilderness Area.

Access

The Funeral Mountains are encompassed by roads on all sides: Highway 190 along Furnace Creek and Death Valley, the Beatty Cutoff and the Boundary Canyon Road to the north, and Highways 95 and 29 along the Amargosa Desert in Nevada. Except around the northern and southern Funerals, these roads are 3 to 8 miles from the base of the range and provide only marginal access.

Several primitive roads supplement this generally poor access by climbing some distance along the fans and sometimes into the mountains, especially from the east side. From around Beatty, Nevada, a road crosses the drainage of the Amargosa River to Chloride Cliff. Further south another one leads from Highway 95 across the same drainage to Indian Pass. This dry drainage is quite sandy and these roads generally require 4-wheel-drive vehicles. On the Death Valley side, a few unpaved roads cross eastward towards the mountains, in particular to Keane Wonder Mill and Red Amphitheater. The rough northern extension of the Echo Canyon Road to the old Echo-Lee Mining District and Nevada Highway 95 is the only road that cuts through the Funerals.

Geology

From Nevares Peak north the long and straight front of the mountains rises along the Keane Wonder Fault, a minor, northwest-trending, 25-mile long fault zone east of, and parallel to, the Furnace Creek Fault Zone. Movements along the Keane Wonder Fault have exposed different types of rocks on either side of it. East of the fault the mountains are one large block of Late to Middle Proterozoic metamorphic rocks (mostly Pahrump Group, Kingston Peak Formation, and Johnnie Formation). West of it the rocks are much younger, mostly Oligocene and Miocene nonmarine sedimentary formations, including the Tertiary alluvial deposits of the Kit Fox Hills. The exposures from the northwestern slope of Winters Peak down to Slit Canyon are Cambrian marine rocks.

The southern half of the Funeral Mountains, from Nevares Peak south to around Death Valley Junction, rises along the Furnace Creek Fault, which defines the drainage of Furnace Creek Wash. The rocks here are largely of marine origin (Ordovician and Silurian). The exception is a long exposure of Pliocene and Pleistocene nonmarine sedimentary deposits stretching from the Hole-in-the-Wall area north to the upper drainage of Echo Canyon. Oligocene nonmarine rocks are also exposed at the very southern tip of the Funeral Mountains.

Hydrology

Because of their low elevation and location in the rain shadow of the Panamint Range, the Funerals are among the driest in the park. Rain, which occurs mostly in the summer, and snow are even more rare than elsewhere. In historical times, summer downpours in the Funeral Mountains produced devastating flash floods, especially along Furnace Creek Wash.

Surprisingly enough, despite this extreme dryness, the largest springs in the park are found at the western foot of the Funeral Mountains. Travertine Springs, the largest of them, produce an average of 2,000 gallons per minute (gpm), while nearby Texas and Nevares springs discharge over 200 and 300 gpm, respectively. The water is believed to originate from a large ground water basin underneath Pahrump Valley in southwestern Nevada. For decades the three largest springs have been a source of domestic water for the nearby resorts. Other springs include Keane Wonder Springs and Navel Spring, which are smaller fault springs, and Monarch Spring, Keane Spring, and Poison Spring.

Hiking

As far as hiking is concerned, the Funeral Mountains stand out for their old mines, deep canyons, springs, and unusual geological formations. The area witnessed the boom and bust of some of the most famous mines in Death Valley—Chloride Cliff, the Keane Wonder Mine, and the Inyo Mine. The Keane Wonder Mine, with its long aerial tramway and mill ruins, is a popular destination, and one of the park's most interesting historical landmarks. The Inyo Mine, deep in Echo Canyon, has extensive mining ruins and one of the largest and best-preserved camps. These abandoned mines and their obsolete machinery add a wonderful dimension to hiking in the Funerals.

The many springs of the Funerals also make good hiking destinations. For short, easy hikes, try the lush Travertine Springs, a short distance up Furnace Creek Wash, or the more peaceful Nevares Springs. For more serious hikes, aim for one of the springs tucked deeper in the mountains—Keane Spring and its small town site, Monarch Spring and its perennial waterfall, or isolated Poison Spring.

Another great asset is the geology. As in the Black Mountains, the unusual variety of rocks, combined with the abrupt uplifting of the mountains, have produced unusual landscapes, quite different from what prevails in the other ranges. A case in point is most of the northern Funerals canyons, which all slice down through strongly folded metamorphic rocks. You would have to travel quite far in the Basin and Range to find anything like it.

Only a few of the Funerals canyons have been named. The longest one, Echo Canyon, is very popular amongst 4WD enthusiasts. The downfall is that on a long weekend it may not be the quietest for hiking. All other canyons are roadless and can only be explored on foot. A few of them can be reached from a primitive road—Monarch Canyon, Indian Pass Canyon, a few nameless canyons near the Hole-in-the-Wall Road, and the two chaotic canyons on either side of Chloride Cliff. Most others, though relatively short, are at the end of long alluvial fans and require a generous gift of time to be visited. Keep them in mind for long day hikes or extended backpacking trips.

■

Route/Destination	Dist. (mi)	Elev. change	Mean elev.	Access road	Page
Suggested Hikes in the Funeral Mountains					
Short hikes (under 5 miles round trip)					
Chloride C. to Big Bell Mine					
via mining road	2.3	1,540'	4,440'	F/6.7 mi	117-118
via cable road	1.7	1,770'	4,640'	F/7.1 mi	117-118
via canyon	1.5	1,390'	4,320'	F/7.1 mi	118
Chloride Cliff-Chloride City	2.2	1,500'	4,880'	F/6.3 mi	115-116
Cyty's Mill	1.2	130'	1,270'	Graded	122-123
Eye of the Needle	1.9	760'	1,800'	P/2.9 mi	146
Furnace Mine (from camp)	0.9	680'	4,080'	F/6.7 mi	147-148
Inyo Mine (from camp)	0.4	320'	3,920'	F/6.7 mi	147
Keane Wonder Springs	0.8	100'	1,280'	Graded	122-123
Keane Wonder Mill & plant*	0.6	400'	1,360'	Graded	132
Keane Wonder Tramway	0.4	420'	1,530'	Graded	133-134
Keane Wonder Mine via rd	1.6	1,720'	2,180'	Graded	133-135
Keane Wonder Mine via cyn	2.4	1,800'	2,260'	Graded	133-135
Monarch Canyon (upper)	1.7	680'	3,160'	P/2.3 mi	106-107
Slit Canyon to the Slit	1.6	850'	2,190'	P/3.7 mi	151-154
Slit Canyon to 1st narrows	2.3	1,450'	2,560'	P/3.7 mi	151-154
Intermediate hikes (5-12 miles round trip)					
Big Bell Ext. Mine via trail	3.4	1,880'	2,170'	Graded	122-126
Big Bell Ext. Mine via canyon	4.7	2,370'	1,920'	Graded	124-126
Big Bell Mine					
from Keane Wonder Mill	3.3	2,660'	2,560'	Graded	133-136
Echo Canyon narrows	2.6	990'	1,920'	P/2.9 mi	146
Indian Pass Canyon (upper)	2.6	945'	2,570'	P/13.1 mi	142
Monarch Canyon (lower cyn)					
via lower trail	4.9	1,840'	2,080'	Paved	108-110
via upper route	3.2	650'	2,200'	Paved	107-110
Nevares Peak	3.5	2,600'	1,130'	Paved	256-258
Slit Canyon (third narrows)	3.4	2,120'	2,920'	P/3.7 mi	151-154
Long hikes (over 12 miles round trip)					
Indian Pass Canyon (lower)	8.9	2,315'	940'	Paved	138-140
Inyo Mine via Echo Canyon	7.1	3,675'	2,750'	P/2.9 mi	146-147
Inyo Mine via Slit Canyon	8.9	4,320'	3,330'	P/3.7 mi	146-147
Keane Wonder Mill/					
Big Bell/Big Bell Ext.*	7.7	5,320'	2,370'	Graded	133-135
to Chloride Cliff	6.0	4,140'	3,290'	Graded	133-136

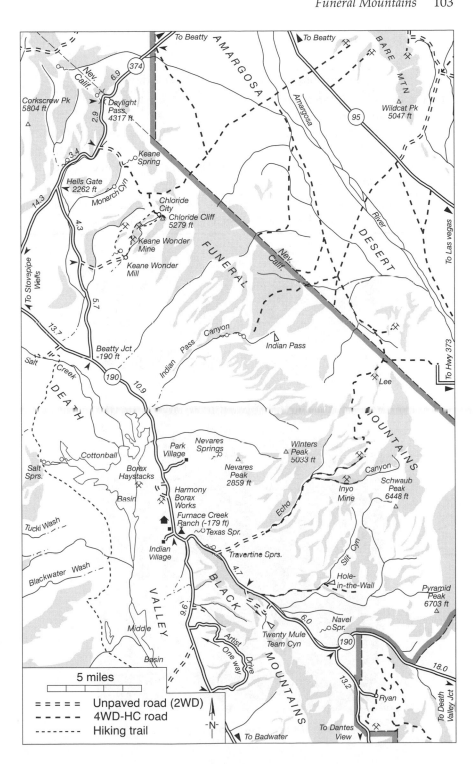

To Beatty

AMARGOSA

To Beatty

BARE MTN

374

Nev. Calif.

6.9

Wildcat Pk
5047 ft

95

Corkscrew Pk
5804 ft

2.9

Daylight
Pass
4317 ft

DESERT

To Las vegas

3.4

Keane
Spring

Hells Gate
2262 ft

14.3

Monarch Cyn

Chloride
City

Chloride Cliff
5279 ft

4.3

Keane Wonder
Mine

FUNERAL

Nev. Calif.

River

To Stovepipe Wells

Keane Wonder
Mill

5.7

Indian Pass Canyon

Indian Pass

To Hwy 373

13.7

Beatty Jct
-190 ft

Lee

Salt

190

10.9

Creek

DEATH

MOUNTAINS

Salt
Sprs.

Cottonball

Park
Village

Nevares
Springs

Winters
Peak
5033 ft

Canyon

Borax
Haystacks

Nevares
Peak
2859 ft

Echo

Schwaub
Peak
6448 ft

Inyo
Mine

Basin

Harmony
Borax
Works

Tucki Wash

Furnace Creek
Ranch (-179 ft)

Texas Spr.

Silt Cyn

Indian
Village

Travertine Sprs.

Hole-
in-the-Wall

Pyramid
Peak
6703 ft

Blackwater Wash

VALLEY

4.7

BLACK

9.9

Navel
Spr.

Middle

Artist

Twenty Mule
Team Cyn

6.0

190

18.0

Basin

Drive

One way

MOUNTAINS

13.2

To Death Valley Jct

Ryan

5 miles

= = = = = Unpaved road (2WD)

- - - - - 4WD-HC road

· · · · · · · Hiking trail

-N-

To Dantes
View

To Badwater

Route/Destination	Dist. (mi)	Elev. change	Mean elev.	Access road	Page
Suggested overnight hikes (over 2 days)					
Keane Wonder Mill to Chlor. City: road/canyon loop*	12.5	7,660'	3,290'	Graded	133-136
Echo Cyn: hwy to overlook	14.5	4,700'	2,590'	Paved	146-148
Echo Cyn: highway to Lee	20.6	6,500'	3,160'	Paved	146-150
Indian Pass Canyon (rd to rd)	11.5	3,260'	1,410'	Paved	138-142
Slit Cyn/Echo Cyn loop*	22.0	8,800'	2,620'	P/3.7 mi	146-154
Key: P=Primitive (2WD) H=Primitive (HC) F=Primitive (4WD) * =Total distance and elevation change (ups + downs) for loops					

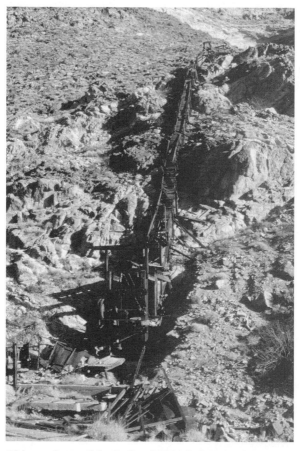

The ore chute of the Indian Mine, in Monarch Canyon

MONARCH CANYON

The most exciting feature of Monarch Canyon is its narrow central gorge, which is bisected by an unscalable drop-off where the canyon's little-known creek spawns what may be the highest waterfall in Death Valley. The upper canyon, with its tortured Proterozoic rocks and interesting gold mine, is the easiest way to see this colorful creek as it winds through a dense oasis. From Death Valley, the lower canyon gives access to the pleasant lower end of the creek and its impressive 110-foot waterfall. Circumventing the drop-off is a great challenge.

General Information

Road status: Roadless; hiking from paved road (lower canyon) or primitive road (upper canyon)
Shortest hike: 1.7 mi, 680 ft one way / easy (upper canyon)
Longest hike: 3.2 mi, 650 ft one way / moderate (lower canyon)
Main attractions: Monarch Spring, creek, waterfalls, narrows, gold mine
USGS 15' topo maps: Bullfrog, Chloride Cliff*
USGS 7.5' topo maps: Daylight Pass, Chloride City*
Maps: pp. 109*, 103

Location and Access

Monarch Canyon is located near the northern end of the Funeral Mountains. Because of the drop-off in the mid-canyon, most people will need to start from different points to see the upper and lower canyon.

The lower canyon used to be reached from the Beatty Cutoff by two mining roads. The upper road, the most direct route, started 0.7 mile south of Hell's Gate. The trail is now just a memory but where it used to branch off the pavement is still the best starting point to the lower canyon. From here Monarch Canyon is the prominent notch in the Funerals to the east, and its mouth is the wide opening below it. The saddle between the Death Valley Buttes is a good marker to find your car on the way back. The second option is the lower mining road, now closed to motorized traffic, which starts 2.7 miles south of Hell's Gate. This longer and more difficult approach is detailed further on.

To get to the upper canyon, drive the Daylight Pass Road 3.4 miles east of Hell's Gate (or 2.9 miles west of the pass) to the Monarch Canyon Road on the south side. This road is unmarked and easy to miss. It is bumpy and gravelly at places, but it is passable with a passenger car until it crosses the wash of Monarch Canyon, a distance of 2.3 miles.

History: The Indian Mine

Like many others, the story of this small gold mine in the heart of Monarch Canyon reflects the frustrated hopes of the many prospectors who once roamed the mountains of Death Valley in search of mineral wealth. It is said to have been discovered in 1903 by a Shoshone Indian named Johnny Hughes, while he was hunting for bighorn sheep. In the wake of the gold rush set off by nearby Keane Wonder, Hughes showed his discovery to a man by the name of Ishmael, who located it in December 1904, aptly naming the richest property the Indian Claim.

The mine was first worked by Frank Durham and Burdon Gaylord, who bonded it in December 1905 for a hefty $20,000. By the following month they had dug a 60-foot tunnel, but all work stopped in April 1906, perhaps due to economic repercussions of the San Francisco earthquake. In the following years, Ishmael sold his claims to the Keane Springs Mining Company, a small outfit that somehow never worked the mine. But Ishmael returned in March 1909, after securing a little financial support, and leased the property back to give it an honest try.

With a partner named Richard Clapp and a team of three or four men, Ishmael extended the existing tunnel and started a second one next to it. Work proceeded at a good pace for nearly a year, in spite of the destruction by fire of the small assay office they had built near the mine. The value of the ore, around $20 per ton, was deemed high enough that in the late spring of 1910 the two men purchased and installed a two-stamp mill on the canyon floor just below the mine. Water was piped from the nearby spring, and by August the small mill began to operate. In October the first gold bullion, representing the production of a few weeks, was shipped out for refinement. Those must have been euphoric moments for the operators of the mine. However, things were actually not running so smoothly. There were minor difficulties with the mill, and this small shipment was probably insufficient to cover costs. The Indian Claim was just not rich enough to make a living. In spite of this encouraging beginning, work at the mine essentially stopped after October. Ishmael gave up first and moved out of the country. Over the next couple of years Clapp tried to raise funding to develop the mine on a larger scale, but his hopes never came true. The small shipment of October 1910 was the only gold that ever came out of the Indian Claim.

Route Description: The Upper Canyon

The Indian Mine. Down canyon from the road the canyon remains wide and gradually deepens, until the first major fall at the confluence with a large side canyon. The old access grade to the mine conveniently bypasses it on the south side. Beyond, the canyon narrows significantly. For a few hundred yards vertical walls uncover giant folded strata of Proterozoic metamorphic rocks, well worth backtracking up into the canyon from the end of the grade for a closer inspection.

The Indian Mine is another 0.4 mile down canyon. It never was a large enterprise but its remains are well-preserved and interesting. They include portions of the mill, the rusted barrels of the mill's stamps, and the ore bin, all located on the canyon floor. Above the mill, the long wooden ore chute that fed the ore into the ore bin still ascends the steep canyon wall to a level area high above the canyon floor. At the head of the chute a narrow gauge track winds its way to the nearby mine tunnel.

The rocks exposed from the fall to around the spring belong to the Crystal Spring Formation. Below the mine and further down canyon there are some great outcrops of staurolite-schist and biotite-schist, in glittering shades of green, silver, and gold.

Monarch Spring and the drop-off. Further down, the canyon is choked in a wall-to-wall oasis of cane, the head of Monarch Spring. In the next few hundred yards you'll have to bushwhack your way through a few thickets to get to the small spring-fed creek. For quite some distance clear water alternatively flows and disappears several times. The creek is particularly colorful, rimmed with crystallites of carbonate salts, carpeted with beds of red and green algae, occasionally forming a shallow pool.

About 0.2 mile below the head of the spring the land breaks away abruptly, giving way to a precipitous drop-off. The wash resumes at its foot, more than 180 feet below, dwarfed by distance. The creek flow is only a few gallons per minute, but it is enough to produce a series of high waterfalls as it leaps over the drop-off. Unfortunately, they are only partially visible from this end. It is still an impressive site.

The drop-off is a serious obstruction, very difficult to bypass, as discussed further on. For most people this is the end of the trail.

Route Description: The Lower Canyon

The approach. For the shortest route to the lower canyon, start where the old road to Monarch Canyon used to branch off the Beatty Cutoff, as described above. You can try to follow it. Near the paved road only traces remain, overgrown with tall creosotes, and you will have to be persistent to not lose it further on, if it is still there. Otherwise just pick a straight route across the fan to the canyon mouth, which is shorter than the old road. To avoid too many ups and downs, aim just to the right of the prominent pink hills located on this side of Monarch Canyon near its mouth. It is a fairly easy, level walk, with good views of the salt pan. The fan supports scattered cholla and beavertail cactus, and it is a treat to be here when they put on their bright floral show, usually around late March. About a third of a mile east of the pink hills, look on the fan for unusual signs of wind and rain erosion. Rocks have been sliced by heat like a loaf of bread, or deeply grooved by differential solution (see *Stretched-Pebble Canyon*). There are also some pretty intricate ventifacts, more deeply gauged than I have found anywhere.

Another possible route is the lower mining road. It is still in place for some distance from the paved road. I have not walked all of it yet but here is what old maps show. After 1.9 miles it used to enter a short canyon south of Monarch Canyon. Further on it turned into a trail, followed the south side to a small mining area, then swung to the north side, crossed over a low saddle, and dropped into Monarch Canyon just above its mouth. The north end of this trail in Monarch Canyon has been washed out, and other portions likely suffered a similar fate. This approach is longer, about 3.4 miles for 1,150 feet up and 200 feet down.

The lower canyon. You have to be patient with this one, as it remains broad for a while and not much happens at first. There are a few monuments marking forgotten claim boundaries on the north side, a few exposures of strongly folded strata, and traces of mining activity near the end of the road. The main side canyon on the south side is narrower and more interesting. It has several pretty, sculpted falls (Crystal Spring Formation), starting with high twin falls that offer one easy and one more challenging climb. Several times this side canyon will trick you into thinking it ends soon, but it actually goes on a fair distance.

Monarch Canyon		
	Dist.(mi)	Elev.(ft)
Upper canyon		
Monarch Canyon Road	0.0	3,520
First fall	0.7	3,260
Indian Mine (Mill)	1.1	~3,080
Monarch Spring	1.5	2,920
Top of drop-off	1.7	~2,800
Lower canyon		
Beatty Cutoff (upper route)	0.0	1,990
Mouth	1.6	2,100
Main side canyon	2.2	2,280
16-ft waterfall	3.0	~2,580
Foot of drop-off (110-ft waterfall)	3.15	~2,640

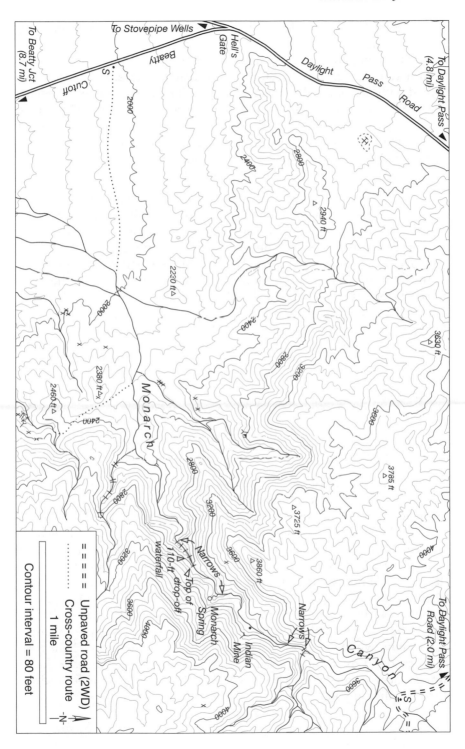

To Stovepipe Wells

To Beatty Jct
(8.7 mi)

Beatty
Cutoff

Hell's
Gate

To Daylight Pass
(4.8 mi)

Daylight Pass Road

2940 ft

3630 ft

2220 ft

2380 ft-x

2460 ft

2400

3785 ft

△3725 ft

△3860 ft

Monarch

Narrows

Top of
110-ft drop-off
waterfall

Monarch
Spring

Indian
Mine

Narrows

Canyon

To Daylight Pass
Road (2.0 mi)

Unpaved road (2WD)
Cross-country route
1 mile

Contour interval = 80 feet

Shortly past this side canyon the main canyon begins to narrow, twist and turn as it enters an erosion-resistant exposure of early Proterozoic metamorphic and igneous rocks. This is the central gorge, from here to the spring a region of tormented metasedimentary rocks veined with pegmatite dikes and small granitic plutons about 1.7 billion years old—among the oldest rocks exposed in the park. The gorge becomes gradually more deeply entrenched and chaotic. The canyon floor is made of crooked beds of polished mosaics cluttered with large boulders. After a few bends you will finally hear running water, and come face to face with a 16-foot waterfall in a small grotto. Pay dirt.

The spring and creek. The final 300-yard stretch, from this waterfall to the drop-off, has one of the most pleasant creeks in the park, flowing along a narrow trench at the bottom of the deepest part of the canyon. At places it passes under low overhangs of mosaics. At others it goes over water-worn lips of travertine, forming waterfalls that plunge 5 to 10 feet down into small pools of algae-covered water. In the heart of one of the hottest deserts on Earth, this is a rare treasure.

The last waterfall is the most spectacular. Backed against a sheer, high escarpment, it is probably the highest perennial waterfall in Death Valley. Only its lower 110 feet are visible from this end, but higher up, within the tight folds of the drop-off, water tumbles down over polished chutes in a series of cascades. The two high, massive curtains of travertine on either side of the fall show that for all its magnificence, this fall is a mere ghost of its former self. Like the thick benches of travertine exposed downstream, they were deposited by the carbonate-rich water when its flow was considerably higher. At one point in time, this area may have looked like a small replica of Arizona's Havasu Falls.

Bypassing the drop-off. Monarch Canyon's 180-foot drop-off is one serious vertical discontinuity. To bypass it is major work, as it is surrounded on both sides by a sheer, 1,000-foot escarpment for quite some distance. Major work, but not outrageous: some of us actually come here for just this kind of challenge. It is more strenuous but easier to find a route from the lower canyon. On the north side just below the fall, a steep talus climbs several hundred feet along the base of a cliff. This may be the least difficult route. On the south side the only route I found involves a technical climb up the cliff about 200 yards from the fall. The beginning is a 5.6 climb at most, but it rapidly becomes exposed, and I don't know whether it goes through. Unless you are an excellent rock climber, don't even think about it. Either route, you will have to go almost clear to the Monarch Canyon Road before being able to drop back into the canyon.

■

CHLORIDE CLIFF

First put on the map in 1871, Chloride Cliff is one of the oldest historical sites in Death Valley. Take a walking tour of its mines and mill ruins, and of the scattered remains of Chloride City, the small town that housed the miners. The dramatic views of Death Valley from high on the crest of the Funerals, if not the wind, will blow you away. For a longer hike, try one of the rough routes down to the Big Bell Mine, hanging on the sheer flank of the Funerals 1,600 feet below Chloride Cliff.

General Information

Road status: Accessed by primitive road (4WD-HC)
Shortest hike: Strolls and short walks / very easy
Longest hike: 2.3 mi, 1,540 ft one way (or more) / difficult
Main attractions: Historic mines, spectacular views, old mining trails
USGS topo maps: Chloride Cliff (15'), Chloride City (7.5')
Maps: pp. 117*, 135, 103

Location and Access

There are several ways to get to the Chloride Cliff area, up on the rim of the northern Funeral Mountains. The shortest but roughest route is the Monarch Canyon Road, which starts at the Daylight Pass Road 3.4 miles east of Hell's Gate (or 2.9 miles west of Daylight Pass). After 5.2 miles, it joins the Chloride Cliff Road. Make a right, and drive 1.1 miles to a junction marked by an old water tank on the right. From here it is 400 yards to the site of Chloride City. If you intend to hike through here, I recommend you start from this junction, which minimizes impact on this fragile area. This itinerary requires a high-clearance vehicle a little past the wash of Monarch Canyon, 2.3 miles from the pavement. Lighter vehicles may also require 4-wheel drive for the last 1.1 mile stretch, which goes over steep and lopsided bedrock.

If you have a standard passenger car, your first option is to drive to Monarch Canyon and walk from there. You can also drive to the junction at mile 5.2 via the Chloride Cliff Road, which heads southeast from Highway 374 just outside of the park boundary. From there it is only a 1.5-mile walk to Chloride City.

Yet the most dramatic way to get to Chloride Cliff, if you have a whole day and energy to spare, is to hike up from the valley floor (see *The Keane Wonder Mine*).

History

The scattered remains dotting the barren hills around Chloride Cliff are the ruins of Chloride City, an area with a patchy, 90-year history of not so successful mining. It started with the discovery of silver-lead ore in August 1871, around what is now Chloride Cliff, by August Franklin, a civil engineer sent to this far frontier to assist in the survey of the California-Nevada boundary. In October, after staking a few claims, he founded the Chloride Cliff Company—reportedly named after the ore he had discovered, silver chloride—thus launching the first mining venture on the east side of Death Valley.

Work started in April 1872. The deposit showed good ore value and progress proceeded at a good pace. By the following year Franklin had several miners working for him, and 100 tons of ore had been stockpiled on the dump. One can only imagine what a lonesome life it must have been to mine in these pioneering days. It was 180 miles across mostly uninhabited country to San Bernardino, the closest sizeable town, with no established road to get there. This long trek was negotiated by trains of pack mules, which left Franklin's mine loaded with ore, and came back weeks later with long-awaited food and supplies. In the process of traveling back and forth across the desert, the mulers painstakingly forged the first route across Death Valley. From Chloride Cliff, it plunged down to Death Valley, continued south across the salt flats to the west side, and left the valley via Wingate Wash. Together with the identification of valuable mineral resources in the Funerals, this was probably Franklin's greatest accomplishment. About ten years later, part of his wagon trail would be used by the Harmony and Eagle Borax Works to haul borax to Mojave. Another 20 years and a couple of lucky prospectors would search the steep slopes below Chloride Cliff and discover what would become the legendary Keane Wonder Mine.

During his own time Franklin faced serious hardships. In spite of his new road, transportation was slow and costly. Franklin ran into the problem that was to plague the Chloride Cliff area its entire lifetime: the ore needed to be processed near the mine to minimize its weight and reduce transportation costs. Franklin may have tried to round up financial support, but the inaccessibility and unknown reserves of his mine probably made it unappealing to investors. The silver rush of 1873 over in the Panamints diverted what little funding was available, and Franklin was forced to shut down after less than two years of operation. But he did not give up. For the next 30 years he dutifully kept his claims alive by carrying out the required annual assessment work. He died in 1904, ironically just missing the rebirth of Chloride Cliff, but his persistence was not in vain. His son George, who continued working his claims after him, would soon reap the harvest of his hard work.

The catalyst for Chloride Cliff's revival was the discovery of Keane Wonder in 1904, just a couple of miles below the cliff, and the Bullfrog soon after. In 1905, as hundreds of prospectors were lured to these two sites, several gold strikes were made in the vicinity of Franklin's claims. By November three companies had been formed, the Bullfrog Cliff Mining Company, the Mucho Oro Mining Company, and the Death Valley Mining and Milling Company. Chloride Cliff was booming all over again.

George Franklin was now working his father's property under greatly improved conditions. The renewed interest meant new roads, supplies at nearby Rhyolite, and better chances to make a profit. The remote region that had seen Franklin's father as sole visitor for decades was all of a sudden hopping. By the end of 1905 all companies were actively developing one or two tunnels each. The miners were housed at Chloride City, a small camp sheltered just behind the cliff. By the spring of 1906 the deepest workings reached several hundred feet, ore values still held up, and two of the companies began looking into ways of milling their ore. In spite of the lingering hardship due to isolation and lack of supplies—water had to be packed in several miles from Keane Spring, and wood from even further—the future looked promising.

The San Francisco earthquake and fire in April that year changed all of that. The destruction of the West Coast financial center seriously jeopardized future support for mining developments and dealt a serious blow to the Chloride Cliff area. The Bullfrog Cliff and Mucho Oro companies shortly suspended all mining activities. The Death Valley Company shut down in July. George Franklin was perhaps happiest of them all. In July he sold the mine that had been in his family for 35 years for a reported $150,000.

It was three years before the area saw its next burst of activity. By December 1907 the Bullfrog Cliff, Mucho Oro, and Franklin mines had been consolidated into the Chloride Cliff Mining Company, and work resumed in December 1909. Gold-bearing ore was discovered soon after, which sparked renewed optimism. As Franklin had found out the hard way decades earlier, the main problem the new company faced was milling and delivering its ore. In the winter of 1910 the company improved the road to Rhyolite for the delivery of a one-stamp mill. The small mill was installed in March just below Franklin's mine, which still had the most productive tunnels. Great plan, but for one minor oversight: the water supply was too low to run the mill, and the mill was never used. After all this work the company had to resort to leasing Rhyolite's Crystal Bullfrog Mill. Using a 12-horse team to transport the ore to the mill, a 100-ton shipment worth about $3,500 was made in August. In the following weeks production was increased to seven tons a day, with as many as 19 miners on the job. Some high-grade ore was shipped to smelters in Needles and Goldfield. But the return was still insufficient, and in mid-October mining was suspended again.

Over the next two years, grand plans were made to build a 4-mile pipeline from Keane Spring to expand milling capabilities, and even to erect a wire tramway to the mill. Developments were initiated at the spring, but funding was insufficient to carry it through. The company began negotiating with a British investor in April 1911. Negotiations dragged on for months and sustained high hopes in the local community. But the mines were just too remote, and the deal never came through. The Chloride Cliff Company closed down for good in June 1912.

Next to Franklin, the most prominent figure in Chloride Cliff's history is J. Irving Crowell, one of Death Valley's most persistent and decidedly most unlucky miners. He was president of the Chloride Cliff Company, and president of the Bullfrog Cliff Company before that. In spite of these two failures he still held on after 1912, mining his property alone off and on. In 1916 he erected a Lane mill and dug a well for it a mile away, but the well ran dry after a few days. He continued assessment work for several years, and finally sold his mine in 1928. Until around 1941 the area was mined intermittently by either the new owner, Louis McCrea of Beatty, or a few lessees. These were the last gold mining years at Chloride Cliff. As before, they produced only small ore shipments. Hard to believe, but in 1941 undeterred Crowell came back

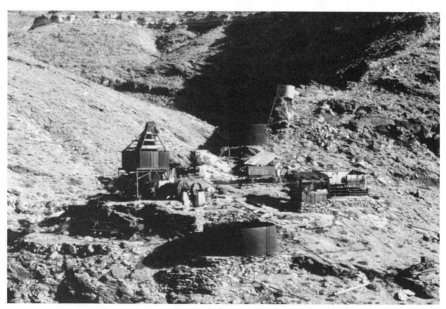

Rusted mining structures in the Funeral Mountains

for more, this time to develop a small deposit of mercury ore (cinnabar) near abandoned Chloride City. A five-ton mercury treatment plant was erected near the mine, but it must not have been Crowell's lucky life: the plant was destroyed by fire after only a small quantity of ore had been treated. Although others poked around here up until the 1960s, this was Chloride Cliff's last significant activity, perhaps for the better.

Hiking Suggestions

Chloride Cliff has four areas of interest, from north to south: the site of the 1941 mercury mining, the ghost town of Chloride City and the 1916 Lane mill, the dugouts, and Franklin's original mines and mill. These sites are fairly small, and each one can be visited with little walking, although covering them all can take half a day. For a more serious hike, try the Big Bell Mine, reached by a steep walk down from the Chloride Cliff area. Three routes are suggested below. The best way is to do a loop hike, going down to the mine one route and coming back up another one. It takes about half a day, including time to smell the roses.

Route Description

Crowell's mercury mine. The mercury mine is at the first turnoff on the right before getting to Chloride City, just below the prominent rusting water tank. The concrete pilings are the foundations of the ill-fated mercury treatment plant, which burnt down shortly after its installation. This is one of the very few cinnabar mines in the park. Here as throughout the Chloride Cliff area, the rocks exposed are mostly staurolite- and biotite-schists, calcite marble, and micaceous quartzite of the Pahrump Group—all of them around the billion-year mark.

Chloride City. The site of Chloride City is at the next junction, about 400 yards down the main road. The town boomed in 1905-1906 and came back to life sporadically during short-lived mining revivals in the 1910s and 1940s. Today few standing structures attest to its historical significance, but it still has some remains, mostly from the later era. The best way to visit it is to walk the half-mile loop around Chloride City. Going down the main road first, look for the floor remains of a house on the left side, which used to be a boarding house. Take the trail that splits off to the right a little further south. It will take you to the humble grave of James McKay (whose life history has been completely forgotten), and to an old wooden shack. The trail then circles westward to a narrow drainage. The ruins on the steep slope below this junction is the site of Crowell's 1916 Lane mill. What is left today are its concrete pilings and a retaining stone wall used to impound mine tailings.

The dugouts. The third area of interest is at the south end of the main road, where three unusual dugouts are lined up along a ravine. These small houses probably housed miners in the later mining period. As their name implies, they were built partially into the side of a hill, which explains why they are still standing. Take a look at pictures of these dugouts in Ruth Kirk's *Exploring Death Valley* (1956), and in Chuck Gebhardt's *Inside Death Valley* (1988) to see how much they have degraded over time, largely due to vandalism. Do your share to preserve them as long as possible by staying away from them.

Franklin's mine and mill. The southernmost area of interest is Franklin's mine. From the dugouts it is reached via the road that circles around the east side of Chloride Cliff. The tunnels at the end of the road are the original group of silver mines Franklin claimed in 1871, the first mines to be operated on the east side of Death Valley. The centerpiece is the tall timber frame of the one-stamp mill erected in 1910, which was unfortunately hardly, and probably never, used. It is still remarkably well-preserved, which is no surprise given its location. Look for it half way down the sheer canyon slope, several hundred feet below the road.

Chloride Cliff. The one thing you don't want to miss is the viewpoint from Chloride Cliff. From this dizzying vantage point you will be looking down the length of Death Valley, more than 5,000 feet below, a breathtaking panorama perhaps surpassed only by Dante's View.

Chloride Cliff and the Big Bell Mine		
	Dist.(mi)	Elev.(ft)
Water tower junction	0.0	4,760
Mercury mine	(0.05)	4,760
Chloride City junction	0.4	4,760
Lane mill loop	(0.7)	4,880
Big Bell Mine (via mining road)	(2.3)	~3,620
Dugouts	0.8	5,010
Big Bell Mine (via cable road)	(1.7)	~3,620
Big Bell Mine (via canyon)	(1.5)	~3,620
Junction	0.95	5,160
Chloride Cliff	(0.3)	5,279
Franklin Mine	1.1	~5,100
Franklin Mill	~1.5	~4,260

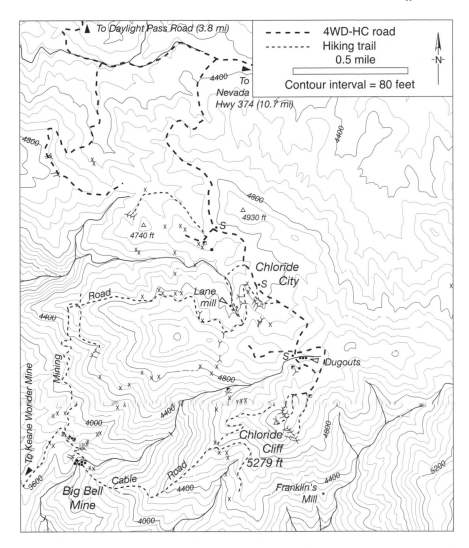

Map legend:
- - - - 4WD-HC road
-------- Hiking trail
0.5 mile
Contour interval = 80 feet
-N-

To Daylight Pass Road (3.8 mi)

4400
To
Nevada
Hwy 374 (10.7 mi)

4800

4800

△
4930 ft

△
4740 ft

S

Chloride
City
S

Road   Lane
mill

4400

Mining

To Keane Wonder Mine

4800

S   ▷ Dugouts

4000

4800

Chloride
Cliff
5279 ft

Cable   Road
4400

Big Bell
Mine

3600

4000

Franklin's
Mill

4400

5200

4000

The Big Bell Mine. This mine is located about 2 miles and 1,600 feet below Chloride Cliff. It can be reached by several routes, none very long but all fairly strenuous. The longest but easiest (though not always well-defined) is the mining road to the Keane Wonder Mill, which starts at Chloride City. Steep at places, it offers spectacular views of the valley. The trail junction to the Big Bell Mine is marked by a shallow, rectangular pit, just past the junction on its south side.

The second route is the cable road. From the dugouts, hike up the road that heads south to Chloride Cliff. In the next 500 yards it forks twice; each time take the right fork. This will put you on a road that circles down and around the west side of Chloride Cliff. The cable road starts on the right in the second left switchback. It is relatively faint at this junction, but you can see it a short distance away going down the ridge, where it is much better defined. This is the shortest route, but it's one hell of a precipitous road. It means spectacular views, hard work for your knees, and slow moving. This road owes its name to the cable that ran along it, which was used to winch a truck, loaded with ore from the mill, up to Chloride Cliff. The road is still lined with remains of the cable and the short metal spikes used to guide it, as well as segments of the pipeline from Keane Spring. The cable road ends at, in fact drops onto, the milling complex of the Big Bell Mine.

The third route to the Big Bell Mine is down the canyon along which it is located. It is the roughest but the most fool-proof. Just head down the wash that runs in front of the dugouts, and you'll eventually run into the mine. At first, and for a short distance, the wash is paralleled by the barely discernable trace of a road. The canyon quickly steepens and deepens, and progress soon requires hard work, with a fair amount of scrambling. From rim to mine, it is a 1,400-foot drop in only 1.5 miles, and as expected there are quite a few falls along the way. The most serious one is about halfway down. It is only a class 4 climb, less than vertical and 15-20 feet high, but it will likely stop people with a fear of heights, especially going downhill.

The Big Bell is an interesting and educational site. The majority of its remains date from the 1935-1937 Coen Company operations (refer to *The Big Bell Extension Mine* for its unusual history). The ore was extracted from several stoped tunnels on the north side of the canyon (staurolite and biotite pelitic schist from the Crystal Spring Formation). It was conveyed by rail to an ore bin on the edge of the canyon. From here it was transported via a short aerial tramway across the wash to the mill, on the south side of the canyon. The milling complex is dominated by the remains of a ball mill and its ore bin, huge water and cyanide tanks in the wash, several tailings and shacks. The processed ore was loaded on the Mack truck that still stands near the mill, and winched up to Chloride Cliff along the cable road, on the steep ridge behind the mill. The mining camp is high above the mines, along the connecting trail to the mining road. Its unusual cluster of small cabins, built on a terraced hillside, was surrounded by a short stone wall for protection against the strong winds. Be aware that the Big Bell Mine is still covered by patented mining claims; it is therefore private land. Respect it accordingly.

Another way to get to this site, which requires no driving on rough roads but more walking, is from the Keane Wonder Mill. This hike is described under *The Keane Wonder Mine*.

■

THE BIG BELL EXTENSION MINE

In this area there is a little something for everyone. One option is an easy walk to scenic springs and the historic remains of Cyty's Mill and cabin. Another one is an offbeat hike up either a steep mining trail or a nameless canyon to the Big Bell Extension, a gold mine once fought over by gunfire. The canyon is pretty, the lore colorful, the geology unusual, and not too many people will be rubbing elbows with you.

General Information

Road status: Roadless; hiking from good graded road
Shortest hike: 0.8 mi, 100 ft one way / easy
Longest hike: 4.7 mi, 2,370 ft one way / difficult
Main attractions: Cyty's Mill, Keane Wonder Spring, a scenic canyon and trail, a remote gold mine, geology
USGS topo maps: Chloride Cliff (15'), Chloride City (7.5')
Maps: pp. 125*, 135

Location and Access

The Big Bell Extension Mine and Cyty's Mill are in the northern Funerals, in the general vicinity of the Keane Wonder Mill. To get there, drive the Beatty Cutoff 5.7 miles north from Highway 190 (or 4.3 miles south from Hell's Gate) to the marked road to the Keane Wonder Mill. This well-graded road is OK for all vehicles. Cyty's Mill is visible from almost anywhere along this road. Look for it in the middle of the extensive area of white rocks at the foot of the Funerals to the northeast. To hike the canyon, park a little before the lowest point in the road, near the sharp left bend about 0.9 mile from the paved road. To hike the mining trail, park at the end of the road, 2.8 miles from the paved road.

History

The intertwined histories of the Big Bell and Big Bell Extension mines revolve around a prospector by the name of Johnnie Cyty, an eccentric, trigger-happy character nicknamed "Johnnie-Behind-the-Gun." Cyty had been prospecting and mining in the California desert for several years when he arrived in the Funerals in 1904, attracted by the Keane Wonder strike. In June, he and a partner, Mike Sullivan, found evidence of gold above the Keane Wonder and located the ten claims that became the Big Bell Mine. At that time or later in the summer, Cyty also filed claims less than a mile away that he called the Big Bell Extension. Cyty did not get involved in these mines right away. Instead, he optioned the Big Bell property to a first party that essentially did not touch it, then to a mining promoter named Walter O'Brien, in November 1905. O'Brien incorporated the Death Valley Big Bell Mining Company and raised a small amount of funding by selling company stock. He had until the following September to exercise his option to buy, and for several months he diligently developed the property, employing a few men to assess its value. A small camp was erected at the site and equipment was hauled down to the mine from Chloride Cliff. In time, rich specimens were exposed, assaying as much as $60 per ton. Spurred by these encouraging results, Cyty and a partner, L. D. Porter, began to work on the Big Bell Extension. They hoped to intercept some of the Big Bell veins, and perhaps even the veins of the Keane Wonder Mine, recognized by then as one of the richest around. Over the next few months, they did expose some valuable ore. These discoveries, just a stone's throw from Keane Wonder, prompted a Rhyolite newspaper to praise the Big Bell as yet another "Wonder". Hopes ran high; O'Brien even talked about a tramway and mill. But when the deadline came around, he and Cyty failed to reach an agreement, and the claims returned to their owners.

Cyty temporarily abandoned the Big Bell Extension to become involved in the Big Bell's new management. Work at the mine continued through 1907, with a long break in the summer to avoid the heat. As usual, a fair amount of activity took place: stock was sold to raise funding, a mine superintendent was hired, and encouraging progress was made. But, also as usual, production was small. By the beginning of 1908 the company had exhausted its funds and work slowed down to a crawl.

The fate of the Big Bell Mine took a Hollywood twist in April, when Cyty lost his 250,000 shares in the company in a night-long roulette game against the owner of one of Rhyolite's gambling halls. The new owner negotiated the sale of the property right away with a prospective buyer from England, who showed a genuine interest for quite some time, but the deal never went through. The Big Bell Mining Company died in the spring of 1911. The property was purchased in the fall by Homer Wilson, superintendent of the Keane Wonder Mine, as additional ore reserves. For some reason the claims were not exploited, even after the Keane Wonder played out the following summer.

With nothing better to do, soon after he lost the Big Bell Mine Cyty returned to prospecting at the Big Bell Extension. However, by then he found that his property was contested by Kyle Smith, recorder of the South Bullfrog Mining District. In the intervening years, Smith had filed claims on some of Cyty's previous sites, thinking Cyty had not properly carried out his required annual assessment work. In the fall, after the dispute had been going on for several months, Smith found Cyty working on the contested site. In a typical movie scene, the two men resorted to their guns, and Smith was shot dead.

Smith was a prominent and popular figure. He had developed several mining claims in this area and over in Echo Canyon. Johnnie Cyty, on the other hand, was generally disliked for his rough manners and fondness for his artillery, and the local press slashed him. He was tried in March 1909, convicted of manslaughter in April, and sentenced to 10 years in San Quentin. Cyty's attorney filed a notice of appeal, which was heard in November. Surprisingly enough, the California court overturned the earlier conviction and ordered a new trial. Cyty went to court again in March 1910, and this time he was lucky. He was acquitted and released on the grounds that on the day of the shoot-out he was defending his property, and that Smith may have fired first.

A year later, in February 1911, Cyty resumed his work at the Big Bell Extension. He hired miners from the Keane Wonder Mine to help bag his ore, with plans to eventually use the Keane Wonder Mill for treatment. After just a few weeks, however, enough valuable ore was in sight—later reported worth $20 to $30 per ton—that he decided to acquire a mill. Once again he was lucky. In those days of instant boom and bust, mining equipment changed hands often, being used for a short time only before being auctioned off to another hopeful miner. Such an opportunity arose just in time for Cyty, who was able to purchase at an auction a second-hand, three-stamp mill for a modest price. In April the mill was hauled to its new home near Keane Wonder Springs, a few miles below the mine. Perhaps because of summer delays, the mill did not become operative until October. By then Cyty's public image had gone around full circle. A Rhyolite newspaper praised him for his perseverance at developing such isolated claims. Unfortunately, in spite of all this work, Cyty's hopes did not materialize. A shipment of unknown value was made in November, but it was the only one ever reported. Operations were probably not profitable, for the Big Bell Extension was never heard of again.

Cyty lived most, and probably all, of the rest of his life in the Rhyolite-Beatty area, following the fortunes of the time. During the Leadfield boom, in nearby Titus Canyon, he built a small hotel in Beatty. For a few years in the mid-1920s he was watchman at the Keane Wonder Mill, which had by then closed its doors. Johnnie-Behind-the-Gun did get in trouble again for assault with a deadly weapon, was convicted, retried and, yes, acquitted once more. He lived to be an old man, probably lucky all along, cherishing fond memories of the gold mine he had in the Funerals—a mine which, he once claimed, "was richer than the Keane Wonder ever dreamed of being."

The Big Bell Mine remained idle all this time, until 1935 when it was acquired and finally developed in style by the Coen Mining Company. The company had ambitious plans and carried them through. It erected a small ball mill near the mine, and installed a pump house at Keane Spring and a pipeline to bring water to the mill. A small rail and short aerial tramway were constructed to transport the ore from the mines to the mill. A very steep cable road was bladed to haul the processed ore by truck nearly 1,400 feet up to Chloride Cliff. It was a commendable effort, but it was unsuccessful. Although no production figures are available, the small amount of gold the company managed to produce was clearly unable to cover expenses. The mine shut down in the fall of 1937. It was reopened for a short period in 1940, but it closed down again the following year, this time for good. Although its ore reserves were once estimated at 30,000 tons, the Big Bell Mine never produced nearly as much as its close neighbor, the Keane Wonder.

Route Description

Access. From the end of the graded road, there are two ways to reach the trail to Cyty's Mill. The fail-safe approach is to hike back 0.25 mile on the graded road to an old, barricaded road on the north side, near the "Mine Hazard" sign. This is the head of the trail to Cyty's Mill. Or walk through the old cyanide plant just north of the parking area, towards the large rusted tank. Just beyond it, look for an old trail heading northwest. It joins the Cyty's Mill trail in about 200 yards. From here it is an easy, level walk along the foot of the Funerals to Keane Wonder Springs. The disjointed pipes along the trail are remains of the pipeline used to deliver water from the springs to the Keane Wonder Mill.

Keane Wonder Springs. Though rarely visited, these little springs are quite interesting. They are made of two small creeks and quite a few smaller seeps. The main creek comes out of a ravine a short distance from the trail, flows among colorful algae and carpets of salt grass, then fans out onto the travertine bench below the trail and disappears over the bench's abrupt edge. This edge marks the location of the Keane Wonder Fault, which runs parallel to the foot of the Funerals for miles. Above the small oasis at the head of the creek, there is a shallow well, probably dug in historical times to tap the spring. At the bottom of the well a rushing stream of clear water flows over pure white travertine. This water has traveled miles along deep faults before finally emerging here, picking up fair amounts of sulfur and heat along the way. The thick fumes emanating from the well are heavily laced with hydrogen sulfide. The NPS sign by the well is not exaggerating; the stuff is nasty. Don't hang around too long.

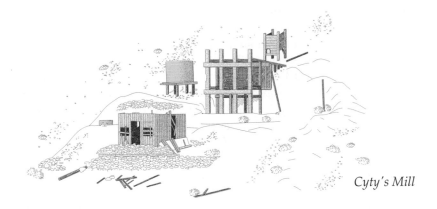

Cyty's Mill

The miniature basins along the creek, the bright terraces of travertine, and the sulfurous drifts are reminiscent of Yellowstone's Mammoth Hot Springs, although on a much smaller scale. Yet at some point in time, perhaps as recently as the Pleistocene, this spring was considerably larger. The travertine mound it left behind at the foot of the range extends for nearly one and a half miles. If you climb the hillside behind the springs or Cyty's Mill and look back, you will see a grand staircase of terraces cascading several hundred feet down to the fan. Although most of this ancient spring has now dried up, if it ever was all active at the same time, it was in fact larger than Mammoth Hot Springs.

Cyty's Mill. The trail resumes just beyond the springs and ends shortly at Cyty's Mill. This site is dominated by the heavy timber frame of Cyty's three-stamp mill, with its ore bin, concrete engine mount, and water tank. The small wooden shack next to the mill was Cyty's living quarters. This area shows numerous signs of turn-of-the-century mining—a rock shelter, trenches dug in the travertine, probably for water reclamation, a well filled with a deep turquoise pool, and raw ore spilling on the slope above the ore bin. The mill itself is a good example of "recycled" mining equipment, recounting the successive hopes and failures of several mining ventures. It was first constructed for the American Mine near Columbia, Nevada. In March 1910, it was sold to the Hayseed Mining Company, which owned gold claims in the Echo-Lee district. After the Hayseed folded, Johnnie Cyty purchased it and moved it here, its final resting place.

The mining trail. The easiest and shortest route to the Big Bell Extension Mine is the mining trail. This trail has been used very little over the last few decades. Its lower portion is faint and a little hard to find. First, look for the trailhead just a few steps to the south of Cyty's Mill, at the head of a manmade trench. From here the trail climbs up to the wide bench above the mill, crosses it to a small wash, then switch-backs up the steep talus on the opposite side to a second bench 220 feet higher. The rest of it is in better shape, although at places it is a little difficult to track when traveling uphill.

Along the first 0.4 mile, the trail crosses extensive exposures of travertine. This rock comes in a variety of forms and colors, from light tan to milky, from finely layered to ceramic-like or covered with convoluted twirls. On the second bench above the mill, the trail passes by a wide open floor of mosaics. These colorful aggregates of small rocks, some coated with desert varnish, others strongly eroded by wind and rain, are probably fan material that was permeated and cemented by hot springs. The trail is steep, but in the cooler months it is a pleasant hike, and you will be rewarded by increasingly fine views of Death Valley. After 1.6 miles the trail reaches a ridge overlooking a deep, nameless canyon. The last stretch to the mine is more gentle, along the abrupt rim of the canyon.

The canyon route. This other way to the mine is longer, but it will take you through a scenic, rarely visited canyon. From the Keane Wonder Mill road about 0.9 mile from the paved road, hike to the narrow slit in the tan bluffs to the north, which is the canyon mouth. The lower canyon goes through a shallow gulch, then opens up for a while. The rock in this area is mostly Miocene arkose and conglomerate. The entrance into the much deeper mid-canyon, which occurs at the Keane

The Big Bell Extension Mine		
	Dist.(mi)	Elev.(ft)
Mining trail		
Keane Wonder Mill	0.0	1,320
Keane Wonder Springs	0.8	1,230
Cyty's Mill	1.2	1,260
Ridge (canyon overlook)	2.8	2,770
First adit	3.1	2,900
Big Bell Extension Mine	3.4	~3,100
The canyon route		
Keane Wonder Mine Road	0.0	730
Mouth	0.6	900
Start of deep canyon	2.1	1,410
9-ft overhang	2.7	1,800
First side canyon	4.4	2,770
Big Bell Extension Mine	4.7	~3,100

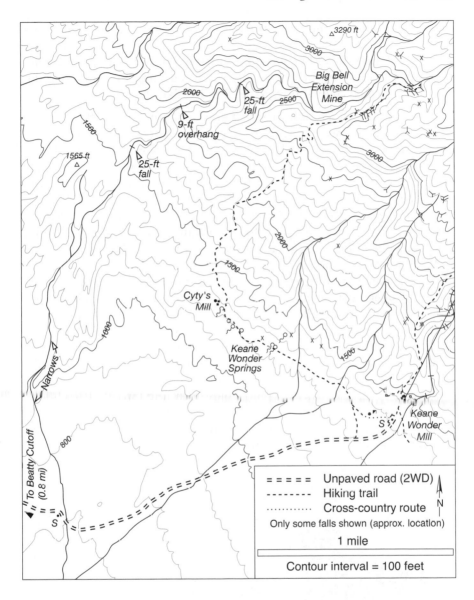

=====	Unpaved road (2WD)
--------	Hiking trail
....	Cross-country route

Only some falls shown (approx. location)

1 mile

Contour interval = 100 feet

Wonder Fault, is quite abrupt. The mountain front was uplifted along this fault, exposing the considerably older Proterozoic metamorphic rocks (Crystal Spring Formation) found along the upper canyon.

This canyon is sprinkled with attractions—a sinuous course, sheer walls of tightly folded rocks, overhangs, several short tight sections, and a generous assortment of falls, the highest ones about 25 feet. The falls are generally easy to climb or bypass, but they still add a modest challenge to this hike. The only exception is a wide, horseshoe-shaped overhang about 9 feet high, which takes a little more effort to either climb (low 5s) or bypass. After much winding around, which may seem to take forever, you will finally reach the first side canyon on the south side, which leads shortly to the Big Bell Extension.

The Big Bell Extension Mine. If you came up the trail, the first historical site you'll encounter is a series of adits, a deep tunnel, and a collapsed stope, starting 0.3 mile past the ridge. This area was mined seriously at some point. Later on, it was converted into living quarters, perhaps for the miners working at the more extensive tunnels down the trail. The shallower tunnels, some of them protected by short rock walls, are still littered with decayed mattresses and other signs of occupation. Two small wooden cabins used to stand a little further along the trail. They have been long since blown over the canyon's rim, and are now reduced to creaking floors.

The main mining area is a cluster of tunnels fanning out into the base of a steep escarpment near the end of the trail. Although not much is left besides the tunnels, it is an interesting site, protected by its poor accessibility and the sheer weight of the few remaining objects. The main tunnel still has a narrow gauge track and remains of an ore car. It ends at a deep vertical shaft; if you must venture into it, don't do it without a flashlight and extreme care. There is also a primitive brick oven constructed with local rocks, a pile of old pipes, and tons of ore—chunks of rust-colored quartz with sparkling mica-schist. This site was probably used well after Cyty's last known activity at the end of 1911, although this part of its history has not been recorded.

■

Petroglyphs (gridiron)
Funeral Mountains

THE KEANE WONDER MINE

With its glorious gold mining past and extensive remains, the Keane
Wonder Mine is one of Death Valley's finest gems. The old mill at the
foot of the Funerals and the mining complex, 1,500 feet up the rugged
scarp of the mountain, are among the best preserved around. The
mining site is reached by a strenuous hike up the old mining road,
offering magnificent views of Death Valley and the mine's unique
aerial tramway. The mines can also be reached via the tortuous, fall-
riddled nearby canyon, through mangled billion-year-old schists.

General Information

Road status: Hiking from a good graded road
Shortest hike: Strolls and short walks/very easy-moderate
Longest hike: 6.0 mi, 4,140 ft one way (and more)/strenuous
Main attractions: Keane Wonder Mine and Mill, a rugged canyon with
       falls, old mining road with spectacular views, geology
USGS topo maps: Chloride Cliff (15'), Chloride City (7.5')
Maps: pp. 135*, 103

Location and Access

The Keane Wonder Mill is located at the foot of the Funeral
Mountains, near the north end of the range. To get there, drive the
Beatty Cutoff 5.7 miles north from Highway 190 (or 4.3 miles south from
Hell's Gate) to the marked road to Keane Wonder Mill. This road dead
ends in 2.8 miles at a small parking area near the mill. It is well graded
and just about anything on wheels can make it.

History: The Great Keane Wonder Mine

In an area where most mines failed to generate anything substantial, the Keane Wonder Mine stands out like a sore thumb. It had
plenty of good ore, enough to warrant the development of one of the
most extensive mining complexes in Death Valley, and for a change, it
paid off. For nearly five years it yielded a steady output of gold, eventually becoming the second largest gold producer in Death Valley.

The gold strike that sparked it all was made in the spring of
1904 by Jack Keane and Domingo Etcharren, two prospectors who had
been searching the area for several months, ironically tracing a small
outcrop of silver. They named their discovery the Keane Wonder and
secured it with 18 claims. News of their strike drew other prospectors to

127

the area, who soon ascertained that the lode was exceptional.

True to their prospecting heritage, Keane and Etcharren looked for a buyer so they could sell out and move on. They first optioned their property in June 1904 to J. R. Delamar, a well-known mining operator who employed a sizeable crew to sink two exploratory tunnels. In the meantime, the Keane Wonder had touched off a feverish gold rush, and the northern Funerals were crawling with prospectors. The Big Bell was discovered, then the rich Bullfrog Hills, and the Chloride Cliff area was reactivated soon after. Delamar's miners carried out enough work to confirm Keane Wonder's wealth, but when the one-year deadline came around Delamar offered to buy the property for less than the amount originally agreed upon. Keane and Etcharren, well aware of the value of their claims, wisely waited for a better offer. Their patience paid off. After an unsuccessful leasing agreement in early 1906, they sold their mine for a reported $50,000 in cash and $200,000 in stock to stock brokers John Campbell and associates, who incorporated the Keane Wonder Company in late March. A few weeks later, Campbell's financial empire collapsed with the San Francisco earthquake, and the mine had to be sold again. It was acquired in June by Homer Wilson, owner of several Mother Lode mines, who set out to develop it for good.

Homer Wilson came to the scene with a prosperous background as a mining promoter and developer. It was largely his effective and visionary management that spelled the success of the Keane Wonder. As the mine was located some 1,500 feet up the steep Funeral Mountains, adequate transportation was needed to haul the ore down to the desert floor. Before mining resumed in early November 1906, Wilson had laid out plans for the two keystones of the mine: a nearly one mile long aerial tramway and an 80-ton milling complex at its lower end.

Construction work focussed first on the mill and auxiliary structures. The foundations were laid down in early 1907, while supplies and machinery were delivered from Rhyolite over Daylight Pass. As construction progressed, the payroll increased to 10 men, then 25, until in the spring even the miners were put to work on the mill. By April the main mill building towered high against the Funerals, and by early summer the mill machinery was essentially installed.

In July the task force was turned to a far greater challenge—the aerial tramway. Plans called for a complex upper terminal, 13 towers 18 to 30 feet high strung down the steep mountain slope, and a lower terminal with connections to the mill. At one place the tramway had to span 1,280 feet across a 500-foot deep canyon. All told, it would require some 75,000 board feet of lumber. To the credit of the men who toiled on this painstaking project, in spite of delays in timber delivery and summer temperatures that restricted work hours to early morning and late afternoon, it took less than four months to complete the job. On October 27, 1907 the first echoes of the mill's 20 stamps bounced off the Funerals. The Keane Wonder was ready to work.

The first gold bullion, worth around $20,000, was delivered to Rhyolite two weeks later. By December the mill was running around the clock, processing on a daily basis 70 to 75 tons averaging $18-20 per ton. The rest is history. Except for a few short interruptions, the mine's two workhorses performed almost flawlessly, and the Keane Wonder produced nearly continuously until the summer of 1912.

There were several reasons for this success. First, it had plenty of valuable ore, a somewhat essential ingredient obviously overlooked by many Death Valley mining ventures. In the early days, just about every new tunnel hit pay dirt. Even a well dug near the mill turned up gold instead of water! Also, the local geology lent itself to mining in horizontal tunnels and stoping directly from the side of the mountain, which is far less expensive than other underground mining methods. As a result, the cost of mining was only around $2 per ton. Tramming, milling, and later on cyanide processing were so effective that they brought this figure up to just over $3. With overhead, the total operational cost was as low as about $10 per ton. The average value of the ore did not exceed this figure by much. Wilson knew at the outset that the Keane Wonder would never compare with the best Mother Lode mines. But by and large it turned out to be, as he predicted early on, "a nice little proposition that will clear good and dependable money every month in the year, and from the looks of things, for many years hence."

Operations, however, did not always run without difficulties. The Financial Panic of 1907 threatened to cut off funding when it was most needed. The local weather periodically threw a wrench in the works, ironically in the winter as well. Record lows froze pipes and freak snow storms delayed operations. In the summer the high water temperature and increased water needs reduced working hours at the mill. The heat made working conditions difficult, even after an ice plant was installed at the mill. Most summers and winters the output dipped noticeably. The scarcity of water was another hindrance, though not as critical as elsewhere. Initially, the mill was run with water from a nearby well. Although waste water was partially recycled, it could support a maximum capacity of only 70 to 75 tons. Over time, new sources of water were discovered, but it was not until September 1910 that the mill was able to run full time at its maximum 80-ton capacity.

The Keane Wonder looked brighter as time went on and new strikes kept on extending its lifetime. In August 1908, the discovery of a large body of high-grade ore was hailed as the largest strike in the mine's history. Less than a year later, the *Rhyolite Herald* announced another strike as "new ore bodies of such immensity that big production is assured for years to come."

In the fall of 1908, with 20,000 tons of mill tailings stockpiled and a payroll of 50 workers, Wilson was ready to install the last piece of the milling complex—the cyanide plant. The mill could retrieve only about two thirds of the gold contained in the ore. Using a chemical process called leaching, the cyanide plant would treat the tailings that had been wisely impounded since the early days of the mine to extract the remaining gold. In spite of a particularly cold winter, the 100-ton plant and its 11 large tanks were ready by mid-March. Over the next three years it steadily went through the huge reserve of tailings, greatly improving the production. The total figure for 1909 reached $220,000, about 50% more than the previous year.

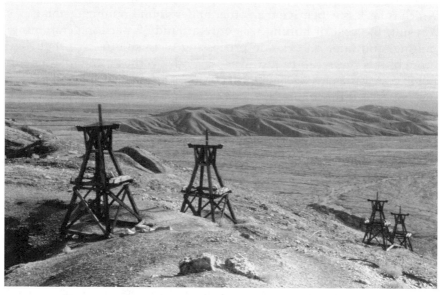

Keane Wonder Mine's tramway, on the edge of Death Valley

One of the largest operating expenses was hauling from Rhyolite supplies for the workers and the huge quantities of crude oil needed to fuel the mill's steam power plant. This task was carried out by two horse-drawn tank wagons, which made about two trips every week. In the summer of 1909, when the heat was too harsh for the horses, an enterprising Rhyolite merchant, Joseph Lane, resuscitated the Old Dinah, a steam traction engine from the borax days, and started to deliver 20 tons of freight once a week. Hitched to four trailers, whistling and puffing its way at 3 to 4 miles an hour, Old Dinah must have been an awkward sight. Lane's business worked well through the fall, but the load and rough road took their toll on the aging vehicle. In November of that year, the Keane Wonder switched back to good old horses when Old Dinah ruptured its boiler and died while climbing Daylight Pass.

In February 1910, the company reached the long awaited landmark of $1,000 a day. By fall, while most of the Rhyolite area had died out, the Keane Wonder was still employing 75 men and looking great. In early 1911 the only other mine alive in the Bullfrog Mining District was the Montgomery-Shoshone. By May it had closed its doors too, and the Keane Wonder remained alone. All previous records were broken the following month with a production of $50,000. For 15 days the production remained at almost $2,000 a day. For the fourth consecutive year the Keane Wonder was the leading gold producer in Inyo County, tying with its rival Skidoo in the Panamints.

But as Homer Wilson had predicted, the wealth of the Keane Wonder was limited. In early 1912 the end of the ore bodies was in sight. In late January the tailings ran out and the cyanide plant was temporarily shut down. While production still ran high through the first half of 1912, parallel efforts were made to assess the reserves of unexplored claims. New ore bodies were discovered, and exploration of the Big Bell claims continued, but nothing substantial turned up. In August the pillars supporting the tunnels were removed to mine the last of the ore. This ultimate effort cleaned out another $10,000 but the mine had been sacrificed, as the unsupported roofs would soon collapse. On August 22 the *Inyo Register* announced that the Keane Wonder had worked out its ore. A small crew was maintained to process the last tailings at the cyanide plant. By the end of 1912 the site was vacant. After five years of glory and nearly one million dollars in gold, the Keane Wonder, one of Death Valley's richest mines, had shut down.

This was not quite the end. For the next three decades its earlier success lured several investors into giving it another try. It was reopened in June 1913 by a Philadelphia company, with Homer Wilson as president. The mill was put back to work, but returns must not have been very high because the property was auctioned off about a year later. In the fall of 1915 new owners expanded the cyanide plant capacity to 300 tons and developed unexploited ore bodies. They were quickly exhausted, and operations were discontinued in July 1916. In 1935 the Coen Mining Company, which operated the nearby Big Bell Mine, obtained mining rights to the Keane Wonder but hardly touched it. The mill finally died in November 1937 when it was sold to a private party who hauled away its machinery and timber for cash. In 1940, under yet another ownership, the tramway and camp were revamped, and a new

150-ton mill was erected on the old mill's foundations. In spite of its magnitude, this effort also did not last. All activity ceased in March 1942, and the mill was dismantled. During all these years, production probably did not amount to one tenth that of the early period. The Keane Wonder had been thoroughly cleaned out during its glory days.

Hiking Suggestions

Depending on your time and ambition, this multifaceted area can be enjoyed in many ways. The most popular activities are browsing around the mill and taking a short walk up the mining road for good views of the tramway and Death Valley. In the same vein of easy walking, try the old pipeline road to Keane Wonder Springs and Cyty's Mill (see *The Big Bell Extension*). For a more serious hike, consider the mining road up to the Keane Wonder Mine, or better yet go up the canyon and return down the road, which takes between a half and a full day.

The best and most challenging hike is to go all the way up to Chloride Cliff. With an early start, the round trip can be done in a day, with just enough time to visit all three mines. There is certainly enough to see for an overnight trip. Hike the canyon on your way up and the road on your way down, as the falls are easier to negotiate going up, and the views from the road are better appreciated going down.

Route Description: The Mill Area

Keane Wonder Mill and the tramway terminal. The area around the end of the road is the site of Keane Wonder's milling complex and camp. The camp, now only betrayed by leveled areas, included the houses of the Wilsons, the mill superintendent and the company vice-president and their wives, a boarding house for the crew, and a general store. The site of the 20-stamp mill is a short distance up the trail beyond the end of the road. Its concrete foundations, three-chute ore bin and huge boiler (part of the steam power plant) give a good idea of its former size. These remains are overshadowed by the massive timber frame of the tramway lower terminal. With the first few tramway towers lined up on the mountain slope behind it, it is an impressive measure of the efforts expended to harvest a million dollars of gold.

The cyanide plant. The barren desert floor west of the trail is the site of the cyanide plant. It is littered with ruins of cyanide vats, tanks, pipelines, and collapsed buildings in a sea of eroded tailings. The largest standing structure is one of the processing tanks, which were used for gold leaching, water storage, or as settling ponds.

Route Description: Mill to Keane Wonder Mine

The mining road and the aerial tramway. The mining road starts on the left in front of the tramway terminal. It is the northern segment of the first trans-Death Valley road, developed by Franklin in the early 1870s (see *Chloride Cliff*). It shoots straight up the Funerals, first ascending over 1,500 feet to the tramway upper terminal in 1.4 miles, then continuing all the way to Chloride City. The road's lower portion follows Keane Wonder's aerial tramway and provides stunning views of one of the mining wonders of Death Valley. The tramway is still surprisingly well-preserved, and most of its original towers continue to defy gravity. At places they are anchored at such unlikely locations that one cannot help wondering how they were erected, or how the heavy cables were strung across them. This hike also offers spectacular 180° views of Death Valley, from the Greenwater Range to the northern Cottonwoods.

The lower canyon. A more adventurous route to the mine is along the canyon that starts just south of the mill. The first couple of falls that soon block the way give a good idea of what lies ahead: a chaotic canyon choked with rocks, high crooked walls of wildly folded strata, shallow whirlpools in polished bedrock, and an impressive collection of falls. The falls vary greatly in composition, degree of polish and color, from dark green mica-schist to marble as white as porcelain. The wash is so sinuous that it often gives little advance warning of what is coming next, which makes for a delightfully unpredictable hike. As you trudge across this broken landscape, hundreds of feet beneath the tramway, you will gain a better appreciation of what it took to haul the heavy timber and machinery across this inhospitable land. You'll pass by many of the tramway ore buckets, half buried in the wash.

There are 11 falls higher than 10 feet, and scores of shorter ones, to the Keane Wonder Mine. Some of them are crumbly and unsafe, while others are quite strong and fun to climb. At least two falls are impassable, and one of them probably exceeds 100 feet. There is always a way around them, often along short bypass trails built in the mining days. Use caution in bypassing the two high falls near the second cable crossing (about 0.6 mile in), which requires scrambling up loose slabs.

The geology is something else to look forward to. Unlike most, this canyon traverses mostly Proterozoic schists, quartzite, and marble (Crystal Spring Formation). The smooth outcrops of marble and quartzite are particularly pretty. Depending on their relative contents of quartz, biotite, and staurolite, the schists cover an amazing spectrum of brilliance and color, from dull to sparkling, silvery to green, purple and gold. At places extensive metamorphism has folded these rocks into oddly distorted formations.

About 1.3 miles above the mouth, the upper end of the tramway is visible 250 feet up on the north rim. Keane Wonder Mine is just beyond it. The easiest way to it is to continue along the wash another 0.5 mile to a side canyon on the right. The old spur road to the left climbs up to the mine in about half a mile.

Keane Wonder Mine. This is one of the park's best examples of an early-twentieth-century gold mining operation. The site is dominated by the imposing remains of the tramway upper terminal, a long structure of heavy timber with some of its original machinery. The tramway was cleverly engineered. The ore was first crushed to 2-inch chunks with a jaw crusher. It was then loaded automatically into buckets, which held about 600 pounds each. Gravity was its engine. When the line was loaded the full descending buckets developed enough traction to pull the empty buckets back up to the mine, and there was enough left-over power to run the crusher. The upper terminal is so well-preserved that it is a satisfying piece of engineering to study.

Although most of the camp buildings have either collapsed or been salvaged, a few are still partly standing, including the walls of a few stone houses. The site is packed with an interesting assortment of

The Keane Wonder Mine		
	Dist.(mi)	Elev.(ft)
The canyon route		
Road's end	0.0	1,320
Mouth	0.1	1,360
Spur to Keane Wonder	1.9	2,880
Tramway upper terminal	(0.5)	~2,840
80-120-ft fall	2.3	~3,200
Big Bell Mine	~3.3	~3,620
Chloride Cliff Road (dugouts)	4.8	4,800
Chloride Cliff	5.25	5,279
The mining road		
Road's end	0.0	1,320
Mill	0.15	1,400
Tramway upper terminal	1.4	2,840
Main mines	1.6	~3,040
Ridge	1.7	~3,080
Junction to Big Bell Mine	2.9	3,800
Big Bell Mine	(~0.15)	~3,620
Chloride Cliff Rd @ Chl. City	5.0	4,840

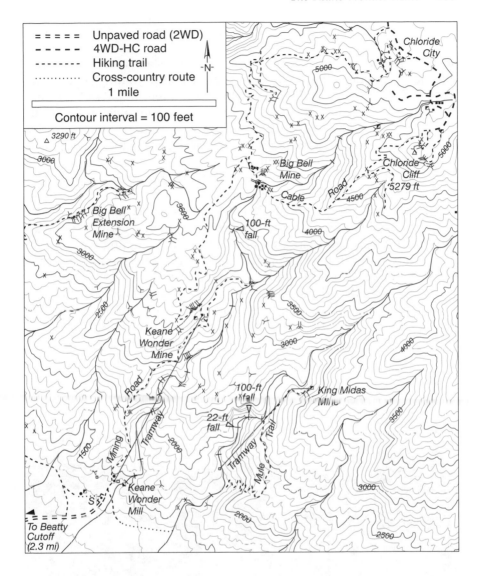

Map legend:
- ≡ ≡ ≡ ≡ ≡ Unpaved road (2WD)
- – – – – 4WD-HC road
- - - - - - - - Hiking trail
- ·········· Cross-country route
- 1 mile
- Contour interval = 100 feet

hoists, rail tracks, tanks, wire cables, ore chutes and bins. And there are, of course, the money makers—scores of prospects, pits, tunnels, shafts, and open cuts pockmarking the nearby hillsides.

Route Description: Mine to Chloride Cliff

This segment of the hike ranks high in scenic appeal, and it will spike your curiosity with two interesting mining sites. The only difficulty is that the two logical routes are both problematic.

The first route is up canyon from the spur road to the mine. Here the wash is gouged into a succession of shallow, narrow troughs in striking greenish or gold schists. Sprinkled with short falls and clogged with large boulders, this is the most chaotic and intriguing part of this canyon. The problem is the impassable 80-120 foot fall about 0.4 mile from the spur. It can be bypassed up the very steep talus on the north side, but it is one long and strenuous climb, and the nearly vertical rocky ledge at the rim takes some doing. At the rim, look for the mining road; it's about 100 yards east, and quite faint in this area. After about 0.6 mile up the road, past a shallow open pit on the right, the road forks. The right fork leads shortly to the Big Bell Mine, back down in the canyon wash (see *The Big Bell Mine*). The left fork winds up to Chloride City.

The other logical route is the mining road. Past the tramway upper terminal it climbs as a foot trail to the main mining area, visible on the cliff up behind the terminal. It takes a little effort to find the trail, but the real problem is that little "No Trespassing" sign posted just past the terminal by the NPS. The reason for this restriction is that the trail soon goes right by a small open pit and partly caved-in mines that are threatening to collapse. You can try a cross-country route around the steep cliff, but in my opinion this is much less safe. To be on the right side of the law, ask the NPS for permission to use the trail.

■

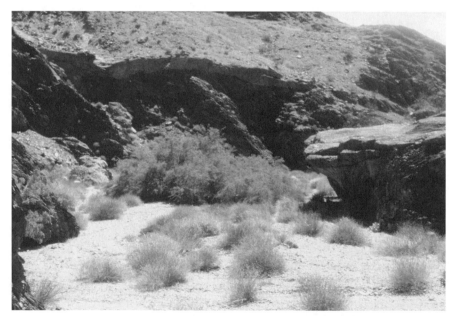

Poison Spring, at the heart of Indian Pass Canyon

INDIAN PASS CANYON

No matter how you go about it, it's a long way to the heart of this isolated canyon. But if you have the stamina, you will find a winding canyon sprinkled with springs and small creeks, falls, old mining claims, an amazing array of mosaic-like conglomerate outcrops, and a deep plunge pool. The grand prize is solitude: there is enough of it here to drive a desert rat crazy.

General Information

Road status: Roadless; extensive hike from paved road, or short hike
    from primitive road (HC)
Shortest hike: 1.1 mi, 320 ft one way / easy-moderate
Longest hike: 11.5 mi, 3,260 ft one way / strenuous
Main attractions: A secluded canyon with springs and short creeks, falls,
    tinajas, mining claims and camp
USGS 15' topo maps: Big Dune, Chloride Cliff*
USGS 7.5' topo maps: Ashton (Nev.), East of Chloride City, Nevares
    Peak*, Beatty Junction*
Maps: pp. 141*, 103

Location and Access

This canyon drains the west side of the central Funerals, starting near Indian Pass. To get to its mouth, start hiking from Highway 190 where the old Table Spring Road used to be (check the 15' map). This is 3.9 miles north of the Cow Creek turnoff (3.9 miles south of Beatty Junction), which is near the south end of the second of three low, sprawling hills parallel to the highway known as the Three Bare Hills. The mouth of Indian Pass Canyon is hidden from view, but from a little further north the pass itself is clearly visible as the lowest point on the crest of the Funerals.

The other option is to start at the head of the canyon. From the end of Highway 374 in Beatty, Nevada, drive Highway 95 south for 14.1 miles and turn right on an unsigned dirt road (look for an opening in the fence). This road ends in about 14.2 miles on the edge of Indian Pass Canyon. There are two junctions along the way. At the four-road crossing 7.4 miles from the highway, make a right. The next junction is in another 4.6 miles. Here the road you want is on the left, but it is extremely faint and easy to miss. Look for it about 0.2 mile beyond the pass, and about 100 feet past the "Mine Hazard Area" sign. The road is well-defined again along the wash 100 yards to the southwest. From here it is 2.2 miles to the end of the road. The first part of this road is a little sandy at places but probably OK for passenger cars, although it would be slow going. The last 5 or 6 miles are bumpy, rutted, and crowded with roadside vegetation, and best tackled with high clearance (4-wheel drive is probably not needed). The ride takes about one and a quarter hours.

From the pass area there are several ways to hike into the canyon. The easiest one is to park about 1.1 miles past the second junction (elev. 3,040'), near a group of mining monuments on the right side of the road. From here you can hike down into either the shallow ravine on the left side of the road (the approach described below), or the side canyon on the right side of the road (fourth side canyon in the chart). A third option is to park at the end of the road and walk down the old mining spur on the right, which drops into the fourth side canyon. These last two routes are the shortest to the upper spring.

Hiking Suggestions

From Indian Pass, it is a relatively easy day hike to the upper spring, out and back. To go to the lower spring is a moderately difficult hike that covers the best of this canyon. With the drive, it makes for a long day. To include the narrower gorge below the 18-foot fall, you may want to consider camping near the pass and getting an early start.

From Death Valley, the lower spring is a fine goal for a day hike, only moderately difficult. However, given the time investment needed to cross the fan, it makes sense to go for the upper spring. A healthy walk, but the grades are unusually moderate and it can be done in a day.

The best is to hike the entire canyon. It's not that bad to do it one way in a day, even going uphill. Because of the springs, this is also a good choice for an overnighter. Count on three days to explore most of the canyon.

Route Description

The fan approach. The lower half of the old jeep road to Table Spring used to be the best route to hike to Indian Pass Canyon, but the little that was left of it was washed out by a storm in the late 1980s. You'll have to do with its approximate route, which is still the best way to go. From the highway, aim for the south end of the middle Bare Hill, circle around its base northward, then keep a course parallel to the long, low ridge to the north. You will probably end up following a broad wash, lined part way on its south side by a 10-foot gravel bank, which is the wash of Indian Pass Canyon. After 2.8 miles (elev. 210'), walk into the wide opening that cuts northeast through the ridge. About 1.2 miles further, the wash opens onto a wider area (elev. 480'). Stay to the left (as opposed to going right towards the more enticing yellowish hills), which will take you shortly into the canyon. The hills along the wash (up to a little past the head of the canyon) are made of conglomerate, micaceous siltstone, and carbonates, fairly young rocks belonging to the Furnace Creek Formation.

This route is a little more complicated than your usual up-the-wash hike. And it's a walk, over more desert gravel than most people get to step on in a lifetime. But the views of Death Valley are good, you'll have trouble not finding pretty rocks in the wash, and if you come here at the right time of year, and on the right year, you'll be walking knee deep in blooming fields of gravelghost and desert five-spot.

The lower canyon. The lower part of Indian Pass Canyon is broad and relatively uneventful. Its highlight is the narrower section a short distance in. Its fluted, mud-covered walls are topped by a few precariously balanced rocks. It is blocked at its upper end by an 18-foot fall (which needs to be circumvented on the north side). Further on there are several pretty exposures of conglomerate bedrock and a small dry spring of mesquite trees, but things don't really pick up until just past the first major side canyon, where the wash squeezes through a small grotto, the beginning of the deeper and more spectacular mid-canyon.

The mid-canyon and Poison Spring. On a good year a little water flows over the small fall inside the grotto. This is the tail end of the lower spring's intermittent creek. Its head is 200 yards further, in a tight trench trapped between a dripping wall and a slick 9-foot fall, graced with small hanging gardens of maidenhair fern. The second spring, a little further up canyon, is the largest. Its creek runs above ground off and on, at times for up to 500 yards. The head of the spring is a thick oasis of arrowweed, tamarisk, and mesquite trees.

In the 1950s, biologists Florence and Ralph Welles spent several years scrambling all over Death Valley to study its bighorn populations, including the Nevares Spring-Indian Pass herd. In their book about the study, they made this interesting comment about Poison Spring:

> The water is brown and bitter the year around, but it is perfectly acceptable to bighorn. Caught there in July without water, we dug a small shaft above the established point of discharge, which filled with clear, uncloudy but exceedingly bitter water, and we drank it with no ill effects whatever—but we thought we knew why it had been named "Poison."

Hopefully you will not have to double check, although a friend of mine did sample the lower spring and at last call was still alive.

The middle canyon has many other treats, including a short, deep gorge and sculpted trenches. Between approximately the lower and upper springs, the walls are composed of the alternating schist and quartzite layers of the Johnnie Formation. The most amazing feature is the countless outcrops of conglomerate and travertine bedrock. Polished over wide areas into smooth slickrock, gouged with potholes sometimes filled with water, they will pique your interest with their ever-changing displays of colorful mosaics.

The upper spring is different again. Set between short vertical walls, it has a denser cover of mesquite trees and a small clump of common cane. Only a few rivulets ooze out here and there. Don't count too heavily on this one for a refill. There is a small mining camp along this spring on the north bench. It is relatively recent, perhaps from as late as the 1950s. Mining in this area was quite limited. It is often betrayed only by the stone monuments erected by miners to mark their claim boundaries—places with romantic names like Queen Azule or Queen of Light. Up canyon from the spring, several of these 4 to 6 foot towers of neatly stacked rocks still trace imaginary lines across the high ridges.

These oases are small and fragile. Even a single careless visitor going back and forth over them once could leave long lasting marks. Stay away from the vegetation and the soft gravel and algae along the creeks. Walk on the surrounding bedrock as much as possible.

Indian Pass Canyon		
	Dist.(mi)	Elev.(ft)
Highway 190	0.0	-220
Mouth	4.1	580
18-ft fall	4.8	780
First side canyon (grotto)	7.0	1,385
Lower spring	7.2	1,435
Second side canyon	8.0	1,780
Middle spring (Poison Spring)	8.5	1,945
Third side canyon	8.5	1,945
Fourth side canyon	8.7	2,020
Upper spring	8.9	2,095
Plunge pool	10.1	2,555
Drop-off	10.4	2,720
Indian Pass road	11.5	3,040

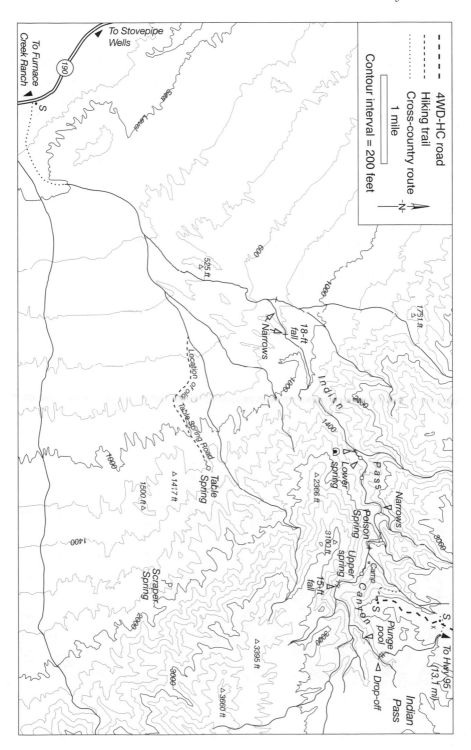

The upper canyon. From the Indian Pass area down to the upper spring, the canyon is fairly windy, shallow at first but it gradually deepens through thick metamorphic rocks (Stirling Quartzite). Many natural tanks (tinajas) occur throughout this area, either as troughs between the broken, tilted metamorphic strata, or as small bowls stream-cut in the bedrock. In the spring, several days after a moderate rain, I saw more water-filled tinajas here than anywhere else in the park.

After about 1.1 miles, past a few forks in the canyon, the wash dead-ends on the edge of a sheer drop-off. About 50 feet high, it controls entry into the mid-canyon. The route continues as a scramble down the unstable talus on the south side, which requires a little care. Check out the huge pit at the base of the drop-off, dug by water when it poured down. Was it made a few years or a few thousand years ago?

Below the drop-off the canyon deepens markedly and goes through a few narrower passages with several slides worn by water, which are probably the most interesting part of this canyon besides the springs. The first one has a very unusual tinaja, a plunge pool of dark water at the bottom of a deep slot chiseled in the bedrock—the only one I found in all of Death Valley. The upper spring is just a little over 1 mile down canyon, past several more polished conglomerate falls and chutes.

■

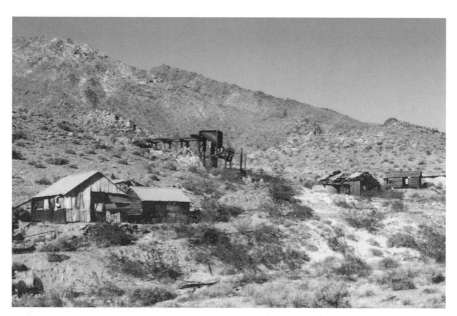

Inyo Mine's camp

ECHO CANYON AND THE INYO MINE

> *Echo Canyon is a scenic canyon that appeals to both hikers and 4WD enthusiasts. The windy lower gorge, with its rugged walls and peculiar arch, is a great target for a short day hike. The canyon road eventually leads to the Inyo Mine and its ghost camp, one of the largest and most interesting in the park, and to petroglyphs in the upper canyon. A rough 4WD road goes up a fork of Echo Canyon past numerous mining areas to the Amargosa Desert—an exciting ride or adventurous backpacking trek clear across the Funerals.*

General Information

Road status: Graded road to canyon; primitive canyon road (4WD-HC)
Shortest hike: Short strolls/easy-moderate
Longest hike: 15 mi, 4,700 ft one way (or more)/difficult
Main attractions: Inyo Mine and camp, natural arch, a narrow gorge,
      petroglyphs
USGS 15' topo maps: Furnace Creek*, Ryan*, Big Dune
USGS 7.5' topo maps: Furnace Creek*, Echo Canyon*, Lees Camp
Maps: pp. 149*, 103

Location and Access

Echo Canyon is the longest in the Funeral Mountains. A primitive road goes through most of it, starting from Highway 190 2.1 miles east of the Badwater Road. It is marked by an inconspicuous sign (the way park signs should be) on the north side of the highway. The first stretch along the fan has a moderate crown and occasional soft gravel. With a little experience and by driving slowly you can make it with a passenger car. After 2.9 miles, just below the canyon mouth, the Echo Canyon Road goes over a rough spot of slanted bedrock, and the gravel is deeper beyond. A high-clearance vehicle, with 4-wheel drive for lighter vehicles, is required past this point.

Hiking and Driving Suggestions

With the right vehicle, it is a smooth and pleasant drive through the gorge to the Inyo Mine, the destination of most visitors in Echo Canyon. From here, one can spend a good part of a day exploring on foot the nearby camp and mines. This ride can be continued on a bumpy backcountry road across the Funeral Mountains to Nevada Highway 95. With a passenger car, if you can drive to the rough spot near the canyon mouth, it's a short day hike through the gorge to the Eye of the Needle. To hike as far as the mine and back in one day is tougher. Most hikers will prefer to make it an overnight trip. The backcountry along the road to Nevada is a wonderful goal for a few days in the desert wild—except during a holiday, the road is not usually very busy.

History: The Inyo Gold

In 1904, after Jack Keane's first discovery of gold in the northern Funerals, dozens of fortune seekers were combing the mountains hoping for new strikes. In January 1905 two prospectors, Maroni Hicks and Chet Leavitt, got lucky and discovered rich gold-bearing quartz veins in Echo Canyon. By May they had staked a total of 20 claims on all the promising ground they could find, and were ready to sell. Over the next few months, several groups of investors became interested in their property, which was rapidly viewed as one of the most promising in the burgeoning Echo-Lee District. In December, after a few false starts, the two men finally fulfilled their dream. A group of Utah mining promoters purchased their entire group of claims and created the Inyo Gold Mining Company, incorporating it with a capitalization of $1 million. Hicks took cash for his half of the property. Leavitt, for better or for worse, retained his interests and became the company's vice president.

For the next two years the company carried out extensive development work. Except for summers, when heat slowed things down to a crawl, the payroll increased steadily, up to around 30 miners. By March 1906 the main shaft was 100 feet deep. A month later several crosscuts had been driven into it, and a second shaft was opened. Soon after, ore worth nearly $300 per ton was uncovered in the new shaft. A third shaft was being exploited in early 1907.

There was good ore in the ground, assessed at one time at $44 per ton, but it was not so good that it could be shipped profitably without milling. It was free-milling ore, which meant it could be milled by simple methods. As usual the main problem was water, which had to be hauled from Greenland Ranch at a prohibitive cost. The company officials had their eyes on the Ash Meadow Water Company, just across the state line, waiting for it to complete a pipeline to the booming Lee area. If and when it did, the Inyo Gold would consider erecting a mill on its property. No ore shipment was made in 1906, perhaps in anticipation that a mill would greatly increase the return on the ore.

The strike had drawn the attention of Charles Schwab, former president of the U.S. Steel Corporation, and one of the wealthiest men in the country. Schwab had invested part of his personal fortune in other mines in the district. By 1907 a town bearing his name had sprung to life less than a mile away, in the north fork of Echo Canyon, a scattering of canvas tents that attracted a population of 200 in two months. During its short lifetime, it had its own post office, telephone, and even daily stage services to Rhyolite. To the east, along the state line, the boom towns of Lee, Nevada, and Lee, California, just a few miles apart, were rivaling for fame and customers. The little camp below the Inyo Gold mines was also keeping pace with its growing number of miners. In the spring of 1907 it had a boarding house, sleeping quarters and several tents, a blacksmith shop, and a store selling groceries and mining supplies.

Around April 1907, the Inyo Gold finally geared up for the construction of its mill, and announced that it would ship out its high-grade ore upon its completion. But it had waited too long. In September, as the summer heat was finally abating and work was about to resume, the funds advanced by the owning partners ran out. The company's debt was over $15,000, and its treasury was empty. To sell the large number of remaining shares, the company officers decided to go public. But this was the fall of 1907, the year of the great financial panic. It hit the area just after the company stocks went up for sale, and investors shied away from this remote district. Had the decision to go public been made a few months earlier, when the area was booming and far less valuable properties were selling like hot cakes, the Inyo Gold would have had a chance. Instead, it faced a depressed market and unavoidable bankruptcy. Mining steadily dwindled down after October and ceased by December. Over the next four years, as the mines remained idle, the company tried every trick in the book to interest investors in either buying, leasing, or sponsoring, but all negotiations failed. In January 1912, the Inyo was finally abandoned. Although the company once claimed to have $650,000 worth of ore in sight, it never shipped any.

But the Inyo Mine had another chance, more than 20 years later. Around 1935-1936, the Inyo Consolidated Mining Company leased the claims from a new owner and worked the old tunnels. It revived the camp and installed a 25-ton ball mill and a small amalgamation and concentration plant, which was run by water hauled from Furnace Creek. The company mined and milled ore averaging $25 a ton, until lack of funds forced closure near the end of 1938. In 1939, a new lessee struck high-grade ore at the bottom of one of the shafts, and made a small fortune shipping 36 tons of ore worth $280 per ton. But there was only so much of this kind of ore, and he gave up shortly thereafter. The mine was leased one last time the following year, to two men who exploited a different area and attempted to treat their ore with a small smelter. Their operation was short-lived, for the mine closed again, this time for good, in 1941. Although little is known about the production of the Inyo's revival era, chances are that it did produce more than an occasional sack of gold—the Inyo Mine was probably, after all, almost rich.

Route Description

The gorge and the Eye of the Needle. The lower canyon is a scenic gorge that starts right away at the mouth and continues with varying degrees of tightness and depth for the next 2.2 miles. It has no true narrows, but it does squeeze through a few tight constrictions, especially along the meandering upper section where the road comes within 6 feet of high-rising walls. The echo is good. Try it in the lower gorge facing one of the sheer walls, and in the meanders of the upper section.

The gorge cuts through thick rock formations deposited at least 500 million years ago in a Cambrian sea. The Bonanza King Formation prevails through most of it. Many of the exposed rocks are cavernous. All over the high walls erosion has carved innumerable caves, spire-framed overhangs and hollows, producing an eerie landscape.

There are several windows in the gorge, often balanced high above the canyon floor. The most striking one is the Eye of the Needle, a triangular, 15-foot tall opening pierced 50 feet above the wash in a narrow fin stranded in a tight bend. From the downhill side one can climb into this shaded observatory for a bird's-eye view of the gorge. The gorge ends at a final constriction 0.6 mile past the Eye of the Needle.

The Inyo Mine's camp. Beyond, the canyon turns into a broad valley all the way to the end of the road. The next 4.1 miles to the Inyo Mine's camp are uneventful, although in the spring the profusion of wild flowers transforms the valley floor into an unbroken carpet of gold.

The Inyo Mine's camp is a cluster of half a dozen wooden houses at the foot of the steep hillside where gold was once mined. It is undoubtedly one of the most scenic mining camps in the park, and one of the very few large enough to qualify as a ghost town. If you are fond of the California gold rush era and its fascinating lore, it will stir emotions which can now be experienced only at a handful of sites.

The large wooden structure at the west end of the camp is the remains of the mill. Although the ball mill itself has been removed, its 30-ton ore bin, the wheels of the jaw crusher, its settling plates and large metal tank, and the diesel engine that powered it are still in place. The small dugout dates from the 1907 mining era. The large house at the east end was the boarding house; the central house with a concrete floor was the cook house. Its kitchen still has parts of the original zinc counter and cast iron stove. Open and shaded, it is an inviting place to sit and rest, and perhaps reflect on what the camp was like when it was active.

The houses are fragile, and being victims of both the elements and vandalism, they are inexorably deteriorating. When I was here a small twister tore off a wood panel from the boarding house, bringing it one step closer to oblivion. The cook house is a mere frame since vandals stripped its siding for firewood. Please do not remove, destroy, or change anything. What would Echo Canyon be without its ghost town?

The Inyo Mine. The main mines are high on the hillside behind the camp and reached by a steep, rocky trail. The local rocks are mostly white quartzite and schists, probably Precambrian in age. The quartzite contains the narrow gold-bearing quartz veins at the origin of the rush. Six parallel veins with lovely forgotten names outcrop on the hillside. The adit level with the top of the large ore bin is the entrance to the main, 700-foot long horizontal tunnel, once known as the Octaroon. At the next level up is a vertical shaft with ladders, the 100-foot deep air shaft that ventilated the tunnel. The tunnel 100 feet above it is the Martha Raye. The next level, at the top of the

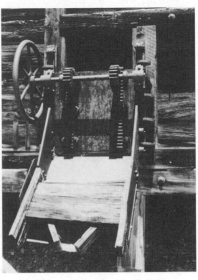

Ore bin trap door, Inyo Mine

trail, is the Upper Ten vein, which was the most extensively mined. A short, rotted tunnel peers into a large cavern supported by huge timber. From here a long inclined shaft drops 100 and 160 feet to two levels of crosscuts, and another 25 feet down to the far end of the Octaroon.

The rock, especially the quartzite, is heavily shattered, and it's a miracle that some adits have not already collapsed. To be safe, you may want to look at all this from the outside, which still leaves plenty to be examined. As if time froze the day of the shutdown, much is left as it was then. At the ore bin a narrow-gauge rail is still awaiting delivery from the main tunnel. The ore bin still holds behind its cogged trap door the last load of ore from the mine. The ladders inside the deep air shaft are still in place, leading down into musty depths. This is a fascinating area, offering a moving glimpse at a forgotten page of history.

The Furnace Mine. The site of the last mining effort of 1940-41, sometimes referred to as the Furnace Mine, is about 0.5 mile northeast of the last shaft, on the far side of the ridge. To get to it, climb the very steep slope north-northeast about 250 feet up, until you overlook the upper drainage. Then follow a contour line (~4,400') along the back side of the ridge to the mine, visible to the northeast. The other approach is to drive or hike the upper canyon road towards Lee. Start at its junction with the saddle cutoff and go 1.9 miles, which should put you at a sharp

90° left bend. A faint trail, starting at a stone platform, winds 400 feet up the steep south slope to a ridge. The cable near the trail was used to literally drag supplies up from the road, which were then lowered down the other side to the mine. The winch drum and engine of the cableway are at the top of the ridge. The main feature at the mine is the small rusted furnace of the smelter. Ore was mined from the timbered, inclined shaft above the furnace, and from a collapsed tunnel, connected to the furnace area by tracks. This is an intriguing site, a repository of obsolete machineries well worth sweating the climb.

The upper canyon. Back in the main canyon, there are petroglyphs past the camp. To minimize vandalism I will only say that I found the

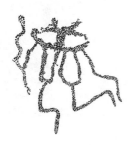

clue that first led me to them in Ruth Kirk's great classic *Exploring Death Valley*. The road dead ends 1.3 miles past the camp, at a minor constriction in the canyon; further progress is on foot. Past a short narrow section, the canyon turns into a broad green valley framed by rolling hills. You can continue a few miles over secluded country to an overlook on the edge of the steep eastern flank of the Funeral Mountains, commanding spectacular views of the Amargosa Desert.

Petroglyph (shaman?)

The upper canyon road to Lee and beyond. From the main canyon road half a mile west of the Inyo Mine's camp, a long and adventurous

	Echo Canyon	
	Dist.(mi)	Elev.(ft)
Highway 190	0.0	405
Rough spot in road	2.9	1,420
Mouth	3.3	1,550
Eye of the Needle	4.8	~2,180
First side canyon	4.9	2,150
End of narrows	5.5	2,410
Upper canyon road to Lee	9.1	3,590
Highway 95	(~25.0)	2,690
Inyo Mine's camp	9.6	3,760
Inyo Mine	(~0.4)	~4,080
Furnace Mine	(~0.9)	~4,400
Road's end	10.9	4,120
Amargosa Desert overlook	14.1	4,770

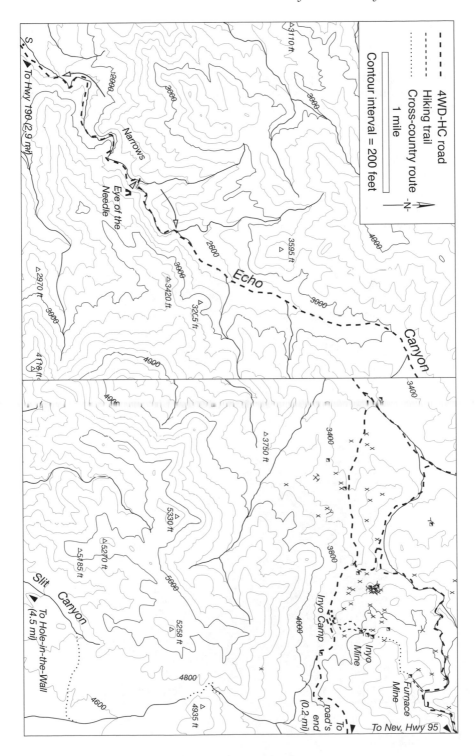

backcountry road winds deep into a fork of Echo Canyon, crosses the divide, then drops to the town site of Lee near the state line. It is then about 13.6 miles to Nevada Highway 95. This route crosses the old Echo-Lee Mining District, a sprawling region of desolate hills haunted by the ghosts of numerous strikes. This area has one of the largest concentrations of mines in the park. Most of the sites of interest are up to just past the divide. Since the road is very rough and requires short-wheelbase 4WD vehicles, it is infrequently traveled and is a great target for a multiple day hiking trek. For a change of scenery, you can return along one of the side canyons of Echo Canyon. There is not much left here besides old tunnels, but seclusion more than makes up for it. There is still gold in the ground, only too diluted to be worth recovering. This thought may spark your imagination as you poke around old tailings along the way.

∎

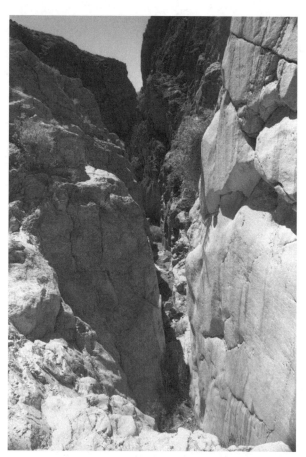

The Slit, along the first narrows of Slit Canyon

SLIT CANYON

Slit Canyon is a little-known canyon beyond Hole-in-the-Wall with several long and beautiful narrows. The nearly mile-long lower narrows, carved in polished gray limestone, are among the nicest and most extensive in the park. It has impressive falls, a shaded grotto, and the canyon's namesake, a straight corridor no more than 5 feet wide. This canyon can be used to access upper Echo Canyon and the Inyo Mine, one of the most colorful mining areas in Death Valley.

General Information

Road status: Roadless; hiking access via primitive road
Shortest hike: 1.4 mi, 590 ft one way/moderate
Longest hike: ~9 mi, 4,600 ft one way/difficult
Main attractions: Good narrows, the Slit, falls, rock climbing
USGS topo maps: Ryan (15'), Echo Canyon (7.5')
Maps: pp. 153*, 149, 103

Location and Access

Slit Canyon, located in the southern Funerals, is the northern-most of several canyons draining through Hole-in-the-Wall. To get there, drive to the Hole-in-the-Wall Road, which is on Highway 190 1.9 miles east of the Zabriskie Point turnoff, near the 1,000-foot elevation sign. Drive this unpaved road 3.7 miles to Hole-in-the-Wall and park. It has loose gravel most of the way but can be negotiated easily with a standard-clearance passenger car.

Route Description

The approach. For this hike I like to start a short distance before Hole-in-the-Wall to better appreciate this majestic gap. The wall itself, 300 to 400 feet high, is a narrow barrier of rock about 2.5 miles long which bisects the alluvial fan of the Funeral Mountains. It is made of upthrusted beds of sandstone and conglomerate from the Furnace Creek Formation, pockmarked with numerous cavities. The beds are folded along a major syncline arching steeply to the southwest underneath Furnace Creek Wash and resurfacing on the far side around Zabriskie Point.

This narrow gateway leads into an almost completely enclosed alluvial fan. This fan is bounded by two major, nearly parallel faults, part of the Furnace Creek Fault Zone. One fault runs along the back side of the wall, the other along the foot of the mountains. Just beyond the wall, leave the road and walk north up the main dry wash. The alluvial fan is cut off to the northeast by a low, elongated hill of yellow and tan mudstones (Furnace Creek Formation) partially covered with darker alluvial debris. Slit Canyon starts where this hill meets the foot of the Funeral Mountains—a gradual, 1.2-mile ascent to the mouth of the canyon.

Grotto fall. Just past the first bend a beautiful area opens up with three falls back to back. The first fall has two parallel, deeply notched chutes in light gray dolomite, 10 to 12 feet at the shallowest. The second fall, banded with black, is around 18 feet high. It is moderately difficult to climb up, worse to climb down as usual, but it gives access to a tall, deeply recessed grotto lined with a pool of fine gravel. This high-ceiling cave is almost completely enclosed and always deeply shaded. At the right time of year, if you stay quiet long enough swallows may come swarming in and out of the shallow depressions in the overhang where they nest.

The third fall, which forms the back wall of the grotto, is about 25 feet high, smooth, vertical, and difficult to scale. To go on you will have to get back to below the first fall and scramble up the talus slope against the eastern canyon wall. The talus is surprisingly stable and this route is safe.

The first narrows. The lower narrows of Slit Canyon, which start just past the third fall and extend for close to 1 mile, rank among the nicest and longest in the park. As they wind deep into the heart of the mountains their character changes, but they are almost continuously

	Slit Canyon	
	Dist.(mi)	Elev.(ft)
Hole-in-the-Wall	0.0	1,860
Mouth	1.2	2,320
Grotto fall (1st narrows)	1.4	2,450
The Slit	1.6	2,700
50-ft fall	1.8	2,850
1st narrows (end)	2.3	3,250
2nd narrows (start)	2.6	3,580
3rd narrows (start)	3.2	3,880
Head	5.4	4,810
Echo Canyon (wash)	(2.6)	3,890
Inyo Mine's camp	(3.1)	3,760

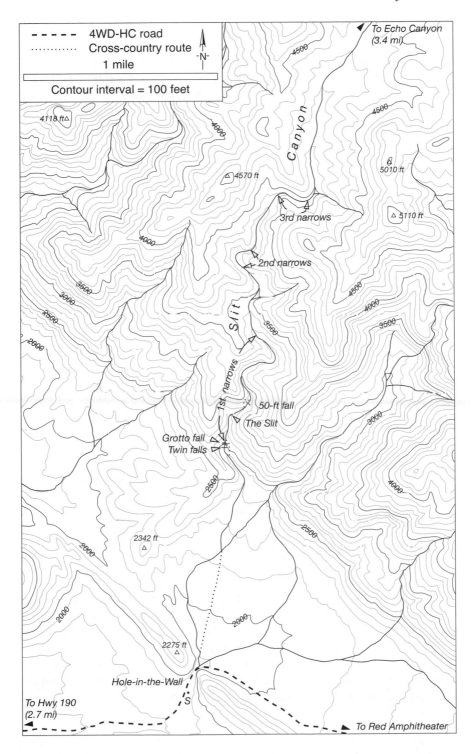

narrow. The dolomite belongs largely to the Nopah Formation, upper Cambrian in age. Generally dark-gray, occasionally as black as jade, it is often polished and undercut into beautiful wavy surfaces.

The Slit, after which I named this canyon, is a straight and narrow corridor occurring a short distance into the narrows. It is a slanted, water-worn trench, 4 to 5 feet wide and 40 to 50 feet deep, slicing through a plug of dolomite. Beginning with a pile of chockstones, it goes on for about 70 feet, so narrow that if you are carrying a pack you may have to wiggle your way through carefully. A 15-foot fall, easy to climb on the right side, closes the far end of this passage.

Less than a quarter of a mile past the Slit the wash dead ends against a majestic fall, a recessed channel polished to a shiny finish and rising 50 vertical feet above the wash. To continue, climb up the steep western talus slope and down the far side. Beyond the fall the narrow wash meanders beneath sheer walls, cut in by a few short falls. The next narrower sections are reminiscent of the lower narrows of Mosaic Canyon. Most of the way the walls are so high and steep that the canyon rims are hidden from view, and the course is so windy that the line of sight often does not exceed 30 feet. This is a rare and exciting place, an enchanted glen of stone for a leisurely, peaceful walk.

The upper canyon. For 1.25 miles past the narrows Slit Canyon remains relatively narrow and very windy. Slanted black walls rise 500 feet or more on one or both sides of the wash. Cottontop cactus grow on the rocky slopes, closer to the wash as the elevation rises. This stretch contains the second and third narrows, both only about 0.2 mile long, relatively shallow but different in character. The more interesting third narrows have several 9- to 12-foot falls and a shallow, 6-foot wide trench. The rest of the way to its head the canyon is broad and shallow. Several prominent peaks frame the western horizon. The canyon ends at a short ridge separating it from the drainage of the next canyon east.

A quiet route to the Inyo Mine. Most people will want to turn around at the second or third narrows. If you wish to explore further, a few cross-country miles will take you to the Inyo Mine (see *Echo Canyon*). This is a quiet approach to a wonderful area that some hikers may prefer to the 4-wheel-drive road via Echo Canyon. The route is fairly straightforward. From the head of Slit Canyon walk down into the next canyon east, then up its broad wash to the ridge at the head of the canyon, a distance of about 1.2 miles. On the other side of this ridge, a steep ravine drops 900 feet in about 1.4 miles to the Echo Canyon Road. The first 200 feet down are steep but the grade is more gentle the rest of the way. The Inyo Mine's camp is 0.4 mile down the road.

■

PART IV

BLACK MOUNTAINS

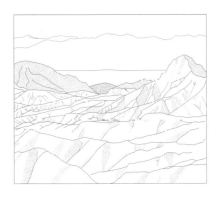

THE BLACK MOUNTAINS border the west side of southern Death Valley, from Furnace Creek Wash down to the delta of the Amargosa River. Of all the park's mountains, they probably offer the greatest diversity of terrain, scenery, and challenges. Somewhere in the intricate folds of this rough range there is a canyon with a 200-foot drop-off, a genuine desert stream, narrows so tight at places you can't see the sky, and at least half a dozen natural bridges. Nowhere else can you get more dramatic views of Death Valley's salt flats, crawl up 40° slopes for several miles, or hike through spectacular badlands—all in one mountain range.

The Black Mountains are about 50 miles long and about 7.5 miles wide on average. They are the second lowest in the park. From the low badlands at their north end they gradually rise to an average elevation around 5,000 feet in their central portion. The main summits are Mt Perry (5,739'), Coffin Peak (5,503'), Funeral Peak (6,384'), and Smith Mountain (5,913'). South from Smith Mountain the range gradually breaks up into lower hills. The topography of the Black Mountains is dominated by their western side, which is extremely steep along most of the range, and often drops more than 5,000 feet to below sea level over just a few air miles.

Part IV also covers the Ibex Hills, located at the very southern tip of the Black Mountains.

Access

The Black Mountains are the most easily accessible mountains in the park, being surrounded closely by a ring of paved and graded roads.

The Badwater Road remains within a mile of the western foot of the mountains along most of their length. At a few locations, graded or primitive roads climb onto the alluvial fan and provide convenient access to the Artist's Palette area and several canyons. At Ashford Junction, most of the way down the range, Highway 178 crosses the mountains eastward to Shoshone, and the Harry Wade Road continues south as a primitive road along the remaining length of the Black Mountains to eventually join Highway 127 just outside the park. The Greenwater Valley Road, graded and suitable for passenger cars, parallels the east side of the Black Mountains along Greenwater Valley. At the north end of this road, a paved spur winds up to Dante's View at the crest of the mountains. Highway 190 closes the loop along Furnace Creek Wash at the northern end of the Black Mountains. Other graded and primitive roads enter into the Black Mountains from their east side, notably into Twenty Mule Team Canyon and Gold Valley.

Geology

The Black Mountains are wedged between two major north-west-trending fault zones, the Northern Death Valley Fault Zone, which runs along the foot of the western escarpment, and the Furnace Creek Fault Zone, which parallels the northeast side of the mountains along Furnace Creek Wash. The two combined faults, which merge into a single fault zone north of Furnace Creek, form one of the longest active faults in California. Over the last few million years, they have contributed significantly to the shaping of the Amargosa Range. The Northern Death Valley Fault is responsible for the steep western front of the Black Mountains. Land east of this fault has been uplifted, while land on the west side (Death Valley) has been sinking. As a result, the fans along the western Black Mountains are generally steep, low, and short. Parts of the mountains are even fan-free, for example along some of the coves south of Badwater. In contrast, the fans on the east side of the mountains, into Greenwater Valley, have long and gentle grades.

As a result of this tumultuous history of faulting and folding, the geology of the Black Mountains is among the most complex and varied in the region. Generally speaking, they can be divided into four areas. The northern part, down to around Natural Bridge Canyon, is primarily made of Quaternary and Tertiary rocks from the Funeral, Furnace Creek, and Artist Drive formations. These soft sedimentary rocks have been deeply eroded into barren terrain, as is dramatically typified by the badlands below Zabriskie Point. The second area is the western escarpment. From Natural Bridge Canyon south to near Saratoga Spring, the majority of this escarpment comprises either late Proterozoic sedimentary rocks or early Proterozoic metamorphic rocks (mostly schist and gneiss). The metamorphism that altered these ancient rocks has been dated at around 1.7 billion years, which makes them the oldest known exposures around Death Valley. The third area is the crest of the central Black Mountains, in particular just west of Dante's View and around Funeral Peak and Smith Mountain. It is made of granitic rocks of Mesozoic age. The fourth area is the eastern flank of the mountains, along the Greenwater Valley. It contains mostly Miocene rhyolite and pockets of Pliocene volcanic rocks, in particular basalt and andesite.

Hydrology

Because the Black Mountains stand in the rain shadow of the Panamints, they are among the driest in the park. The average annual precipitation has been estimated at 3 to 5 inches. This general dryness is reflected in the absence of a pinyon pine-juniper community in the high Black Mountains. Springs are also few and far between. Most notable are Lemonade Springs on the slopes of Mount Perry, Greenwater and Sheep springs in the central Black Mountains, and Scotty's, Virgin, and Montgomery springs further south. Yet, paradoxically, some of the largest springs are found in this range. Willow Creek, east of Mormon Point, is one of the longest perennial streams in Death Valley. At the southern tip of the Ibex Hills, Saratoga Spring feeds several large perennial ponds and a substantial oasis, a green haven for water fowl matched by no other in the park.

Hiking

The Black Mountains offer what is probably the most diverse and extensive collection of canyons in the park. With few exceptions, they are comparatively short, roadless, and easy to get to. Also, they almost completely lack marine sedimentary rocks, in particular the limestone and dolomite formations so common elsewhere. This basic difference makes the topography of many areas in the Black Mountains quite different from just about anywhere else around Death Valley.

Although every area has its own character and appeal, the most scenic canyons in the Black Mountains are perhaps at their northern end and along their western escarpment. The northern area is a vivid celebration of the stark beauty of badlands, and it offers countless avenues for exploration in a relatively gentle setting. On the other hand, along the western escarpment, from Artist Drive to Mormon Point, the combination of rapid uplifting and flash flood erosion has produced deep, tight, and precipitous canyons, generally obstructed by high falls. This includes archetypical Bad Canyon, but also Natural Bridge and Scotty's canyons, and quite a few others not included here for lack of space, in particular Hades, Twin, and Coffin canyons. They are all reached by a short walk from the Badwater Road, but they quickly turn to tight narrows with high falls. The surface of the surrounding slopes is often covered with loose rubble, which makes bypassing the falls difficult. Travel through these places can be extremely challenging, requiring rock climbing experience and endurance, although it forms the basis for some of the most rewarding canyoneering around. At the southern end of the mountains, a few historical sites add another dimension to hiking, including Ashford Mine and the Desert Hound Mine.

The Ibex Hills offer a different kind of hiking experience. Their more subdued topography of lower desert hills and wider washes is particularly scenic and riddled with interesting old mining sites. Saratoga and Ibex springs, and the talc mines in their vicinity, are great examples of what that remote corner of Death Valley has in store for those who take the time to venture there.

■

Suggested Hikes in the Black Mountains					
Route/Destination	Dist. (mi)	Elev. change	Mean elev.	Access road	Page
Short hikes (under 5 miles round trip)					
Artist Drive Area					
Canyon at first dip	0.7	670'	1,280'	Paved	180-181
Canyon at second dip	0.5	470'	1,100'	Paved	181-182
Artist's Palette #1	0.5	240'	720'	Paved	182-184
Artist's Palette #2	0.7	350'	780'	Paved	184
Ashford Mine's camp	2.1	1,130'	1,670'	H/2.8 mi	213-216
Bad Canyon (lower canyon)	1.2	950'	210'	Paved	189-190
Desolation Canyon	1.8	770'	230'	Graded	176-178
Dante Peak	0.4	230'	5,590'	Paved	191
Golden Cyn (Manly Beacon)	1.4	820'	360'	Paved	161-164
Golden Cyn (Red Cathedral)	1.4	530'	270'	Paved	161-164
Gower Gulch borax mines	1.9	440'	430'	Paved	166-168
Ibex Spring and camp	<1.0	<100'	1,130'	F/2.3 mi	229-230
Moorehouse Mine	1.3	810'	1,370'	F/2.3 mi	230-232
Natural Bridge Cyn (to fall)	0.7	470'	660'	Graded	186-188
Pleasanton-Monarch mines*	2.5	1,100'	1,300'	F/2.2 mi	230
Twenty Mule Team Canyon	1.7	680'	1,540'	Graded	173-174
Virgin Spring	2.4	1,030'	1,900'	F/1.3 mi	221-222
Willow Creek (lower cyn)	2.3	1,020'	290'	Paved	204
Willow Creek (upper cyn)	1.8	1,240'	2,920'	Paved	201-204

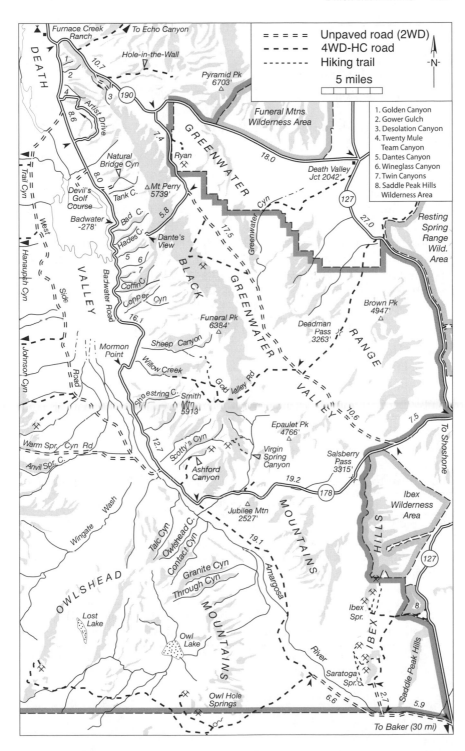

Route/Destination	Dist. (mi)	Elev. change	Mean elev.	Access road	Page
Intermediate hikes (5-12 miles round trip)					
Ashford Mine (tramway)	3.0	1,660'	1,860'	H/2.8 mi	213-216
Ashford Peak	2.9	2,510'	2,130'	H/2.8 mi	213-216
Bad Canyon (to drop-off)	5.3	4,130'	3,890'	Paved	191-194
Desert Hound Mine					
via Ashford Canyon	4.4	2,950'	2,580'	H/2.8 mi	213-216
via Scotty's Canyon	5.1	3,440'	2,130'	H/2.8 mi	207-210
Gower Gulch (to mouth)	2.6	740'	370'	Paved	166-168
Gower Gulch-Golden Cyn*	6.2	1,960'	290'	Paved	161-168
Ibex Spring and camp	2.6	300'	1,030'	P/3.2 mi	228-230
Moorehouse Mine	3.2	660'	1,090'	P/3.2 mi	228-232
Pleasanton-Monarch mines*	6.9	1,450'	1,120'	P/3.2 mi	228-230
Natural Bridge Cyn (to head)	3.1	3,180'	2,060'	Graded	186-188
Scotty's Spring	3.0	~1,430'	1,530'	H/2.8 mi	207-209
Sheep Spring	4.0	2,370'	980'	Paved	195-198
Long hikes (over 12 miles round trip)					
Desert Hound Mine (old site)					
via lower Virgin Cyn trail	6.9	2,630'	2,700'	F/1.3 mi	221-226
via upper Virgin Cyn trail	8.5	2,630'	2,700'	F/1.3 mi	221-226
Scotty's Canyon (to head)	6.6	4,500'	2,880'	H/2.8 mi	207-210
Sheep Canyon (to head)	9.0	5,920'	2,740'	Paved	195-198
Timpapah Spring	3.8	2,350'	1,850'	H/2.8 mi	207-210
Virgin Spring Cyn (to head)	7.2	2,410'	2,590'	F/1.3 mi	221-226
Willow Creek, rough spot					
in road to drop-off	7.2	3,100'	3,210'	P/7.1 mi	201-204
Overnight hikes (over 2 days)					
Sheep Canyon					
to Gold Valley Road	10.2	5,860'	2,650'	Paved	195-198
to Willow Creek drop-off	15.1	8,160'	2,680'	Paved	195-204
Virgin Spring Canyon					
to Greenwater Valley Rd	12.8	3,590'	2,860'	F/1.3 mi	221-226

Key: P=Primitive (2WD)   H=Primitive (HC)   F=Primitive (4WD)
* =Total distance and elevation change (ups + downs) for loops

GOLDEN CANYON

Golden Canyon is one of the most easily accessed and busiest hiking destinations in the park. It provides an easy path to explore the striking badlands of the Black Mountains, formed just a few million years ago when a lake filled Death Valley. The ultimate goal is Red Cathedral, a long, 400-foot cliff, deep red and beautifully carved by erosion, looming over the head of the canyon.

General Information

Road status: Roadless; easy access from paved road
Shortest hike: 0.25 mi, 85 ft one way / very easy
Longest hike: 1.4 mi, 530 ft one way (or more) / easy
Main attractions: Scenic canyon, badlands, geology
USGS 15' and 7.5' topo maps: Furnace Creek
Maps: pp. 167*, 159

Location and Access

Golden Canyon is a short drainage near the northern end of the Black Mountains. For the easiest access, drive the Badwater Road 2.1 miles south from Highway 190 to the signed Golden Canyon turnoff. For a slightly longer approach via the upper canyon, hike from Zabriskie Point, off Highway 190 4.6 miles east of Furnace Creek Ranch. The signed Golden Canyon trail starts at the north end of the parking area.

Route Description

The narrows. Just above its mouth Golden Canyon goes through short narrows. The lofty walls of this tight passage are made of a hodge-podge of dark sedimentary and volcanic rocks, including large chunks of basalt and tuffs, all lake deposits from the Furnace Creek Formation. Since it was deposited between 6.3 and 5.3 million years ago, this formation was tilted by uplifting and broken by frequent faulting. What once were horizontal lake beds today lie at odd angles. This helped form Golden Canyon by providing weaker fault planes for water to flow and erode the rocks. Throughout the narrows and further up canyon, look for evidence of this past geophysical activity, particularly in the abrupt breaks in the walls on the north side, and in the strongly tilted strata on the opposite side. For more details about the local geology, use the Golden Canyon trail guide (available at the trailhead and Visitor Center), which is keyed to markers along the canyon.

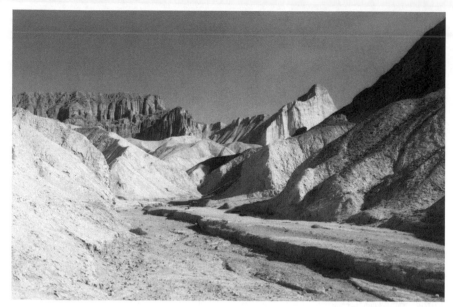

Golden Canyon, with Red Cathedral and Manly Beacon in the distance

A road used to go through Golden Canyon. It dates back to 1929, when a one-time gold seeker named Bob Eichbaum first opened Death Valley to tourism. Three years earlier, he had graded the first road down Towne Pass into the valley, the Death Valley Toll Road (now Highway 190), and developed Death Valley's first resort, a group of bungalows at Stovepipe Wells nicknamed "Bungalette." Golden Canyon was targeted as a tourist attraction for its scenic value and proximity to the oasis of Greenland Ranch (now Furnace Creek Ranch). The canyon road used to go nearly to the end of the canyon. Today, all that is left of it is a few sections of of sheared pavement in the narrows.

The mid-canyon.   After 0.25 mile the scenery changes abruptly as the dark narrows open up onto a bright, gold-colored corridor. The rocks exposed from here on are mostly siltstones and mudstones, also from the Furnace Creek Formation. These soft lake sediments, impermeable to water, have been severely eroded, even by the scant local rains, to produce the spectacular badlands that prevail along the rest of the canyon: a primitive, desolate landscape, deeply gullied and barren as neither soil nor plants get a chance to develop. Only two of the hardiest perennials manage to grow in the wash: honeysweet and desert holly.

These badlands can be leisurely explored along the gentle grades of Golden Canyon. Look for gypsum and borax interbedded in the mudstone. They occur in white veins between a fraction of an inch and several inches thick. The borax is milky; the gypsum is translucent and conspicuously fibrous. These evaporites indicate that this land was formed under a lake, and that the climate was then hot enough, at least periodically, to sustain a high evaporation rate (see *Twenty Mule Team Canyon*). More spectacular evidence is provided by ripple marks left on the rocks by waves on the lake. They resemble the patterns imprinted on silt at the shallow edge of a lake. Ripple marks are common on the flat, tilted walls forming the south side of the canyon, for about 400 yards past the narrows, and along the narrows as well.

One of the best but often overlooked features of Golden Canyon is its half a dozen or so short side canyons. Their often tight passages lead to colorful hillsides dissected into sharp pinnacles. Throughout this canyon, stay in the washes to preserve the fragile hills and ridges.

Red Cathedral. After about 1 mile the wash passes below Manly Beacon, the prominent spire looming on the south side. Shortly after, the canyon splits into two forks, at what used to be the end of the canyon road. The next goal is Red Cathedral, the spectacular 400-foot cliff to the east visible from most of Golden Canyon. It can be reached via either fork, or either one of the two side canyons that branch out a little earlier. These four short canyons, bright against the colorful background of Red Cathedral, are perhaps the most scenic part of this drainage. They are all much tighter than the main canyon, occasionally clogged with boulders and falls, and a lot of fun to explore. This area is also far less congested than the lower canyon. The main fork, straight from the old parking area, has collapsed a short distance in. This is a comparatively recent event—look for the torn steel ladder still buried under the small landslide. You will have to crawl or wiggle through to reach the end, the foot of the sheer wall of Red Cathedral. The other three forks give access to different parts of Red Cathedral. There are delightful places to discover

Golden Canyon		
	Dist.(mi)	Elev.(ft)
Mouth	0.0	-140
End of narrows	0.25	-55
Trail to Zabriskie Point	1.0	150
Foot of Manly Beacon (trail)	(0.4)	~680
Gower Gulch (trail)	(1.3)	500
Zabriskie Point (trailhead)	(1.7)	640
Fork	1.2	250
Red Cathedral	1.4	~390

in this area—soaring walls, deep grooves shooting up to the sky, and fluted pillars of stone, like shrines from a distant past.

The massive deposits of Red Cathedral belong to the Funeral Formation. They are the remnant of an alluvial fan that once spilled out of the mountain range onto the older Furnace Creek Formation. A dry climate clearly prevailed in the late Pliocene when this formation was deposited. The fan material was cemented into a fanglomerate, a fairly resistant, cliff-forming rock. The deep red stain results from weathering, which oxidized the iron of the original rock.

The Golden Canyon trail. This scenic trail, indicated on the south side of the canyon a little before the fork, leads to Zabriskie Point in 1.7 miles. It first climbs to the foot of Manly Beacon, where it offers excellent views of the badlands and Red Cathedral. Golden Canyon perhaps best deserves its magical name when viewed from this area around sunset, when the hills turn to a fiery gold. The trail continues up and down several ravines to eventually reach Gower Gulch, the next canyon south. From here you can either continue up the trail to Zabriskie Point (the trail is not the faint path climbing the hill straight ahead, but up the side canyon to your left). Or you can return down the eerie wash of Gower Gulch. This is a beautiful loop, about 5.4 miles long, one of my all-time favorites in Death Valley (see *Gower Gulch*).

■

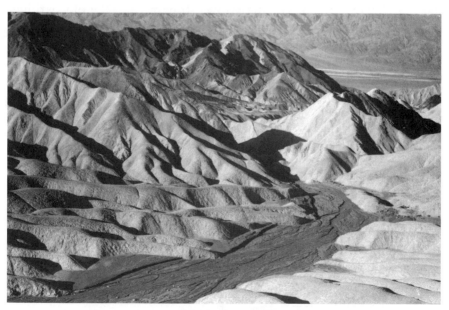

Gower Gulch from Zabriskie Point

GOWER GULCH

Starting from famed Zabriskie Point, an easy walk down the gently sloping wash of this scenic canyon will take you through an other-worldly landscape of brilliant naked hills with intriguing side canyons. You'll eventually reach abandoned borax mines and a nar-rower gorge on the edge of Death Valley. This hike can be extended into a half-day loop by returning via nearby Golden Canyon.

General Information

Road status: Roadless; easy hiking access from paved road
Shortest hike: 0.4 mi, 160 ft one way / very easy
Longest hike: 2.6 mi, 800 ft one way (or more)/easy
Main attractions: Scenic badlands, borax mines, geology
USGS 15'and 7.5' topo maps: Furnace Creek
Maps: pp. 167*, 159

Location and Access

Gower Gulch is the prominent wash below Zabriskie Point, in the northern Black Mountains. To get to this popular viewpoint, drive Highway 190 4.6 miles east of Furnace Creek Ranch. Hiking down from the observation platform to the gulch on the steep trails that have developed in recent years is not recommended, as the scenery is becoming increasingly scarred by such use. Instead, take the marked Golden Canyon trail, which starts at the west end of the parking area.

To hike in from the other end, start from the Badwater Road 0.6 mile south of the Golden Canyon turnoff, at the concrete-lined dip where the wash of Gower Gulch crosses the road. Follow the north side of the wash 0.25 mile to the Golden Canyon-Gower Gulch connecting trail, and use this trail to bypass the fall at the mouth of the gulch.

Geology: Gower Gulch or Furnace Creek?

In 1941 a major portion of the surface flow of normally dry Furnace Creek Wash—the wide wash parallel to Highway 190—was diverted into Gower Gulch to avoid episodical flooding of the Furnace Creek Inn resort. The diversion is a short gravel dike across Furnace Creek Wash, visible just uphill from the Zabriskie Point turnoff. Gower Gulch originally drained only about 2.5 square miles of low elevation, low precipitation terrain. The artificial diversion made it the recipient of the 100 times larger and higher elevation drainage of Furnace Creek. For all intents and purposes, Gower Gulch has become Furnace Creek.

The increased volume of water and debris brought in by flash floods over the last few decades has produced major changes in Gower Gulch. Much of the wash has been widened, deepened, and coated with gravel from Furnace Creek Wash. Below the mouth of the gulch, 2.5 miles downstream, the deep wash gouged in the fan is also the result of artificially increased erosion. This rapid evolution illustrates that in a barren desert environment, erosional processes can produce sizeable changes over periods of time insignificant compared to geological times.

Route Description

The upper canyon. The main appeal of Gower Gulch is the unique terrain it crosses, a strikingly barren world of rounded hills deeply chiseled by erosion. Most of the way you will be wandering through a strangely empty and magnetic landscape composed of simple forms and monochromatic colors—gold hills against blue sky, blinding during the day, richly colored and filled with shadows in the early and late hours of the day. Devoid of the common characteristics of Earth's landscapes, it conjures up pictures of alien worlds. This setting has in fact been used on several occasions for science fiction movies. The winding side canyons and ravines branching out from the gulch are wonderful avenues to explore this stern and surreal terrain.

The badlands of Gower Gulch were eroded in the soft mudstones deposited at the bottom of Furnace Creek Lake, which covered much of this area in the late Miocene (see *Twenty Mule Team Canyon*). The dark brown layers capping the hills to the south and west are fan gravels, rich in volcanic rocks, which are locally retarding erosion of the softer underlying mudstones. This entire area is made of extremely soft

Gower Gulch		
	Dist.(mi)	Elev.(ft)
Golden Canyon trailhead	0.0	640
Gower Gulch wash	0.4	500
First borax mines	1.2	310
Main borax mines	1.9	200
Narrower canyon	2.1	110
Mouth (40-ft fall)	2.6	~-80
Badwater Road	(0.4)	-170
Mouth of Golden Canyon	3.5	-140
Back via Golden Canyon	6.2	640

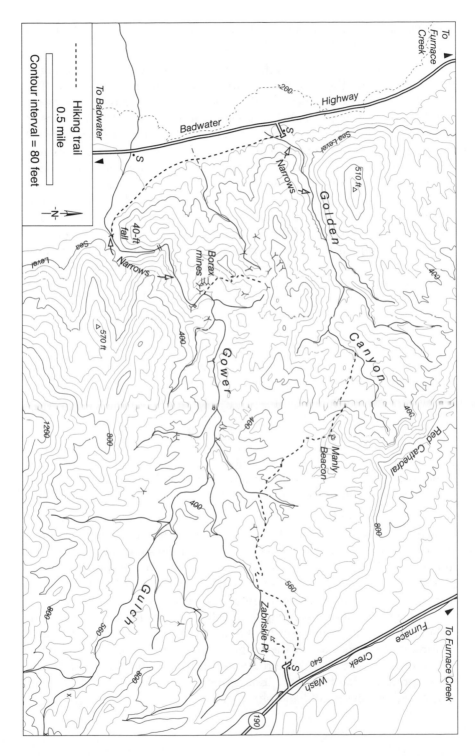

Contour interval = 80 feet

0.5 mile

Hiking trail

To Badwater

Badwater

Highway

200

Sea Level

Golden

510 ft

Narrows

40-ft fall

Narrows

Sea Level

Borax mines

570 ft

400

Gower

400

Canyon

400

500

Red Cathedral

800

Manly Beacon

1200

800

400

560

Gulch

800

560

800

560

Zabriskie Pt

640

Furnace Creek Wash

190

To Furnace Creek

To Furnace Creek

rock. Do not walk on the hills or ridges, even if they have a trail. Stay in the washes to avoid leaving unsightly marks on these graceful badlands.

Borax mines. Gower Gulch had a brief history of borax mining in the 1880s, around the time the 20-mule-teams were first put to use. The Pacific Coast Borax Company, which eventually owned just about every borate deposit in the area, held ten claims in the gulch. The segment of Golden Canyon trail from Zabriskie Point to the gulch is in fact part of the wagon road the company built to access its claims. Little borax came out of Gower Gulch because it was abandoned when more accessible deposits were discovered further east (see *Twenty Mule Team Canyon*).

The mining area starts 1.2 miles from the trailhead and continues for about 0.8 mile. It is marked by several short tunnels, rock mounds, and remnants of timber. Borate ore, mostly colemanite and ulexite, outcrops a little bit everywhere, usually as white, powdery stains on the hillsides and snow-white chunks near the mines. The rock mounds, common near the mines, are made of weathering piles of borax bricks. Their purpose is no longer known. Some of them may have been windbreaks or shelters, others tent platforms or simply stockpiles.

The main mining area, on the north side at a wide left bend in the wash, has half a dozen tunnels and several rock mounds. The wooden stakes lined up on the ridge across the wash from the mines mark old property lines. In front of the tunnels a weathered trail switchbacks up the lava talus to dead end in 0.2 mile at a saddle. There are a few prospects down the steep ravine beyond the saddle, but the real payoff is the good panoramic views of the surrounding badlands.

Just down canyon from the main mines there is a last tunnel on the opposite side, with shredded wood lying around and signs of a tent or house site. This area may have been the end of the wagon road, where a small assaying office stood in the 1880s.

The lower gulch. The lower part of Gower Gulch is a narrow passage twisting between steep high walls, with a few constrictions and a couple of short falls in hard conglomerate. On the south side there are a few long and high flat walls, tilted at 45°, on which well-preserved ripple marks from ancient Furnace Creek Lake are recorded. One of them is just down canyon from a prominent green hillside on the south side.

This passage ends abruptly at a 40-foot fall on the edge of Death Valley. A trail safely bypasses the fall to the right, drops to the fan, and continues along the foot of the range to the mouth of Golden Canyon, which offers a nice alternative route to return to Zabriskie Point. In the early spring the fan below the trail is often covered with vivid displays of gravelghost, desertgold and phacelia.

■

TWENTY MULE TEAM CANYON

> *This scenic canyon is a good place for a short drive through the color-*
> *ful badlands of the Black Mountains. Along the way, short walks lead*
> *up to the many tunnels made by the turn-of-the-century prospectors*
> *who mined this area for borax and gypsum. The upper canyon is road-*
> *less and ideal for an easy hike, spiced with short narrows, falls, inter-*
> *esting geology, and more exciting tunnels.*

General Information

Road status: Good graded road (lower canyon); roadless beyond
Shortest hike: Short walks/very easy to easy
Longest hike: 1.7 mi, 680 ft one way/moderate
Attractions: Scenic badlands canyon, borax mines, history, geology
USGS 15' and 7.5' topo maps: Furnace Creek
Maps: pp. 173*, 159

Location and Access

Twenty Mule Team Canyon is a short side canyon of Furnace Creek Wash draining the east side of the northern Black Mountains. A one way road follows the wash of the lower canyon, starting at the marked junction on the west side of Highway 190, 5.7 miles east of Furnace Creek Ranch. It returns to the highway 1.7 miles east of its starting point. It is graded and suitable for all passenger cars.

Geology: Furnace Creek Six Million Years Ago

The large borate deposits of the region occur mostly in the lower part of the Furnace Creek Formation. This formation was deposited between about 6.3 and 5.4 million years ago (late Miocene). At the time, faulting of the Basin and Range, which eventually produced the north-trending valleys and mountains of Nevada and eastern California, had been going on for several million years. In the Death Valley region, initial extension of the crust had created long troughs separated by slowly rising ranges. One such elongated basin stretched southwestward from today's Salt Creek Hills down to Furnace Creek Wash and along the east side of the Greenwater Range. It was flooded under Furnace Creek Lake, a huge body of salt water covering at least 600 square miles. The Furnace Creek Formation was deposited in this lake—mostly alluvia washed down from the surrounding ranges and volcanic rocks.

The rocks of the surrounding ranges contained small amounts of boron. Underground water, heated by renewed volcanic activity, dissolved borates and other salts as it passed through the rocks, then resurfaced as hot springs and flowed into the lake. The area enjoyed an arid climate with a mean temperature around 60°F, much like today. As the lake had either limited or no outlet, continuous evaporation caused intermittent precipitation of the boron salts. Only trace amounts of boron are contained in rocks, but the volume of rocks is so enormous that this slow concentration process produced millions of tons of borate.

After this borate-rich formation was laid down, sedimentation continued through the Pliocene, burying it under around 2 miles of rocks. The increased temperature of the deeply buried borate deposits altered them into rich colemanite. Block faulting continued—it is still active today—eventually resulting in the opening of the Badwater Basin, Death Valley's deepest trough. Because this new basin is oriented at an angle to the old Furnace Creek trough, it cut right through it and helped erosion dig up the Furnace Creek Formation's colemanite, now exposed in the northern Black Mountains.

History: Borax Mining

Borax mining played a significant role in the history of Death Valley, which first gained popularity from the colorful 20-mule-team wagons used around the turn of the century to transport borax ore across the desert. The 20-mule teams starred in a nationwide advertising campaign for borax, and the image of these long trains painstakingly crossing the barren desert flats is an enduring symbol of the Death Valley days. This awkward means of transportation was conceived during the early borax mining efforts, spearheaded by William Coleman, to haul to Mojave ore scraped from the valley floor and processed at his Harmony Borax Works plant just north of Furnace Creek Ranch (see *Harmony Borax Works*). At the time, it was generally thought that borate only occurred in salt flats. Nearby Monte Blanco, in what is now Twenty Mule Team Canyon, is a conspicuous white hill high above Furnace Creek Wash, but it took imaginative observers to suspect that it contained borax. In 1883, in the early days of Harmony, a party of three men aware of the value of borax and of the simple flame test to identify it, applied the test to a rock sample from Monte Blanco and realized what it was—a whole mountain of borate.

Within a year other major discoveries of boron ore were made further east, near the Greenwater Range, in particular on the Biddy McCarthy and the Lila C. claims, the latter named by Coleman in honor of one of his daughters. Coleman acquired all of them, including Monte Blanco, and soon owned most of the known borate deposits in the region. They contained a new, rich borate ore later named colemanite, but the need for expensive underground mining, the lack of a simple method to process it, and the success of the Harmony Borax Works, all combined to hinder the early development of these claims.

Harmony was operated until the late 1880s. In 1890 Coleman's financial empire collapsed and his assets were acquired by Francis Marion "Borax" Smith, who formed the Pacific Coast Borax Company and became the new borax tycoon. The company first opened not its richest but its most accessible deposits, starting with the Lila C. The 20-mule teams were once again put into service, until 1907 when a 7-mile rail spur was constructed from the newly completed Tonopah and Tidewater Railroad. The Lila C. played out in 1915. Mining was then shifted further west to the Biddy McCarthy and other claims in the Ryan area. A new spur, the Death Valley narrow gauge, was constructed to serve these mines. The plan was to extend it to Monte Blanco after Ryan played out, but it never materialized. Ryan kept on producing until 1928 when a new borate deposit was discovered at what is now the sprawling mining complex of Boron, southwest of Death Valley. It was an enormous lode, more accessible and economical to mine, and it spelled the temporary closure of the Death Valley borax mines.

So it was that in spite of its nearly 3-million-ton reserve, Monte Blanco was spared from development. Claims in nearby Corkscrew Canyon were worked in the mid-1950s, but only to fill small special

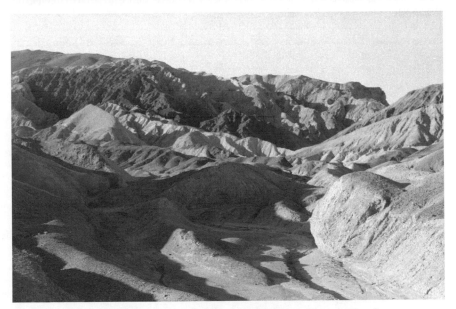

Eroded hills along the Twenty Mule Team Canyon Road

orders. Twenty Mule Team Canyon underwent extensive prospecting in the early 1900s, but it probably never saw the hooves and wheels of the famous mule teams.

Route Description

The canyon road. Whether you hike, bike or drive through this canyon, you will find its short road offers a scenic trip along a narrow wash and colorfully stained badlands. Both canyon walls, made mostly of mudstone of the lower Furnace Creek Formation, are crawling with prospects, some in plain view, others hidden in short side canyons or on ridges. The tunnels near the crest of the eastern ridge explored minor deposits of gypsum and borate, while the deposits on the west side contained only borates. The few visitors who venture out of their cars all seem to get involved in the same activity: crawling into the tunnels. Of course, I would not advise anything so foolish; much too dangerous. Besides, most of the prospects were obviously not winners and are pretty boring. But then again, in the beam of your flashlight some tunnels may come alive with a thousand sparkles from faceted ore, or a cavity full of colemanite crystals may shine back at you.

After 1.8 miles the road climbs slightly out of the main wash and turns left, while the wash of Twenty Mule Team Canyon veers off to the right. Keep track of the mileage, as this old junction is easy to miss. The old access road to the Monte Blanco mining area used to branch out at this point and continue up the wash, but it is now completely erased. On the left side of the road is the site of the Monte Blanco assay office, a large wooden house shaded by a verandah built in 1883 to serve local

Twenty Mule Team Canyon		
	Dist.(mi)	Elev.(ft)
Twenty Mule Team Canyon Road		
Highway 190	0.0	870
Road leaves wash	1.8	1,200
Highway 190	2.8	1,190
Roadless canyon		
Road leaves wash	0.0	1,200
Monte Blanco mines	0.3	~1,290
15-ft fall	0.7	~1,420
Slot side canyon	0.9	1,500
Fork	1.1	1,710
Head	1.7	1,880

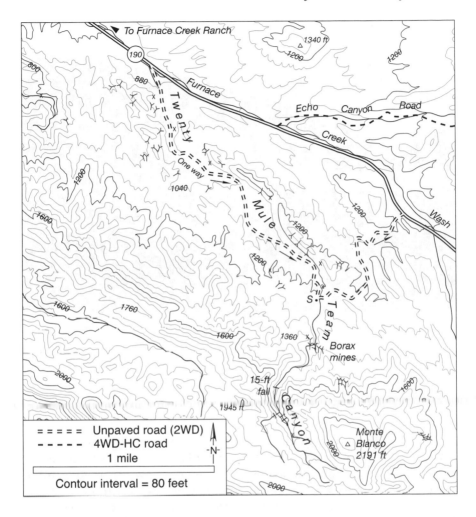

miners. The original house was moved to Furnace Creek Ranch in the 1950s to house the Borax Museum. It is still there today, and has gained the respectable title of the oldest house in Death Valley. Now only the wall-lined underground cellar betrays its former location. Nearby and across the road are traces of tent sites marked by slightly depressed flat areas and scattered stones. If you continue along the road, you will soon ascend the ridge on the east side and wind your way up and down scenic hills back to the highway.

The upper canyon. As usual, the best part lies beyond the road. From the old junction, the narrow wash leads in 0.3 mile to the foot of Monte Blanco, the golden hill covered with white, vertical streaks of snow-like borate ore. This is the site of the first discovery of colemanite

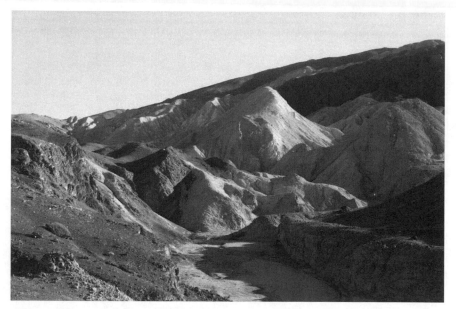

Monte Blanco and the roadless section of Twenty Mule Team Canyon at sunset

in Death Valley. The wooden posts lined up along the wash are remains of the fences strung out by the Pacific Coast Borax Company around 1916 to discourage encroachment. Some of the best tunnels, rock mounds, tailings, and loading platforms are found around here, on either side of the wash and in the small side canyon nearby.

Past the mines the scenery changes rapidly as the narrowing wash cuts successively through the colorful layers of the Furnace Creek Formation—golden mudstone, then purple lava flows crumbling from ancient exposure to sea water, conglomerate, sandstone, more volcanic rocks, and finally mudstone in the upper drainage. In the mid section a 15-foot slanted fall, easy to negotiate, then two slightly more difficult boulder jams, complicate matters a little. But try to go on. Somewhere in there you will find a deep and narrow slot canyon, high cliffs and color-ful hills, a beautiful orange slickensided boulder, and ultimately an eerie landscape of eroded dune-like hills topped with pointed turrets.

■

DESOLATION CANYON

In more ways than one, Desolation Canyon is a fairy tale version of the larger canyons found in the badlands of the Black Mountains. A good part of the way it is narrow and twisted, punctuated with short falls and inviting side canyons—a pleasant playground for hikers of all ages to take a closer look at the desert.

General Information

Road status: Roadless; easy access on short graded road
Shortest hike: 1.1 mi, 340 ft/very easy
Longest hike: 1.8 mi, 770 ft (or more)/easy
Main attractions: Narrows, geology, easy hiking
USGS 15' and 7.5' topo maps: Furnace Creek
Maps: pp. 177*, 159

Location and Access

Desolation Canyon is in the northern Black Mountains, between Golden Canyon and Artist Drive. To get there, drive the Badwater Road 3.7 miles south from Highway 190 to the graded road to Desolation Canyon. This road used to go to just below the mouth of the canyon, but it was washed out by a flood in August 2004, and only the first half a mile has been re-graded. Park at the small parking area at the end of this good road. The mouth of Desolation Canyon is the wide opening in the side of the mountain less than half a mile to the east.

Geology

Desolation Canyon cuts through the sedimentary rocks of the Artist Drive Formation, deposited in a lake in the late Miocene (see *Artist Drive Area*). The deposits were later uplifted and dissected by erosion into the tormented badland topography typical of the northern Black Mountains. The late Miocene was a period of volcanic activity, and ashes were periodically blown across the lake. They reacted with the trace chemicals dissolved in the water and produced new compounds, which now stain the hills along the open wash with green and pink hues. As sulfates present in the lake periodically precipitated, gypsum (a hydrated calcium sulfate) was also formed. Thin veins of this translucent to white, fibrous rock are exposed in the mudstone along the canyon walls.

Route Description

The main canyon. The trail that heads east from the parking area
follows the route of the old access road for 0.25 mile. At its end, head
down into the wide wash of Desolation Canyon 100 yards northeast,
then follow it uphill to the canyon. This is nice preamble to the canyon
hike itself, in full view of the colorful front of the Black Mountains.

Desolation Canyon starts as a broad gulch, but after a short distance it tightens considerably, and remains narrow most of the way. This
is a colorful place, framed by hills and walls painted in pastel shades of
gold, pink, and blue-green by volcanic minerals. At a few places, it
squeezes through short twisted passages no more than 6 feet across,
trapped between sheer walls. It is along these barren corridors, completely devoid of plant life, that Desolation Canyon best justifies its
name. Even the wider areas support little vegetation, mostly scattered
desert holly. There are a few falls along the way, all under 8 feet and
easy to climb, and a few side canyons, the largest ones on the east side.
Always follow the right fork if you want to stay with the main canyon.

This is a miniature canyon where all dimensions—length,
width, wall height, even the grade of the wash—are oddly scaled down.
Take your time exploring it. It has more to offer than may appear at first
glance. Look for thin veins of gypsum, for undercuts dug by flood water
in tight bends, and for thin layers of mud, like wax drippings on a candle, deposited on the walls by rain water. There are other signs of active
erosion, such as the unusual conical piles lined up along the wash
underneath overhangs. Each of them is made of fine debris which, when
loosened by the wind from the high walls above, fall over the lip of an
overhang, always at the same spot, like sand in an hourglass. You will
probably witness a few such minor slides during your short visit here.

	Desolation Canyon	
	Dist.(mi)	Elev.(ft)
Road's end/trailhead	0.0	-55
End of trail	0.25	0
Canyon wash	0.3	-10
Start of narrower canyon	0.8	130
7-ft fall	1.1	270
Side canyon	1.2	320
Side canyon	1.5	510
18-ft fall	1.8	700
Head	2.3	1,440

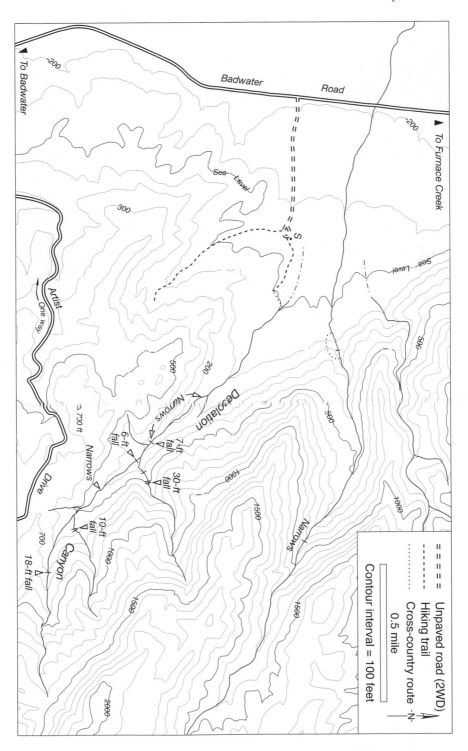

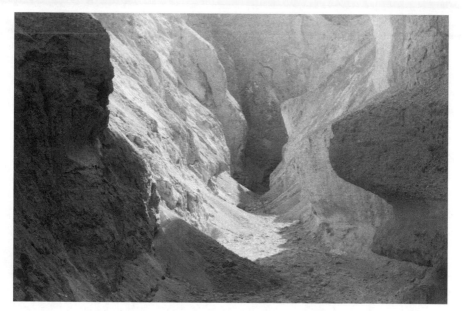

A narrow passage along Desolation Canyon

Near its upper end, past a long talus of dark volcanic ash, the canyon is blocked by an 18-foot fall carved like a stairway. The brittle rock makes the climbing tricky and unsafe—this is essentially the end of the trail.

The side canyons. If you are hungry for more, explore the short tributaries on your way back. They will take you into deep and tight places where you can gaze up soaring walls to a blue ribbon of sky, until you eventually reach an impassable fall.

A word of caution. Desolation Canyon is small, and it weaves through soft desert fabric; even a little abuse can do lasting damage to it. Please respect it. Do not walk on surrounding hills and taluses. Stay in the washes and ravines. They recuperate relatively fast. Don't put up cairns—it's useless in a canyon where one would have to work hard to get lost. This is a great place for children, but make sure they obey these elementary rules and understand why.

■

ARTIST DRIVE AREA

> *These short hikes—under two hours each—explore narrow, chaotic canyons brightened by colorful volcanic rocks, all easily accessed from Artist Drive. Some of them are very easy, while others take a lot of scrambling and climbing. From children to desert rats, just about everyone will find a place matched to their expectations.*

General Information

Road status: Roadless; very easy hiking access from paved road
Shortest hike: Short walks / very easy
Longest hike: 0.7 mi, 670 ft / moderate
Main attractions: Short colorful canyons, narrows, volcanic rocks, falls, rock scrambling
USGS topo maps: Furnace Creek (15'), Devil's Golf Course (7.5')
Maps: pp. 183*, 159

Location and Access

The short, unnamed canyons suggested here drain the western foot of the Black Mountains. They are all accessed from Artist Drive, the one way road that starts on Badwater Road 0.6 miles south of Highway 190. The canyons and their location are described from south to north, in the order they are encountered along the road.

Geology

The canyons found in this area all cut through the Artist Drive Formation, a pile of jumbled blocks which is perhaps the most colorful formation in Death Valley. Stretching for about 10 miles along the west side and crest of the Black Mountains, approximately from Desolation Canyon south to Natural Bridge Canyon, it was first noted and named for its striking exposures along Artist Drive. This is a relatively young formation, deposited from 8 to 6.3 million years ago. The presence of fresh water fish fossils in its lower tuff beds suggests that it was laid down in a large lake, with volcanic materials and basin sediments deposited concurrently.

The Artist Drive Formation is divided into two massive pyroclastic layers separated by three well-stratified sedimentary layers. The latter generally consist of mudstone, sandstone, and conglomerate. The pyroclastic members are vivid tuff-breccia, blue-green to pale orange and pink. Together with the upper sedimentary member, which also

contains volcanic detritus, they are responsible for the colorful exposures prevailing in much of this area. The brown felsite and dark basaltic
rocks scattered throughout the formation add yet different hues to the
scenery.

When the Artist Drive Formation was accumulating, the north
end of the Black Mountains was probably low land and the rest of the
Black Mountains and the northern Panamints were already in place,
although not yet separated by Death Valley. During the subsequent
uplifting of the northern Black Mountains, the formation broke off from
the underlying Precambrian basement and slipped down, perhaps as
much as a mile, to the foot of the mountains, producing the jumble of
blocks that prevails in this area today.

Route Description

Canyon at first dip. For this action-packed hike, start at the first
pronounced dip along Artist Drive, 3 miles from the Badwater Road
(park at the small turn-outs on either side of the dip). The canyon is up
the wash that crosses the road at the bottom of the dip. It is a chaotic and
multi-colored place, deep and narrow a good part of the way. The walls
come together almost right away, and for the next half a mile progress is
repeatedly challenged by falls and rock jams. The first high fall, less than
1000 feet in, is about 11 feet high, nearly vertical, and an effective people
filter—many hikers cannot go past it. There is another fall a little further,
higher but easier, then comes the first high dam, an impressive, 30-foot
jam of huge chockstones. It marks the lower end of a long landslide of
large volcanic blocks that crashed down from the north wall and crowds
the next stretch of canyon. To continue, the easiest route is to scramble
up the steep landslide, staying on the north side of the wash. It is hard
work, periodically rewarded by a look back at the blinding salt flats
shimmering in the distant wedge between the canyon walls—improbable visions of order in a world of chaos. Look for slickensides on some of
the block surfaces. They point to fault planes where the walls scraped
against each other before the collapse. The other route, up the wash
itself, is spiked with falls and more difficult. Although the rock is
crumbly just about everywhere, rock climbers will enjoy the exercise.
The wash eventually reaches a second towering dam that must also be
bypassed, above which the two routes converge.

Shortly past this second natural dam and a couple of other falls,
the canyon levels off into a straight corridor rimmed by high walls. In
another quarter of a mile the wash veers left and fizzles out abruptly at
the base of a cleavage of sheer falls and chockstones totalling about 40
feet in height. This is the end of the trail for most people. But if you don't
like to give up this easily, cheer up. You can still try to explore this last

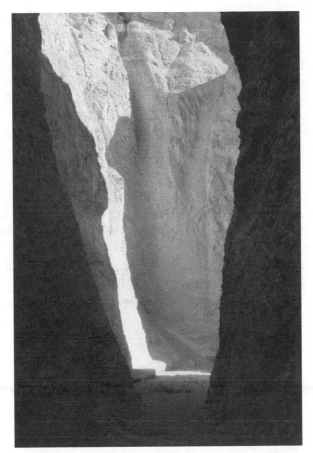

Narrows at the upper end of the "second dip" canyon

obstruction, or look for a route around it via the deep gullies chiseled in the face of the nearby wall.

Canyon at second dip. This deep, short canyon is my favorite in this area. While it has much the same character as the canyon at the first dip, it is more colorful, overall a little more accessible, and blessed with beautiful tight narrows. Start at the second dip in the road, 3.5 miles from the Badwater Road. There is a small turn-out to park at the top of the rise just past the dip, on the right side. Hike up the wash at the bottom of the dip. The short pink fall 50 yards from the road is the entrance to a very pretty, cathedral-like passage that gradually deepens. It is graced by pale, blue-green tuff boulders stranded along the wash. Look for overhangs, for mud drippings on the walls, and for crumbling slickensides on boulders and higher up on the polished walls. Other than the geology and the scenery, the main attraction of this hike is the challenge of the half dozen tall dams of large boulders jammed across the wash, the highest one being about 25 feet. A little scrambling is needed to get over them, but none is as difficult as in the canyon at the first dip (even my mom made it!). If this is near the limit of your capabilities, several times you will think you have reached the end, only to be thrilled seconds later after finding you can actually make it a little further.

The crowning glory of this short canyon is the beautiful narrows hidden beyond the last of these obstructions, an eery corridor that folds beneath vertical walls rising well over 100 feet. When the sun manages to reach into it, this tight passage is suffused with a deep orange glow. It ends (much too soon) at a dark, claustrophobic cul-de-sac closed off by a 20-foot fall and huge chockstones wedged high between the walls. This is as far as most people will be able to go. Rock climbers will find a worthy opponent in this and the following few falls.

Artist's Palette. If you have children, you may want to take them on one of several easy hikes from Artist's Palette. This scenic viewpoint is 4.5 miles from Badwater Road. The most accessible hills in this area are wearing down fast from overuse. To avoid further damage, stay away from the soft ridges, and walk in the washes only.

Artist Drive Area		
	Dist.(mi)	Elev.(ft)
Canyon at first dip		
Artist Drive	0.0	940
30-ft jam (foot of landslide)	0.3	1,190
40-ft fall	0.7	1,610
Canyon at second dip		
Artist Drive	0.0	860
25-ft fall	0.15	1.035
Narrows	0.3	1,120
20-ft fall	0.45	1,330
First canyon at Artist's Palette		
Artist Drive	0.0	600
Narrows	0.4	730
25-ft fall	0.5	840
Second canyon at Artist's Palette		
Artist Drive	0.0	600
Narrows	0.2	630
High fall	0.75	950

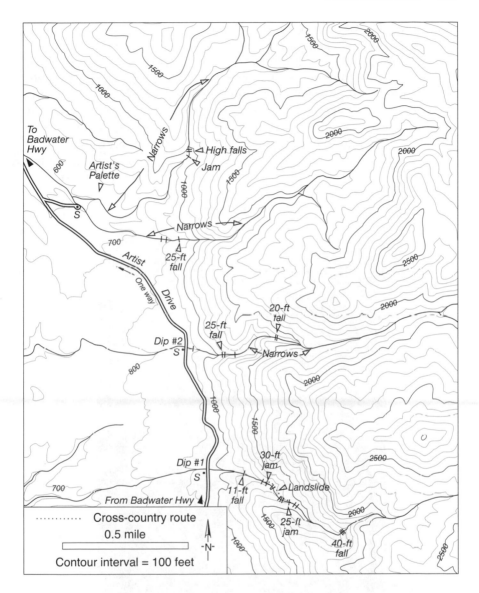

To
Badwater
Hwy

Artist's
Palette

Narrows

High falls
Jam

Narrows

25-ft
fall

Artist

One way

Drive

20-ft
fall

25-ft
fall

Dip #2

Narrows

800

Dip #1

30-ft
jam

700

11-ft
fall

Landslide

From Badwater Hwy

25-ft
jam

40-ft
fall

.... Cross-country route

0.5 mile

N

Contour interval = 100 feet

    The common starting point is the confluence of the two shallow
washes just below the viewpoint. The first canyon, up the wash closest
to the viewpoint, starts in about 0.4 mile at a high portal. What follows
are short, windy narrows with hollowed-out walls. Nothing Earth shattering, but again kids will have a great time, provided they get a little
help to climb the two crumbly, 7 to 8-foot falls along the way. The narrows end in 700 feet at an impassable 25-foot fall in a small circular

amphitheater. Do not miss the unusually long and narrow slot that branches out on the north side, about 80 feet from the foot of the last fall.

The second canyon, up the furthest wash, is comparable in length but quite different in character, and it offers the longest nearly unobstructed walk. After about 0.2 mile up the wash, the canyon begins to narrow and twist between sheer ochre walls. The scenery, reminiscent of Golden Canyon, gradually improves as the walls gain height. Most people will turn around after about 0.6 mile, just past a group of large boulders, where the wash is interrupted by a high fall. Above the fall the main canyon squeezes through an enticing slot, but the rock is crumbly and the climb difficult.

∎

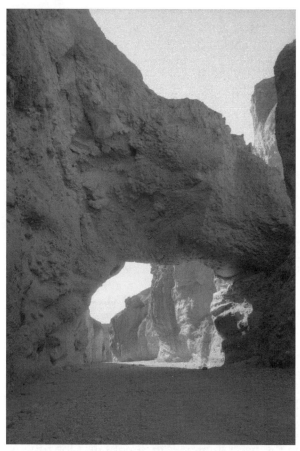

This massive bridge spans the sheer walls
of Natural Bridge Canyon

NATURAL BRIDGE CANYON

> *The short hike to the massive bridge in Natural Bridge Canyon, the largest in the park, is quite easy and one of the most popular. Past the bridge the sheer canyon walls come together to form shaded narrows, with interesting hanging canyons and fluted falls, up to a vertical 15-foot fall. Hardly ever visited, the fall-ridden upper canyon above it is a challenging place for the adventurous rock climber.*

General Information

Road status: Roadless; easy access via good graded road
Shortest hike: 0.35 mi, 180 ft one way / easy
Longest hike: 3.1 mi, 3,180 ft one way (or more) / strenuous
Main attractions: Natural bridge, geology, narrows and falls, technical
        rock climbing
USGS 15' topo maps: Furnace Creek*, Ryan
USGS 7.5' topo maps: Devil's Golf Course*, Ryan
Maps: pp. 187*, 159

Location and Access

Natural Bridge Canyon is in the northern central Black Mountains. It is accessed by a good, well-marked graded road branching off the Badwater Road 13.1 miles south of Highway 190, or 3.5 miles north of Badwater. It is 1.8 miles up the fan to the small parking lot at the mouth of the canyon (the road ends sooner than indicated on the 7.5' maps). In the summer this road is usually closed, and you will have to walk from the Badwater Road. The NPS exhibit on the local geology at the parking area is well worth reading before hiking in.

Geology: Turtlebacks

Natural Bridge Canyon is near the northern end of the Badwater turtleback, a giant dome of uplifted and arched rock stretching for miles along the western front of the Black Mountains. Its curvature is clearly visible from the Badwater Road, especially from a mile or so north of the canyon road. As you drive this road, look for the smooth, gullied surface of the mountain just south of the canyon. This is the faulted front surface of the turtleback, mostly made of the very old Precambrian metamorphic core of the mountains. Over the last few million years, as the mountains were being uplifted, the younger deposits that rested on top of it slid down the dome of the rising turtleback towards the valley, piling up at its base and exposing the underlying Precambrian core. These younger deposits are the lighter-colored rocks now resting against the base of the mountain. They belong to the late Miocene Furnace Creek Formation. Mostly lake deposits, they are much softer and more deeply gullied than the metamorphic rocks. The lower portion of Natural Bridge Canyon was eroded into this formation and is well-behaved. In contrast, where the canyon eventually penetrates into the Precambrian core of the turtleback it becomes considerably steeper and difficult to negotiate.

Route Description

The bridge. Up to a little past the bridge, the canyon is not very narrow but has impressive walls soaring vertically from the gravel wash. It is an easy and pleasant walk along this well-defined corridor to the popular natural bridge, located only a third of a mile from the parking area (I once saw a woman in dust-covered 3-inch heels returning from it). The bridge is a massive arch of rock joining the canyon walls 35 feet above the wash, about as thick as it is high. This is one of the few bridges in the park, and the largest I know of. While standing under it, look for the deep recess in the north wall 8 feet or so above the wash. Before the bridge was formed, the water flowed along this old channel, diverted from a straighter path by the harder rock plug above you. In time, water washed out the gravel from beneath this plug and dug a new channel underneath it, thus forming the bridge.

Dry falls, hanging canyons and dripping wax. Although most visitors turn around at the bridge, there is much more to see just a little further. Erosion has etched several unusual falls in the canyon walls. The most striking one is on the south side, about 100 yards past the bridge. It is a 25 to 30 foot high vertical tubular groove deeply recessed in the wall, gouged by storm water pouring down from the small side canyon just

Natural Bridge Canyon		
	Dist.(mi)	Elev.(ft)
Parking area (mouth)	0.0	420
Natural bridge	0.35	600
Small side canyon	0.5	700
15-ft fall	0.7	890
20-ft fall	0.85	1,030
Saddle (Tank Canyon)	1.9	2,740
Head	3.1	3,600

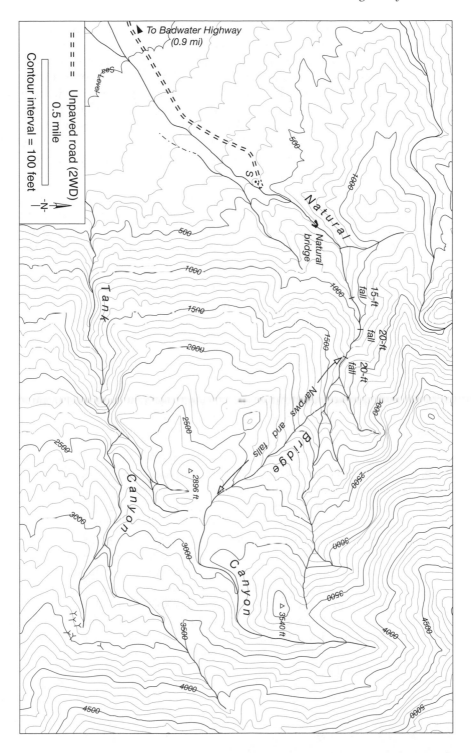

To Badwater Highway
(0.9 mi)

Unpaved road (2WD)
0.5 mile

Contour interval = 100 feet

-N-

Sea Level

500

1000

Natural
bridge

Natural

15-ft
fall

20-ft
fall

20-ft
fall

Narrows and falls

Bridge

Tank

Canyon

Canyon

2500

3000

3500

4000

4500

△ 2896 ft

△ 3540 ft

above it. Stream erosion has dug down much faster and deeper in the main canyon than in this little side canyon, which was left hanging well above the main wash. Even in the driest of North American deserts, stream erosion is still quite active. The peculiar, cream-colored beads covering the walls around the fall, like wax drippings on a candle, are signs of recent erosion. After a storm, the hanging side canyon fills up with an ephemeral stream that picks up mud and redeposits it on the walls. As you walk up canyon, look for other dry falls, hanging canyons and panels of "wax." High on the north wall, along a small diagonal fault, there is also a dark cave excavated by erosion.

A small side canyon. If you came here with children, you may want to take them into the small side canyon on the left side, 250 yards past the bridge. Fairly narrow, filled with boulders easy to climb, it's a place children seem to enjoy exploring—with a little assistance from above.

The narrows. Along the way the canyon gradually narrows down and changes character. If you have never experienced the excitement of canyon walls closing in on you, this is a good place to do so. The wash runs into short cascades of polished bedrock, then passes under a giant boulder almost as wide as the canyon. The increasingly numerous exposures of harder bedrock in the walls and wash hint at the proximity of the Precambrian rock. About 0.3 mile past the bridge, the wash finally runs into what is essentially the boundary of the turtleback, and bumps into the first occlusion, a 15-foot vertical fall—for most people, the end of the road.

The upper canyon. This first fall has good holds but it is fairly high, and the climb down is tricky. Unless you are a good rock climber, I don't recommend going any further. Besides, the upper canyon above it is as wild and challenging as the lower canyon is tame, and progress rapidly becomes increasingly difficult. Just 250 yards further there is a second fall, about 20 feet high, topped with a huge chockstone. Not very difficult, maybe only a 5.7, but exposed again, and there are more falls just beyond. Bypassing them is difficult and dangerous, as the surrounding high terrain is steep, slippery with loose stones, and the few rocky outcrops one would normally use to hold onto are rotten. Only excellent rock climbers have a chance to make any kind of progress through here safely, and have fun doing it. You'll need to set up protections for safety, so bring a rope and a full rack. Don't come here alone, and be even more cautious than usual.

■

BAD CANYON

Bad Canyon is a deeply encased chasm that drops nearly 6,000 feet in less than 7 miles from Dante Peak to Badwater. At its core is a spectacular, mile-long, deep and narrow passage riddled with high falls, divided by a vertiginous 200-foot drop-off. Getting close to these narrows is a serious challenge. The lower canyon, easy to reach from Badwater, is an oppressive place trapped between stunning vertical walls. To reach the narrows from this end requires technical climbing. The hike from Dante's View down to the drop-off, over rough terrain and falls, is one of the most demanding hikes suggested in this book.

General Information

Road status: Roadless; hiking from paved road
Shortest hike: 1.2 mi, 950 ft one way / moderate
Longest hike: 5.3 mi, 4,150 ft one way / grueling, with rock climbing
Main attractions: Narrows, drop-offs, falls, spectacular views, technical
      rock climbing
USGS 15' topo maps: Bennetts Well, Funeral Peak
USGS 7.5' topo maps: Badwater, Dantes View
Maps: pp. 193*, 159

Location and Access

Bad Canyon drains the central Black Mountains, from just north of Dante's View down to just south of Badwater. About two thirds of the way down, a 200-foot precipice, essentially impossible to bypass, splits it in two. To see the lower canyon, the starting point is the parking area at Badwater, on the Badwater Road 16.6 miles south of Highway 190. The upper canyon is accessed from Dante's View.

Route Description: Lower Bad Canyon

A cathedral-like passage. From the Badwater parking area, walk south along the road for 100 yards to the foot of the steep fan and start climbing it. You will be following to your left a two-step vertical offset in the fan gravel, 10 to 15 feet in height. This is a segment of a long escarpment that can be traced off and on along the foot of the Black Mountains from near Furnace Creek to Mormon Point. It was created by the last large earthquake that rumbled through Death Valley, about 2,000 years ago. That quake meant business. All along the east side of the valley the ground sank vertically around 20 feet, about half of which was taken up

189

by this escarpment. The nearly vertical face of the Black Mountains behind it is the rising edge of a giant dome of Precambrian rocks known as the Badwater turtleback (see *Natural Bridge Canyon*).

At the top of the fan you will reach the mouth and very wide wash of Bad Canyon. Above its mouth, the canyon cuts a straight trench through compacted alluvial deposits that have slipped down the front of the turtleback. The grade is steep, littered with rocks of all kinds. The vertical walls, strangely blistered with huge boulders trapped in the ancient alluvia, progressively deepen to 100 feet. I do not know why this canyon was named Bad, whether for the proximity of Badwater, its roughness, or some other reason, but in the morning darkness of the looming walls its oppressive atmosphere more than justifies its name. It always makes me think of an austere cathedral dedicated to a forgotten cult. Beyond two sharp curves filled with large boulders, the wash dead-ends abruptly at the base of a 30-foot fall—the lower end of the narrows.

The lower part of the narrows. Above this first fall there is a deep and narrow passage, an intriguing place trapped between distorted walls, lost in perennial dimness—Bad Canyon at its best. Unless you are a rock climber, you probably don't want to try getting in there. The technical climb up the 30-foot fall is fairly easy, maybe 5.6, but if you fall from near the top you are history. The climb up the crumbly chimney just to the right of the fall is only marginally safer. Either way, you'll need to set up a rope and protections, which is not easy. Just above the first fall there are two others, easy, then a fourth one, about 60 feet high and unscalable. From here you can climb out to the south rim. From your point of exit, you can walk up along the rim for a few hundred yards. This area offers spectacular views of the deep narrows, of the 200-foot canyon walls below, and of the blinding expanses of salt flats.

To get to the rim without climbing the first fall, walk back from the fall about 75 yards to a steep ravine on the south side. After scrambling up it for about 100 yards, you will go through a U-shaped gateway, cross a narrow wash, and scramble up the wall on its far side (which can only be climbed at a couple of places). This first wall is made of large, loose boulders, so apply extreme caution. You will then cross two minor washes before getting to the rim of Bad Canyon. This is only about 0.3 mile, but it involves scrambling on steep slopes strewn with loose rocks, which can be treacherous, especially coming back down.

Passage through Bad Canyon from here on up is extremely dangerous and not recommended. Access down into the canyon would require difficult technical rappels, and there are more high falls ahead. Further progress along the rim is equally difficult and dangerous as the grade steepens markedly. If you want to see the upper canyon, try the route from Dante's View described below.

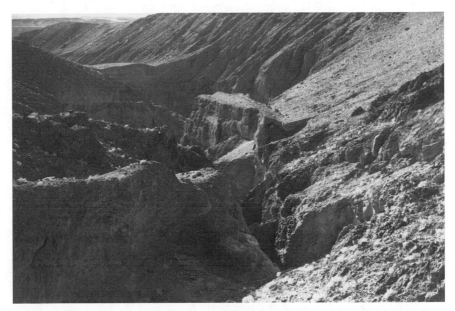

The lower portion of Bad Canyon's narrows

Route Description: Upper Bad Canyon

The ridge. From Dante's View, the easiest way to reach Bad Canyon is to follow the primitive trail that climbs the ridge north of the parking area. It leads in 0.5 mile to Dante Peak, then continues as a dimmer track along the crest of the Black Mountains. From the peak and the trail, the views of the gaping void of Death Valley provide a strangely primordial experience. You can look straight down at the salt flats (-282') just west of Badwater and at Mount Whitney (14,494') 90 air miles away, the lowest and highest points in the contiguous United States. The edge of Badwater is 2.6 miles away by line of sight and over one mile down—as steep as the Grand Canyon at the south rim, and a little deeper. Dante's View was named by officials of the Pacific Coast Borax Company (see *Twenty Mule Team Canyon*), who were said to have been inspired by Dante's vision of purgatory. They obviously had it all wrong: this is paradise, with the minor bonus that you're still alive.

From Dante Peak, continue on the crest trail at least to the prominent 5,190' saddle (~1 mile). From here the general idea is to climb westward down to the wash of Bad Canyon. Several routes are possible, none easy, all hopeless to describe. The shortest one starts at the 5,190' saddle. You can also continue northward on the ridge until you find a ravine or ridge you feel has a manageable slope (routes get a little easier, though longer, further north). The route shown on the map and distance chart is the longest but least painful. Most ravines have high falls and boulders. You may need to cross into the next ravine over until you find one you can handle. This is difficult hiking, especially the end, which involves sliding down loose talus slopes, but it is full of fun scrambling.

The upper canyon. Bad Canyon starts as a straight, V-shaped valley. It follows the Hades Fault, a minor southwest-trending fault that slices through the south end of the turtleback. It marks the boundary between two geological formations, granitic rocks on the west slope, and Miocene volcanic rocks on the east slope. The variety of local formations is reflected in the unusually eclectic assortment of minor mineral treasures found in the wash. The fault is clearly visible at the lower end of this straight valley, where the wash veers sharply right: erosion has carved a prominent notch right into the fault at the crest of the south wall. If you climb to the top of the notch, you will be rewarded with great views on the far side of rugged Hades Canyon as it drops along the southern continuation of this fault all the way to the valley floor.

The falls. The next stretch, between the fault and the narrows, is one of the most interesting. As it winds down steeply between vertical walls, the moderately narrow wash goes over several attractive falls. The most striking ones are smoothly polished in white marble finely veined with gray and pink. All but one fall can be climbed down or bypassed relatively easily. The exception is the third and highest fall, about 25-feet high, which can be circumvented on a 2-foot wide ledge high above it to

	Dist.(mi)	Elev.(ft)
Bad Canyon		
Lower canyon		
Badwater Road	0.0	-270
Mouth	0.4	-20
Narrows (30-ft fall)	1.2	680
60-ft fall	1.25	760
Upper canyon		
Dante's View	0	5,475
Dante Peak	0.4	5,704
Leave ridge	1.9	5,150
Wash	~3.1	3,960
Sharp bend	3.8	3,480
25-ft fall	3.9	3,370
60-ft drop-off	4.9	~2,360
200-ft drop-off	5.3	~1,800

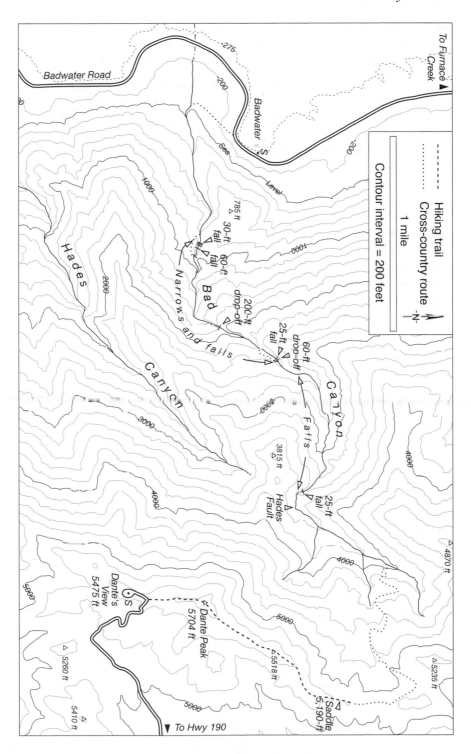

the left (there may be another, less hairy way around it). Further down, giant panels of Precambrian gneiss are exposed in the walls, streaked with wild black and white folds and oddly-shaped inclusions.

The upper part of the narrows. The wash is eventually interrupted by a 60-foot drop-off, which marks the head of Bad Canyon's narrows. Below it the canyon turns into a long and deep slot. The least difficult way to reach into it is to climb onto the steep southern wall and follow it at constant elevation for about 0.2 mile, to a giant stairway of narrow benches cascading down to the narrows floor. Although a moderately difficult descent, it is made treacherous by the brittle rocks and should be attempted with great care. The slot, only 10 to 25 feet wide and about 0.4 mile long, is punctuated with short falls and chockstones. Its upper end is closed off by a 25-foot fall and the impressive 60-foot drop-off just beyond it. The lower end comes to a screaming halt on the brink of a second drop-off, a blood-chilling precipice so deep a stone thrown over its edge takes four long seconds to hit bottom. That's a staggering 170-230 feet, the deepest continuous fall I have seen in Death Valley. For most people this awesome abyss is the end of the trail.

A few words of caution. Getting down to either drop-off is one of the two or three most difficult hikes suggested in this book. It involves more than 4,000 feet of elevation change in just over 5 miles, several falls and steep, unstable slopes, and it should only be attempted by experienced desert hikers in top shape. Remember that if you run out of energy at the drop-off, continuing on down to Badwater is *not an option*. All around and below the drop-off the terrain is so steep and unstable that it makes the first part of this hike seem like a walk in the park. An accidental fall here would almost certainly be deadly.

On one of my trips here, a friend and I were so absorbed by the narrows that we lost track of time. It was late when we realized we could not make Badwater and turned around. We were still scrambling out of the canyon at dusk, struggling on all fours up fluid talus with a flashlight clenched in our teeth at dark, and we reached Dante's View several hours after sunset. The hike to the drop-off and back takes one long day. No matter where you go in this canyon, be extremely careful. Bring a walking stick and a rope, just in case. Come prepared for plenty of action, preferably not alone.

■

SHEEP CANYON

> *Although not as narrow as some canyons, Sheep Canyon is deep and tortuous, and it provides access to a series of small springs with a little water and shade. Beyond the springs, more extensive routes lead to scenic Gold Valley and upper Willow Creek, or clear across the Black Mountains to Greenwater Valley.*

General Information

Road status: Roadless; access from paved or primitive road (HC)
Shortest hike: 4.0 mi, 2,370 ft one way / moderate-difficult
Longest hike: 9.0 mi, 5,920 ft one way (or more) / difficult
Main attractions: Springs, a deep and windy canyon, bighorn sheep
USGS 15' topo map: Funeral Peak
USGS 7.5' topo maps: Gold Valley*, Funeral Peak
Maps: pp. 197*, 159

Location and Access

The easiest hiking access to Sheep Canyon is from the Badwater Road 13.4 miles south of Badwater (or 16 miles north of the Harry Wade Road). This is 0.4 mile south of where the road straightens out to cross a deep cove. The mouth of Sheep Canyon is due east, at the top of the fan.

A more tedious access is from Gold Valley, on the east side of the Black Mountains. To get there, drive the Greenwater Valley Road 17.5 miles south from the Dante's View Road (or 10.6 miles north of Highway 178) to the Gold Valley Road. Drive this road 9.4 miles (2.4 miles beyond the pass) to a mining trail on the right just past a prominent hill, and hike from there. Refer to *Willow Creek* for road conditions.

Route Description

The lower canyon. Although fairly short, the Sheep Canyon fan is rough and the walk up to the canyon is somewhat tedious. In the canyon the wash is steep, uneven, and littered with large rocks, and the walking is not any easier. The saving grace is that from about a mile above its mouth to Sheep Spring, the canyon is a deep gorge winding beneath peaks hundreds of feet high. The walls often shoot vertically, even overhang in some outer bends. The canyon constricts a few times, although it is never very tight, about 25 feet at best. It is impressive, however, especially when hiking downhill. There is a small boulder jam and two rock slides along the way, none of which constitutes an obstacle.

Most of what is exposed is diorite, probably Mesozoic in age, an igneous rock made of hornblende (the black component) and plagioclase (white). Its composition varies from fine to coarse-grained and even large exposures of its individual constituents, such as white walls of massive plagioclase. The wash contains a much wider variety of rocks, including volcanic rocks washed down from higher formations.

Sheep Spring. This spring has five small seeps, in close succession along a 0.6-mile stretch of canyon starting 2.9 miles above the mouth. Each of them supports a cluster of low mesquite trees at the base of the steep hillside along the wash. They differ mostly in size and tree maturity. The third seep, the largest in area, has a small stand of common cane and is shaded by a few tall mesquite trees. Some old maps label this canyon as Sheep Creek, but the seeps rise from a shallow fault and have minimal surface water. Only on one of my visits, in the winter, did I find surface water, in the form of a small puddle at the first seep. The surface flow is greater at times, as indicated by calcareous deposits in the wash, but it is not a perennial creek.

Nonetheless, these tiny seeps demonstrate the power of water in the desert. They manage to keep alive small carpets of grass so green that they seem out of place. Signs of bighorn sheep are plentiful around the spring and all along the canyon—hoof prints where they pawed through the mud to get to the water, droppings, prints and trails in the gravel, sometimes bone fragments and partial skeletons. Biologists sometimes come here to study the local bands. Other wildlife is attracted by the springs. I saw birds, lizards, and one fat chuckwalla. Most people will find Sheep Spring the highlight of this canyon. The best time is after late spring, when the green foliage of the trees offer welcome pools of shade to cool off a little.

Sheep Canyon		
	Dist.(mi)	Elev.(ft)
Badwater Road	0.0	-220
Mouth	1.1	220
Side canyon #1	2.5	1,150
Sheep Spring (lower seep)	4.0	2,150
Main side canyon	4.7	2,560
Gold Valley Road	(5.5)	3,700
Side canyon #4	5.0	2,660
Side canyon #5	6.1	3,420
Head	9.0	5,700

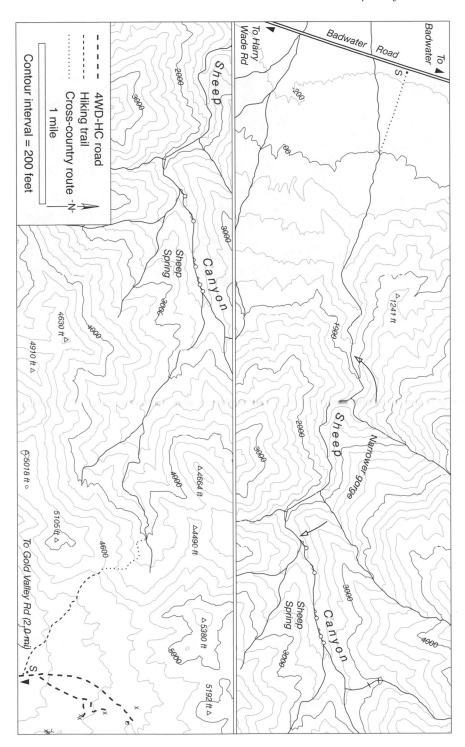

Legend:
- ▬ ▬ ▬ 4WD-HC road
- ─ ─ ─ Hiking trail
- ·········· Cross-country route
- |‑‑‑‑| 1 mile

Contour interval = 200 feet

Sheep Canyon

To Badwater

Badwater Road

To Harry Wade Rd

1241 ft △

Narrower gorge

Sheep Canyon

Sheep Spring

4630 ft △

4910 ft △

5018 ft ○

5105 ft △

4664 ft △

4490 ft △

5380 ft △

5192 ft △

To Gold Valley Rd (2.0 mi)

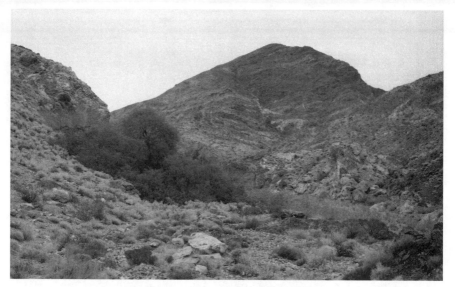

The largest of the seeps at Sheep Spring

The south fork to Gold Valley. Sheep Canyon is shallower past the first seep, and opens up to a V-shaped valley past the main fork. A good three-day hike from here is up the south fork along the old Sheep Canyon route to Gold Valley, then down into the exciting stream-fed narrows of Willow Creek. If you want to see upper Willow Creek but cannot drive the rough Gold Valley Road, this route is actually a little shorter and more scenic. The trail shown on the USGS maps along Sheep Canyon is no longer visible anywhere between the road and the fork, and it was probably never more than a cross-country route. It may still be in place in the upper part of the south fork.

The upper canyon. Above the main fork, Sheep Canyon (the north fork) remains wide for a little over 2 miles, with the exception of a couple of tighter stretches. Above 4,200 feet, the uppermost canyon is significantly narrower most of the way to its head. This area is drained by quite a few side canyons. Some of them, like the one just above the fork, are narrow at places and have good falls for climbing. These places are largely unknown and far more challenging than the main canyon.

The head of Sheep Canyon is a deep notch just below Funeral Peak, overlooking wide and barren Greenwater Valley. For a moderate, two-day backpacking trip, you can return down the unnamed wash on the east side of the pass into the Greenwater Valley. A little further on you will pick up an old road, not shown on the USGS maps, which eventually connects with the Greenwater Valley Road.

∎

WILLOW CREEK

Willow Creek is one of the finest canyons in the park. The upper canyon, reached by a long, rutted road, is a lush and narrow chasm irrigated by a half-mile long creek with several waterfalls, a distinction shared by few in arid Death Valley. The lower narrows have numerous falls that add challenge to their charm, until progress is interrupted by a 70-foot drop-off. The impressive lower end of these narrows is best reached by a pleasant walk from the Badwater Road.

General Information

Road status: Roadless; access from paved road or primitive road (4WD)
Shortest hike: Short stroll/very easy
Longest hike: 1.8 mi, 1,240 ft (or more)/difficult, with rock climbing
Main attractions: Desert stream, waterfalls, springs, narrows, history
USGS topo maps: Funeral Peak (15'), Gold Valley (7.5')
Maps: pp. 203*, *159*

Location and Access

Willow Creek is located in the southern Black Mountains. To get to the upper canyon, drive the Greenwater Valley Road south from the Dante's View Road for 17.5 miles (or 10.6 miles north from Highway 178), to the Gold Valley Road. This road crosses Greenwater Valley westward, climbs to a pass, then drops into Gold Valley, the upper drainage of Willow Creek. It ends in about 12.5 miles at Willow Spring. The Greenwater Valley Road is graded and suitable for passenger cars, but the Gold Valley Road has a high crown, rocks, and rough stretches. Without good clearance, and 4-wheel drive for lighter vehicles, you'll probably have to quit about 0.4 mile before the pass, where the roadway is steep and strongly canted, and walk the remaining 5.4 miles. The next best option is to come in via Sheep Canyon, a four-day backpacking trip.

The lower canyon is easy to reach from the Badwater Road. Hike in from about 14.3 miles south of Badwater (15.1 miles north of the Harry Wade Road). This is near the south end of the deep cove north of Mormon Point. Willow Creek is up the short fan to the southeast.

History: Three Strikes and Out

In August 1906, as the copper rush in Greenwater Valley was reaching its full swing, latecomers exploring unclaimed ground in outlying areas stumbled upon secluded Gold Valley. What they first discovered was not ore but Willow Creek, one of the most plentiful and reliable streams in the region. In a short time, however, signs of copper were found around the spring, and it sparked a disproportionate frenzy. Almost overnight, Willow Creek became the new mining utopia. Despite the lack of signs of sizeable deposits, promoters and prospectors poured into the area. In November the camp that had been established near the spring was organized into the town of Willow Creek, with lots advertised for as much as $250. By the end of the year five companies had been formed, involving millions of dollars of capitalization.

It was only in the winter, after the dust of the initial rush had settled, that the companies started seriously looking around for copper. The wealth of the deposits had been grossly exaggerated, and little valuable ore was found. The momentum of the rush, however, was not impeded by such minor details, at least not right away. Several more companies were created before things slowed down a little.

In May 1907, as the interest in copper was slackening, one of the companies discovered high-grade silver-lead ore on its holdings, and the rush started all over. Copper companies came back to assess their properties for silver. In the following weeks new locations and discoveries were made. They were fairly small, but local newspapers magnified them to such proportions that more miners joined the crowd. In anticipation of an unprecedented rush, the ground was surveyed to make Willow Creek a sprawling 31-block city.

Everything changed again in June when gold was discovered at the southeast end of the valley. The ore assayed at $200 per ton, and it drew even more excitement. In just a few weeks the area was advertised as another Goldfield. The *Inyo Register* asserted that "the surface showing is the richest ever discovered in this desert region, if not in the world." Again miners streamed in and new companies were created, reaching a total of 13 by fall. Willow Creek quickly died as the town of Gold Valley sprang up near the site of the strike. Many one and two-man operations were working the hills, and by the end of the year dozens of small gold and silver strikes had been made. Gold Valley, approved by the county to cover some 96 blocks, included a lodge, a barbershop and the obligatory saloon. In February 1908 the collapse of Greenwater brought in a new wave of miners and merchants. A few buildings were moved from Greenwater to the new town, which boasted a population of 70 by March. A few frame buildings were under construction, and application for a post office was underway.

But even in Death Valley illusions don't last forever. In the aftermath of the Panic of 1907, financial backing was scarce and development slow. In the beginning of 1908 only a few companies were active. In May the first ore shipment was finally made, about 250 tons estimated at

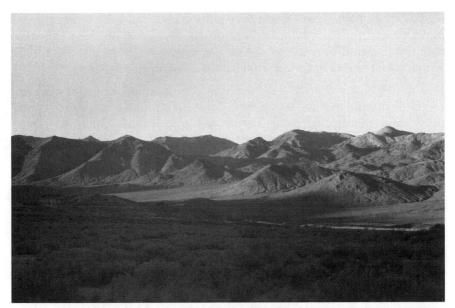

Gold Valley at sunset

$75,000. Ironically, it coincided with the end of the boom. There was just not enough ore to justify the hard labor and high costs of transportation and living in this remote location. Over the next few months the companies folded one by one. By early 1909 most miners had left. The boom had survived two and a half years and involved hundreds of people, but probably less than $100,000 worth of ore had come out of the ground.

Route Description: The Upper Canyon

Gold Valley. This is a beautiful high-desert valley enclosed by low hills. It preserves the gentle topography that prevailed prior to the uplifting of the Black Mountains. Little remains of the short-lived attempts at mining this far corner of the desert. The town site of Gold Valley, at the end of the left fork in the road about 0.6 mile east of the pass, shows only a few tent sites. The tunnels and tailings from the 1907-1908 gold rush are scattered in the hills to the south. Willow Creek, just before the end of the road on the right side, is marked by a large stone platform, the site of the only real building the district ever had.

Willow Spring. Oases are rare in Death Valley, but somehow this canyon inherited five of them, and several smaller ones. The first one, Willow Spring, starts at the end of the road. It is a narrow, 1000-foot long grove of willows surrounded by cane and arrowweed, too thick to enter. Further down there are two other springs, back-to-back and similar. They have running water, usually more than Willow Spring. To make your life easier, bypass them on the right, up on the rocks and along trail segments made by sheep. The canyon is then clear for a little while, until the fourth spring—the headwaters of Willow Creek.

Willow Creek and the wet narrows. The next stretch—the wet narrows—is unique to this canyon. For about half a mile a vigorous stream flows through a heavy cover of brush, willow, and mesquite trees, over polished bedrock, creating waterfalls and shallow pools in the deep shadows of the high canyon walls. Over time, the heavily mineralized water has deposited small travertine channels in the creek bed, thin ivory drapes over the falls, and lacy terraces around the pools. Like all oases this is a magical place, full of hidden secrets. This one, far from the world of humans, conquered only with a generous expenditure of time, is even more special. Look for colorful algae and tiny watercress thriving in the stream, for fern and mosses on the walls, and for prince's plume and stream orchis on the banks. Listen to crickets in the evening. On one of my visits I saw a band of six bighorn sheep. This is one of their best strongholds in the park, and evidence of their presence is everywhere.

There are several falls in this area. Like the rest of the gorge, they are cut mostly into diorite, a hard, granite-like rock, and they are generally sturdy enough for safe climbing. However, a few of them are high enough to warrant caution. The most difficult one is a triple waterfall, 35 feet high. It can also be circumvented by a tedious but safe,

	Dist.(mi)	Elev.(ft)
Willow Creek		
Upper canyon		
Willow Spring	0.0	2,635
Second spring	0.35	2,455
Third spring	0.4	2,420
Fourth spring (Wet narrows)	0.8	2,200
35-ft waterfall	0.95	~2,030
Wet narrows (end)	1.2	~1,880
Fifth spring (Lower narrows)	1.55	~1,680
70-ft drop-off	1.8	~1,400
Lower canyon		
Badwater Road	0.0	-220
Mouth	2.0	410
Lower narrows (end)	2.1	475
40-ft fall	2.3	800

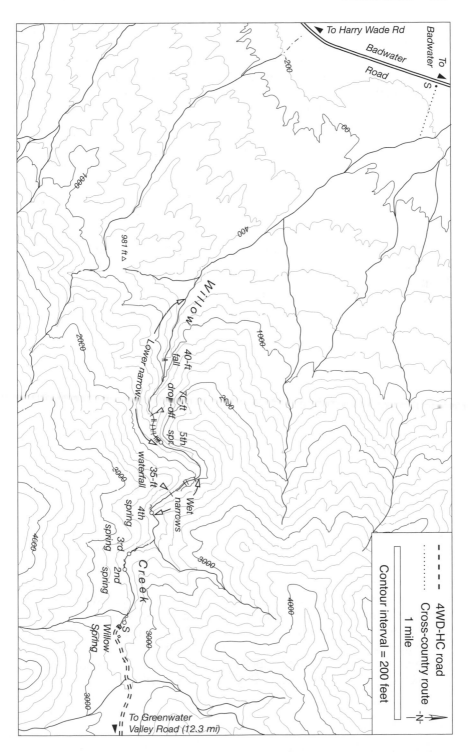

0.2-mile scramble on the north side. Further down there is a tricky 13-foot fall topped with a chockstone to bypass on steep slickrock.

This is one of the most unusual oases in Death Valley, but there is a price for it. It is a rough place. The amount of water and vegetation varies greatly over the years, but much of the canyon is usually overgrown with brush and trees, making progress slow and strenuous.

The lower narrows. The creek eventually vanishes underground and the canyon opens up a little. A third of a mile further there is a fifth spring, a dense stand of spindly tamarisk. It marks the beginning of the lower narrows, a dramatic gorge that plunges straight down through the Black Mountains nearly all the way to the valley floor. This is a spectacular place, deep, constricted and dark, as silent as a tomb. Its sinuous course is dotted with pockets of water, tight polished bends, and isolated tamarisks in tiny gravel-filled basins. There are also many falls, all fairly easy (never worse than 5.6) and relatively safe to negotiate. Progress is eventually stopped on the brink of a vertiginous 70-foot drop-off bounded by sheer walls. The bighorn sheep seem to be doing all right with it, squeezing by along a hairy foot-wide ledge on the right side of the fall. But most humans would need a rope for this one. Between here and the 40-foot fall in the lower canyon lies a nearly half-mile long chasm so difficult to access that it may still be unexplored.

Route Description: The Lower Canyon

From the Badwater Road it is a moderate walk up the gentle incline of the fan towards the canyon. Along the first mile, look for a series of conspicuous beach cliffs etched by ancient Lake Manly on the hillside to the south, a few hundred feet up (see *The Badwater Basin*). The second half is along a coarse wash between increasingly high fanglomerate walls to the mouth of Willow Creek.

The narrows start just into the mouth of Willow Creek. The gray, high-rising diorite walls form a deep V so closed that this place lies in deep shade most of the time. In about 0.2 mile the wash runs into a split-level fall with a total height of at least 40 feet. The lower, 12-foot fall has good holds but the last move is too tricky for most people. The upper fall is slicker, twice as high, and only for experienced climbers. If you can't climb it, you may want to look for a bypass. If you like boulder scrambling, try the very steep chimney on the north side just below the lower fall. Some hikers will find it a strong incentive to know that the narrows above may never have been visited. Even if you do not succeed, the deep narrows make this half-day hike well worth it.

■

SCOTTY'S CANYON

> *Once the hideout of Death Valley Scotty, this canyon is, much like the famous con man, two-faced. The lower canyon is gentle and easy to walk. Ornate with sculptured conglomerate beds and beautiful mosaics, it leads to Scotty's Spring, where a tiny creek wanders among carved grottoes and mesquites. The third grotto is the threshold to a very different upper canyon. Its wild narrows, windy and rugged, blocked by numerous falls, are a thrilling destination for the adventuresome hiker and experienced climber, with tantalizing goals like Timpapah Spring and the Desert Hound Mine—perhaps Scotty's "fabulous" mine.*

General Information

Road status: Roadless; hiking from primitive road (HC)
Shortest hike: 3.0 mi, 1,430 ft one way / moderate
Longest hike: 6.6 mi, ~4,500 ft one way (or more) / very strenuous
Main attractions: Springs, grottoes, mosaics, narrows and falls, rock
    climbing, gold mine
USGS 15' topo map: Confidence Hills
USGS 7.5' topo maps: Shoreline Butte*, Epaulet Peak, Gold Valley
Maps: pp. 215*, 159

Location and Access

Scotty's Canyon is in the southern Black Mountains, on the south side of Smith Mountain. To get there, drive the Badwater Road to the Ashford Canyon Road, which is about 27.4 miles south of Badwater (or 2.1 miles north of the Harry Wade Road). It is just across from the marked turn-off to Ashford Mill, on the east side of the road. Drive the Ashford Canyon Road 2.8 miles (bear left at the fork 0.7 mile in) to the top of the rise at the mouth of Ashford Canyon, where the road ends (see *Ashford Canyon* for road conditions). The hike starts here. To get to Scotty's Canyon, walk the cut-off trail that starts as a beat-up jeep road dropping on the left, just before the top of the rise.

If you cannot drive the Ashford Canyon Road very far, your other option is to park at the Badwater Road and walk the old Scotty's Canyon Road (now closed to motor vehicles), which starts just to the left of the Ashford Canyon Road. It is about 2 miles on this road to the wash of Scotty's Canyon, then 1.3 miles up the wash to the canyon mouth.

History

The namesake of this canyon is Walter Edward Scott, of Scotty's Castle fame, a would-be prospector who played a major role in the history of Death Valley. A hike here can be greatly enhanced by a little knowledge of this man's amazing life history. Scotty's involvement in the area started in 1902, when he began to claim he had discovered a fabulously rich gold deposit somewhere in the inferno of Death Valley, and to use this imaginary mine to live off investors. Scotty was a skilled liar and manipulator, and he came up with clever tricks to keep investor after investor interested in bankrolling him, supposedly to work his lode, while endlessly discouraging them from taking a look at his mine. He invoked the unbearable temperature and extremely rough terrain of Death Valley, made up stories of attacks by dangerous armed gangs out to steal his mine, and even staged ambushes. Yet he periodically produced samples of high-grade ore obtained from other mines to keep them interested. This was an incredibly dubious plan, but it worked well and for a surprisingly long time. He impressed people so much, and on such a scale, that he became a national figure and remained in the limelight for the best part of a decade. He was perceived by the media as an eccentric man—flashing his temporary wealth, lighting cigars with $100 bills, and establishing railroad speed records across the country—a man as mysterious as his secret mine.

There is much more to the fascinating life story of Walter Scott—the subject of several entertaining books—but this is the part that relates to Scotty's Canyon. When Scotty visited Death Valley, he made this canyon his headquarters, camping in the shelter of an overhang near the spring. "My main camp was in a high mountain," Scotty said. "Sort of a hole in the rock. Other overhanging rocks almost came together at the top leaving just a small opening. I had it fixed nice—even a bath tub and a steamer chair. Whenever I wanted to disappear, I headed for 'Camp Hold Out,' as I called it." A visitor later wrote that the walls were literally covered with pictures of famous actors, actresses, and prominent men, and that it took "fully one hour to look them over."

Scotty and a partner actually had a mine in this area—some claims on a ridge several rough miles above Camp Hold Out. Years later, it became the Desert Hound Mine, but it never produced much (see *Virgin Spring Canyon*). Scotty's Canyon was in fact originally named Greyhound Canyon, an interesting connection with this mine. But whether this was Scotty's "fabulous" mine has never been established. Scotty managed to keep everyone guessing for many years. It was not until 1912, pressed by investors and the law, that Scotty finally confessed his mine was a hoax. He fell into disgrace and came out penniless, but during this period he had unknowingly secured a comfortable future for himself. Ironically, one of the investors he had conned was Albert Johnson—the man who, a few years later, would build the mansion in Grapevine Canyon that somehow became Scotty's Castle.

It has been said that through his tall tales Scotty may have made a more significant contribution to Death Valley's mining industry than any other individual. After he died in January 1954, an editorial writer for the *San Francisco Chronicle* wrote these befitting words about Scotty: "Some say he was a fraud; we disagree. He was a purveyor of wonderful nonsense, whose medium was not a pen or a brush, but life itself."

Route Description

The approach. Starting about half a mile from the paved road, both canyon roads circle two large hills of brown to red rocks partly buried in sand. Try to take a little time to explore this unusual formation, known as the Amargosa Chaos. It occurs almost exclusively in the southern Black Mountains, and the particular sequence exposed here, called the Jubilee phase, is the least common (see *Virgin Spring Canyon*). Along the eastern side of the northernmost hill, three types of rocks are exposed, all Tertiary in age: giant breccia of quartz monzonite and granite, the deep-red, fine-grained conglomerate specific of this phase, and andesite. They often occur in well-defined blocks with sharp boundaries, pockmarked with countless cavities of all sizes. In the spring, the fan south of the road is often graced with colorful mats of sand verbena.

If you start from the mouth of Ashford Canyon, take the cutoff trail to Scotty's Canyon mentioned earlier (about 0.6 mile). It drops steeply to the wash of Ashford Canyon, and resumes on the other side as a hiking trail. From there it winds northwest into the hills to eventually come out through a narrower, colorful passage at the wash of Scotty's Canyon, within sight of the canyon mouth.

The lower canyon. Scotty's Canyon begins as a relatively wide wash beneath red-brown hills. Plant life in the wash is dominated by *Eriogonum*, the most common genus in the park. The small bushes that resemble miniature flat-topped trees are Rixford eriogonum. Their tight network of thin purple branches, most striking when the plant is bare, produces small white flowers in the spring. The desert trumpet is also unmistakable for its barren stems swelling to conspicuous "trumpets." In the spring, the thin end branches bear clusters of tiny yellow flowers.

Past the narrow constriction about 0.5 mile in, the gravel is replaced by fine silty sand and the wash turns into a surprisingly smooth compacted floor. Many types of rocks are exposed up canyon, often just a few yards from each other, from sedimentary (limestone, dolomite and conglomerate) to igneous (granite) and metamorphic (schists and gneiss). At one place the drainage is obstructed by a large polished boulder of greenish gneiss. The majority of the exposures are Proterozoic in age, some of the oldest rocks in the park.

An interesting feature here is the beds of conglomerate. These massive exposures, oddly rounded like frozen flows of concrete, have been gouged by erosion into oblong basins and smooth chutes, narrow passages, intriguing overhangs and caves that invite exploration. Their polished surfaces form extensive panels of mosaics, eclectic kaleidoscopes of rocks of different sizes, forms, and colors bound in a grayish matrix. The variety, abundance, brightness and aesthetic appeal of these mosaics are unique. Whoever named Mosaic Canyon was obviously unaware of this place!

Camp Hold Out and Scotty's Spring. As the elevation rises the canyon gradually tapers down between rough walls. The first signs of the spring are a cluster of dwarf mesquite trees in the wash and a small channel in the sand where a trickle of water flows. The long overhang in the south canyon wall, across from the mesquites, is Camp Hold Out, Scotty's first hideout in Death Valley. A clever location: easy access, shaded most of the time, and a stone's throw from running water. Just beyond Camp Hold Out is the first grotto, a horseshoe-shaped and overhanging white wall, grotesquely blistered, sometimes haunted by the hypnotic sound of dripping water.

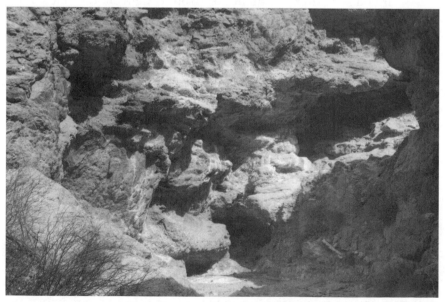

Grotto at Scotty's Spring

This grotto can be easily circumvented on the south side, starting a little below the lower end of the creek. Beyond, the canyon is narrower still. A little further on there is another seep in a second grotto, beginning with a deep, 50-foot long overhang guarded by a thorny mesquite tree. This grotto dead-ends at a high travertine-stained chockstone with a tiny waterfall. The third grotto, a short distance away, is trapped between high walls and a 20-foot fall. Its walls are coated with white and spiny carbonate crystals. If you come here on a hot day, look forward to the deep and refreshing shade of the grottoes.

The upper canyon. For most people the third grotto is a fine goal for a day hike. For more adventurous hikers it may be just the beginning. The upper part of Scotty's Canyon is one deep, constricted, and enticing narrows, often blocked by falls, as tough going as the lower canyon is easy. For a taste of what to expect, here is what happens at first. The fall at the third grotto can be bypassed on a narrow ledge high up on the right side of the fall, but there is little point, as there is a difficult 20-foot vertical fall just above it, and about half a dozen more falls beyond. The only practical route is to bypass this first section of narrows, which can be done by climbing into the first steep gully on the north side just before the third grotto (look for cairns or pick your own route). Several faint sheep trails lead up canyon along the steep, rock-strewn rim, with plunging views of the narrow windy canyon below. In about 0.25 mile a steep talus leads back down to the wash. The next 1,000-foot stretch is another chaotic narrows. Past five manageable falls,

Scotty's Canyon		
	Dist.(mi)	Elev.(ft)
Trailhead at Ashford Canyon	0.0	1,090
Wash of Scotty's Canyon	~0.6	930
Mouth	0.9	950
End of old road	1.4	1,140
First side canyon	2.6	1,730
Scotty's Spring (first grotto)	3.0	1,980
Second grotto	~3.1	2,020
Third grotto	~3.3	2,180
South fork	3.7	2,720
Desert Hound Mine	(1.4)	~3,990
Timpapah Spring	3.75	2,770
Head	6.6	4,820

it dead-ends at an unscalable fall at least 30 feet high, a deep cleft in a sheer wall with a little water trickling at its base.

This is just a sample. Things go on like this up to the fork, then either left to Timpapah Spring and beyond, or right to the Desert Hound Mine. To explore this chaotic area requires a combination of climbing, short scrambles, and wider bypasses around intractable falls. It is strenuous. Yet I cannot stress enough that this area of tight canyons, with its many forks, seeps, chockstones, mesquite clumps and chimeric, hollowed-out and blistered walls, is truly wild and thrilling. The crowning glory of this hike is the Desert Hound Mine, lost on a high, wind-swept ridge—Scotty's brainchild, perhaps the mysterious lode that inflamed so many imaginations (see *Virgin Spring Canyon*).

Progress in the upper canyon is very slow. If you come here for just a day, after the long drive and the hike up the lower canyon, there may not be much time left to do justice to the narrows, let alone to reach the Desert Hound. To make the most of it, camp at the trailhead or at the canyon mouth and get an early morning start, or backpack in.

■

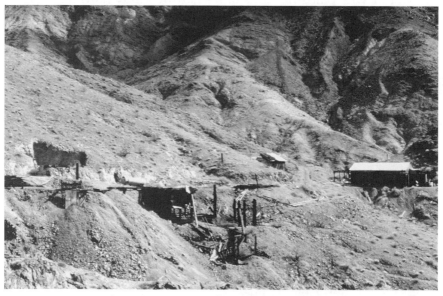

Old buildings at Ashford Mine's camp

ASHFORD CANYON

> *For most people, the highlight of this hike is the Ashford Mine, located in a scenic canyon graced with extensive exposures of colorful mosaics and sparkling schists. With its old cabins, troglodytic rooms and mining structures, the well-preserved camp and surrounding mines provide an interesting glimpse of life in a remote gold mine. Strong hikers can try to go on either to Ashford Peak or all the way up to the Desert Hound Mine. Solitude and awesome views are guaranteed.*

General Information

Road status: Essentially roadless; access by primitive road (HC)
Shortest hike: 2.1 mi, 1,150 ft one way / moderate
Longest hike: 4.4 mi, 2,950 ft one way (or more) / strenuous
Main attractions: Mine and camp, mosaics, falls, geology, peak climbs
USGS topo maps: Confidence Hills (15'), Shore Line Butte (7.5')
Maps: pp. 215*, 159

Location and Access

Ashford Canyon is in the southern Black Mountains, just south of Scotty's Canyon. The starting point of this hike is the same as for Scotty's Canyon. Drive the Badwater Road about 27.4 miles south of Badwater (or 2.1 miles north of the Harry Wade Road) to the marked turnoff to Ashford Mill ruins. Take the dirt road on the east side of the road, across from the turnoff. Drive it 2.8 miles (make a left at the fork 0.7 mile in) to its end at the top of a rise at the mouth of Ashford Canyon. The hike starts down into the canyon wash to the east.

This access road is decent for about half a mile, worse along the next mile (sometimes there is a little sand past the fork), and the rest of it gets gradually steeper and rougher, with lots of rocks and wash crossings. It's no problem with a high-clearance vehicle, but if you are driving a normal passenger car, how far you go will depend on your skill and determination. I usually give up after 2 miles and start walking.

History: The Golden Treasure of the Ashford Brothers

The main fame of this area is the Ashford Mine, a sprawling mining complex with a sad story that reflects the frustrated hopes of countless miners in the Death Valley days. It started in January 1907, when Harold Ashford prospected around the Desert Hound Mine, a little north of the canyon that now bears his name. The Key Gold Mining

Company had already claimed most of the land surrounding the Desert Hound (see *Virgin Spring Canyon*), but it had failed to carry out the annual assessment work required to validate its claims. Ashford became aware of this and relocated some of them. He worked the claims for nearly two years before the company realized it and took him to court. It took a while, but Ashford eventually won title to the property, in January 1910—for better and for worse.

Until 1914 he and his two brothers worked their grounds sporadically. They failed to produce the bonanza they had hoped for, but the ore they had exposed was probably promising enough that they were able to option their property. In November 1914, the mine was leased to Benjamin McCausland, an oil industrialist from Los Angeles, and his son Ross, who proceeded to develop it in earnest. By February 1915 a road had been built up the canyon to the mine. A 40-ton mill— today's Ashford Mill—was erected on the valley floor below the canyon to treat the ore prior to shipment. For a short time, mining and milling employed as many as 28 men. But after more than $125,000 in investment, several months of hard work, and 2,000 feet of tunnels, only about $100,000 worth of ore had been taken out of the ground. This production was up a few notches from typical Death Valley mines, but still not good enough to break even. The ore was just not as rich as the McCauslands had thought, and they quit in September. After they failed to pay their year's lease, the Ashfords filed suit. The property and equipment were returned to them, but they never got their money back.

Such as they were, those were the heyday of the Ashford Mine. The property remained idle until 1926, was worked episodically and probably minimally for a short time, then was idle again for many years. In 1935 it was reopened under a lease agreement with the Golden Treasure Company. It worked the mine for a few years, eventually cleaning out mostly high-grade pockets to minimize transportation costs. Instead of being processed at the mill, the raw ore was trucked to the Tonopah and Tidewater Railroad at Shoshone. But even this ultimate effort was not enough to make it. They gave up in 1938, after reportedly shipping only $18,000 worth of ore.

The property and equipment were again returned to the Ashford brothers. They inherited a gutted mine, but they were persistent. They worked it for a little while, until they somehow managed to lease it again. This time the new company constructed a short aerial tramway above the mining camp to collect the ore mined at the many tunnels scattered up the steep mountain slope. It probably took a lot of work—at one point in time ten men were employed—but they also eventually found the deposit too poor to be worth mining. They discontinued their operations in 1941.

Although the Ashfords held on to their claims for quite a while longer, they apparently never worked them again themselves. In the 1950s when the property was finally idle for good, Harold Ashford estimated the total footage of workings around 4,000 feet. But the total production had sold for $135,000, about half as much as was invested.

Geology

The dominant rocks along Ashford Canyon are mica-schist and gneiss from the Archaean metamorphic core of the Black Mountains—among the oldest rocks exposed in Death Valley. The schists come in an amazing variety of colors and textures, from gray to green, sparkling with inclusions of mica, strongly layered and interbedded with gneiss or folded veins of milky quartz and feldspar. The gold mined in the past occurred in veins of granitic gneiss, in association with copper ore. Fine samples of the most common copper minerals (malachite, azurite, chalcopyrite, chalcosine, bornite, etc.) have been found in this mine, and are on display at the Borax Museum.

As in Scotty's Canyon, massive beds of conglomerates are extensively exposed all along the lower canyon. Large areas of billowing conglomerate bedrock have been carved by erosion into natural basins and polished into beautiful mosaics. One of the pleasures of hiking this canyon is to search for prize exposures of both mosaics and ancient metamorphic rocks.

Route Description

Along the access road. While driving or walking the old mill-to-mine road, you will pass by the low hills separating the drainage of Ashford and Scotty's canyons. They are part of the Amargosa Chaos (see *Virgin Spring Canyon*). Refer to *Scotty's Canyon* for further detail on these colorful hills, which are well worth checking out.

The lower canyon. When you reach the wash, you'll have two options: the old canyon road or the wash. The road climbs out of the wash on the left side (it is washed out a short distance up) to bypass a 0.3-mile stretch of canyon. It is easier going than the canyon route, but you'll miss much of the fun. The portion of canyon that the road bypasses has good narrows encased between steep walls, short but action packed if you like rock climbing. There are four falls near the end of the narrows, offering very different climbs, low 5s to 5.8, with one overhang move. The first two falls can be bypassed, so even with no climbing you can inspect the narrows up to the last two side-by-side falls.

Along the next mile above the narrows, discontinuous segments of the old road remain. These segments were constructed higher than the wash to circumvent a few falls, and they were spared by floods. If you prefer, you can use them to bypass the falls, which are one of the highlights in this canyon, especially the next one above the narrows, with its polished lip of vivid mosaics. The two side canyons on the north side are also worth a side trip. In fact the first side canyon offers a good shortcut to the camp. It is more scenic, narrower, and has more interesting carved formations than the main canyon.

The Ashford Mine and camp. The road resumes on the right side shortly after the second side canyon. It crosses the wash, swings around, and climbs up to the mines and camp. Only a little over 2 miles of walking so far. A pretty good deal: scattered all around here there are more prospects, mine shafts, tailings, cabins, and pieces of mining equipment than you can explore before the next rain.

The highlight is the small camp of the Ashford Mine, overlooking the deep gash of the canyon. Stolid under the searing sun, oblivious to time and humans, it is one of the most eloquent tributes to Death Valley's fortune seekers. At the time of this writing, the camp still had three wood cabins with partial furnishings—a closet, a gutted refrigerator, shelves, spring boxes, an old 1950s stove. Outside the largest house (the cook house and office) a table and two chairs seemed to still be expecting visitors. Low wooden doors give access to a couple of troglodytic rooms carved in the rock walls. Try them on a hot day; they provide effective natural air conditioning.

The mining structures a short distance down the road from the camp include remnants of a headframe and a few tunnels. This is the site

Ashford Canyon		
	Dist.(mi)	Elev.(ft)
Mouth (knoll on road)	0.0	1,100
Road bypass	0.3	1,220
End of road	0.5	~1,430
First side canyon	1.2	1,780
Second side canyon	1.6	2,060
Road	1.8	2,240
Ashford Peak	(1.1)	3,547
Ashford Mine's camp	2.1	2,230
Mining area/end of road	2.2	~2,200
Upper tramway mines	(0.8)	2,670
Desert Hound Mine	4.4	~3,990

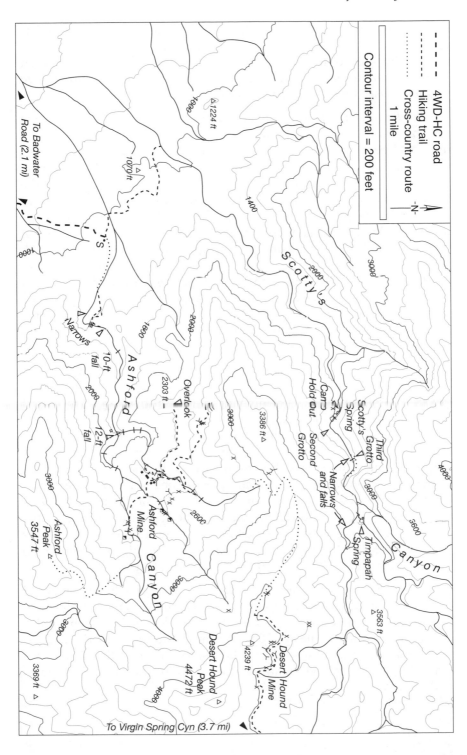

of the lower terminal of the aerial tramway built around 1938, which has unfortunately long since collapsed. The road ends just a little further on, at the deep wash of the first side canyon. Most of the tunnels exploited in the past are a short distance up and down this wash, and up the two washes crossed by the road before the camp.

The tramway mines.   The area around the end of the road is the starting point of several old mining trails, which can be fun to follow to their final destination. The longest one is the trail to the tramway mines. To find it, walk up canyon along this side of the wash; you'll pick up the trail shortly as it follows the wash. After about 250 yards, it drops to the wash, resumes a little further up the wash on the opposite side, and ascends the steep hill 0.7 mile to the mines and ruins of the tramway upper terminal. Spurs along this trail descend to the slender towers of the tramway. The ore at the dumps is pretty—lots of quartz stained with green copper ore.

Another trail starts on the far side of the wash from the end of the road. Work your way across the wash a little further up canyon, then follow this easy, nearly level trail about 0.5 mile to a good overlook on a saddle ridge (elev. 2,280'). Look for the old tramway buckets and pulleys scattered on the nearby slopes.

The Desert Hound Mine.   For a more challenging hike, try the leg-endary Desert Hound Mine (see *Virgin Spring Canyon*), located just north of Desert Hound Peak, the prominent peak east of the camp. The easiest approach from this drainage is up the first side canyon from the camp After a few falls and bends, this open canyon splits into several ravines at the foot of a steep, high slope. From here the objective is to reach the ridge 700 feet above, which separates this drainage from Scotty's Canyon to the north. I made it by climbing up one of the ridges between the ravines, moving to the right towards friendlier slopes about half way up. It takes a lot of hard scrambling, but the rest of the route, up the ridge to the mine, is much easier. Of the three approaches to this remote mine suggested in this book, this is the shortest, but given the terrain, to make it there and back in one day is still no mean feat.

Ashford Peak.   For a little easier hike with almost equally grand views, try Ashford Peak. The route suggested on the map is up the main canyon to the side canyon on the south side (elev. 2,520'), then up this side canyon to the saddle at 3,280', and finally up the steep ridge to the peak. Ashford Peak offers the best bird's-eye views of the Confidence Hills, the Narrows of the Amargosa River, and the Owlshead Mountains to the southwest.

■

VIRGIN SPRING CANYON
AND THE DESERT HOUND MINE

> *If you enjoy hiking through wild, desolate areas, put Virgin Spring Canyon at the top of your list. You can check out an unusual forma-tion known as the Amargosa Chaos, rest by a remote spring, or hike the long, rugged trails to the Desert Hound Mine. Located on the high spine of the Black Mountains, it is one of the most isolated mines in Death Valley.*

General Information

Road status: Roadless; access by short primitive road (HC)
Shortest hike: 2.0 mi, 750 ft one way/easy
Longest hike: 7.5 mi, 2,330 ft one way (or more)/strenuous
Main attractions: Virgin Spring, the Desert Hound Mine, geology
USGS 15' topo maps: Confidence Hills, Funeral Peak
USGS 7.5' topo maps: Epaulet Peak*, Funeral Peak, Shore Line Butte
Maps: pp. 225*, 159

Location and Access

Virgin Spring Canyon is in the southern Black Mountains, where it drains south between Desert Hound Peak and Epaulet Peak. The primitive road that used to go part way into it was completely washed out years ago. It was rerouted, washed out again in 2004, and re-established to the starting point of this hike. This road starts from Highway 178 about 0.4 mile west of Jubilee Pass. Drive it 1.3 miles to its end at a small parking area, where a little sign will confirm that you are at the right place. Park and walk from here. The mouth of Virgin Spring Canyon is the wide opening 0.5 mile to the northwest, across the open wash. Starting 0.2 mile from the highway, the road has a few nasty sand traps. If you are driving a low-clearance vehicle, you are likely to get stranded, so you might want to play it safe and walk from here.

Geology: The Amargosa Chaos

The geology of Virgin Spring Canyon is well-known for the Amargosa Chaos, a rare geological phenomena characterized by highly disordered blocks ranging in size from tens of feet to a good fraction of a mile. Adjoining blocks are commonly made of rocks as widely different as dolomite, sandstone, lava, marble, quartzite, and granitic rocks. The term "chaos" was coined by Levi Noble, a prominent geologist who carried out extensive field work in this region beginning in the 1930s and first recognized its geological complexity. Although he and many geologists after him have tried to decipher the origin of this puzzling feature, many questions still remain unanswered.

The Amargosa Chaos is divided into three units, called phases, differentiated by the type of rocks they contain. The Calico phase is mostly Tertiary rhyolitic lava and tuff. This particularly colorful unit occurs extensively in the northeastern reaches of Virgin Spring Canyon, and around Calico and Epaulet peaks just east of it. The Virgin Spring phase, exposed in the lower canyon and on the south flank of Ashford Peak to the west, is made of late Precambrian to Cambrian formations. The Jubilee phase is an even more bewildering hodgepodge made of just about any formation deposited between the late Proterozoic and the Tertiary. This phase, which occurs at lower elevations, is now largely buried under Quaternary alluvia, and it is more poorly represented. Its best exposures are along Jubilee Wash and between the roads to Ashford and Scotty's canyons.

All three phases rest on top of the much older crystalline Precambrian basement. A thrust fault roughly follows the contact between them. The chaos is believed to have resulted from intense folding in the early Tertiary, followed by movements along this fault in the middle or late Tertiary. In the process, the original rocks were thoroughly faulted and shattered into today's complex mosaic. Many of the blocks were deeply fractured and show signs of friction from grating over the basement rocks during transport.

History: The Desert Hound Mine

Two mining areas are associated with Virgin Spring Canyon. The first one, in the vicinity of Virgin Spring, witnessed two short-lived strikes, neither of which left very much behind. The first one took place in the fall of 1906, probably spurred by the copper boom in nearby Willow Creek. The usual scenario: a euphoric prospector, probably hallucinating from a sunlight overdose, found indications of copper; a few men worked hard at sinking a small shaft under the support of a brand-new company; the showings turned out to be pathetic, and the mine was abandoned two months later. This effort was followed by a second one, in the spring of 1908. This time it was a small gold strike, but it was equally short and unsuccessful.

The second mining area, the Desert Hound Mine, is historically far more significant. This mine is actually located in the upper drainage of Scotty's Canyon, but while active it was associated with Virgin Spring Canyon, being reached by trails originating in this canyon. The story of the Desert Hound is connected with Walter Scott, more widely known as Death Valley Scotty, a con artist and would-be prospector who put Death Valley on the map by his tall tales and outrageous conduct. Around the turn of the century, soon after he first came to Death Valley, Scotty began claiming he had a gold mine, of course nothing short of fabulously rich, and in the most remote part of Death Valley. The idea was to convince investors to finance him—in principle to work his mine, in practice to skip the work and make an easy living. Since his mine was probably imaginary, it was key to his success to keep its location secret. A difficult task, but Scotty was resourceful (see *Scotty's Canyon*).

In the fall of 1905, pushed by his creditors, perhaps realizing his credibility was wearing thin, Scotty agreed for the first time to show his mine. The lucky man was Azariah Pearl, a self-promoted mining investor from New Hampshire who probably could not tell fool's gold from the real thing. Scotty took Pearl to some claims he and an Indian friend named Bill Keys owned, assuring Pearl they were "just as rich" as his secret mine. The claims, originally discovered by Keys, were located in the rugged heart of the Black Mountains, in a hard-to-reach place now called Scotty's Canyon. As usual, Scotty complicated matters. So that Pearl would believe thieves were after his mine, Scotty asked a couple of friends to stage a little gun play while he and Pearl were in the canyon. As planned, the two men beat a hasty retreat before Pearl had a chance to look at Scotty's "real" mine.

In spite of all this, in earnest or perhaps because he became Scotty's accomplice, Pearl was impressed. In the following months, he managed to interest a group of investors in raising funds to purchase Keys' claims. One of them was a newly formed venture called the I. E. Du Pont de Nemours Powder Company. Contingent on its involvement, however, the company requested that one of its mining experts, Daniel Owen, be taken to the mine to assess its value. Put on the spot again, Scotty prepared a second expedition to his mine. The party included Owen and other investors or their representatives, Scotty's brothers Bill and Warner, Bill Keys, and Scotty's friend Jack Brody. The party left Daggett, south of Death Valley, late in February 1906, rode to Panamint Valley and up the Panamints on its way to Death Valley. To scare off his party, Scotty arranged another ambush, but this one backfired. As the party was crossing Wingate Pass, Keys and Brody, waiting in hiding, fired a few shots at the leading men, failed to miss, and wounded Scotty's brother Warner. The expedition was successfully aborted, but Scotty had indirectly injured his brother and had to face the law, if not his guilt. The following month warrants were issued for Keys' and Scotty's arrest on charges of assault with a deadly weapon. Keys, Pearl, and Scotty were soon arrested, but not for very long, as charges were dismissed at the end of April on a mere technicality.

The Battle of Wingate Pass, as Scotty's staged skirmish became known, made headlines nationwide. Its publicity spiked the curiosity of the investors, who decided to go ahead with the claims and formed the Key Gold Mining Company in May 1906. Keys' claims were purchased for $25,000—not a bad tag considering no one had ever seen them. Over the following months the company acquired as much of the surrounding ground as possible, eventually controlling nearly two square miles of claims. One such transaction, made in the early part of 1907, involved claims reported the previous summer by two prospectors. It was the only one of Du Pont's sprawling property that would return a little gold and excitement. It was called the Desert Hound.

Although in its early stages the Desert Hound was managed by Bill Keys, development didn't start until October 1907, when a new manager took charge. The mine soon employed six men, and in a few weeks about $20,000 worth of gold ore was ready for shipment. By the end of 1907, the workings included a 120-foot tunnel and a 70-foot shaft. Things looked good enough that in February 1908 two experts were brought in from Boston to assay the ore. For the occasion a 600-pound furnace was hauled up the long, steep trail to the mine. The experts' report was so enthusiastic that the company immediately planned for a small on-site mill and a fancy aerial tramway to take the ore down to it. In January 1909, a wagon road was being built from Death Valley Junction to improve access, but water was so scarce and the site so remote that this project was never completed. In February another mine was opened, and a plentiful supply of ore worth $80 to $100 a ton was reported. The company steadily increased its task force to about a dozen people by fall. A year and a half later, in April 1911, the main tunnel reached an impressive 1,300 feet. Around that time 40 tons of ore worth about $12,000 were shipped to the smelter in Needles, California. Here more than anywhere else, isolation was a tough enemy. Only the best ore could be profitably shipped out, and there was only so much of it. Mining continued through at least the beginning of 1912, at which point the Desert Hound was shut down—and not re-opened for more than 20 years.

The mine saw its second and last period of activity during the Depression, when a one-man operation brought it back to life for a few years. The enterprising man built (or refurbished) two trails to the mine from Virgin Spring Canyon, and worked some of the old tunnels. The ore was treated at a small mill near Virgin Spring, 4 miles and 1,600 feet below the mine. Judging by the small size of the tailings and the scarcity of remains at the mill, he probably spent more time building trails than mining. By the time the Desert Hound was abandoned for good in the late 1930s, it is doubtful that it had produced much more than $30,000.

Good old Scotty had indeed fooled them all. By then he was savoring his success from the comfort of Albert Johnson's mansion, the lavish castle that would soon bear his name. Even then he was still fueling speculations that he might indeed have had a rich mine all along.

Route Description

The lower canyon. Though wide and mostly straight, the lower part of Virgin Spring Canyon is quite colorful and varied because of its unusual geology. The Virgin Spring phase of the Amargosa Chaos occurs on the west side all the way up to the main fork, except for a 1-mile stretch of crystalline basement starting 0.3 mile in. The sweeping cliff framing the west side of the wash about 0.2 mile past the mouth is a good example. It has a few small faults, shattered rocks, and old slickensides. Other good examples are found in the two short side canyons around the spring and in the longer one past it, all on the west side. The latter, flanked by golden, eroded slopes capped with black volcanic rocks, is the most brightly colored.

The ancient basement, mostly gneiss, mica-schist, migmatite, and quartzite, is exposed on the east side almost up to Rock House Wash, but outcrops are few and not striking. Better exposures are found further up canyon, and at the Desert Hound where miners worked hard to dig them up for us. The metamorphism that altered these rocks was

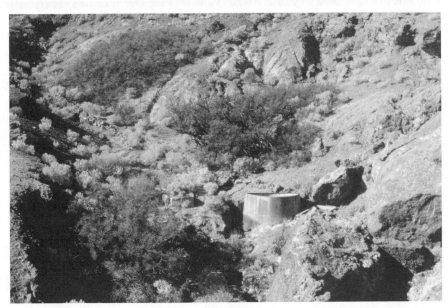

Virgin Spring

dated at 1.7 billion years. The original rocks, deposited prior to this event, are even older, and among the oldest rocks exposed in the park.

Virgin Spring. The first route to the spring is up the short side canyon on the west side, just before a lone, 8-foot high, cubic boulder in the wash. The second route is up the next side canyon, 250 yards further, marked a short distance in by a similar boulder. This is where the lower trail to the Desert Hound Mine used to start. About 0.1 mile in, on the left side, are the small, studded concrete foundations of the mill and the small tailing from the 1930s revival of the Desert Hound. A little further, the wash makes a sweeping bend to the right. Towards the end of this bend, look for the old spring trail climbing up to the low saddle on the left. The trail disappears on the saddle. Just walk across it to the edge of the next side canyon south, which overlooks the spring.

Virgin Spring is small and pleasant. A few dwarf mesquite trees grow in a steep, shallow ravine, among colorful outcrops of blue-gray shale and a conglomerate made of igneous rocks. The spring caved in and dried up years ago, but the Park Service dug it up recently for the benefit of bighorn and other wildlife. Now water from the old pipe collects in a brand new tub. It is a marginal spring, judging by the tub overflow—maybe 10 drops a second, on a good second. Yet even in the hot season this is enough to keep the tub full, and a few chirping birds happy. The remains scattered around—a large, bottomless water tank, drum, rusted pipes, and small prospect—date from the small copper and gold rushes of 1906-1908. Although some people will doubtlessly argue it is not worth the walk, if Virgin Spring is as far as you go it will likely be the highlight.

Rock house ruins. Back to the main canyon, about 0.8 mile past the turnoff to the spring and on the left side of the wash, stand the ruins of four stone houses and a tent site. This small camp was probably used by miners working on the copper claims near the spring in 1906. As of 1992, three of the houses had crumbled to short walls. The largest house, built against a large outcrop and the most protected, still had some of its original walls, doorway, and chimney. It is one of the largest ruins of a stone structure in the park.

The short side canyon just east of the ruins, referred to by Noble as Rock House Wash, is a good spot to check out the Amargosa Chaos. The tall dolomite boulder (Virgin Spring phase) standing at the mouth of the wash is a typical chaos block, well striated from grinding against other blocks during the formation of the chaos. The vivid Calico phase is exposed up the wash—yellow, red, and brown rhyolite and tuff a short distance in, light purple andesite and dark basalt flows further on up.

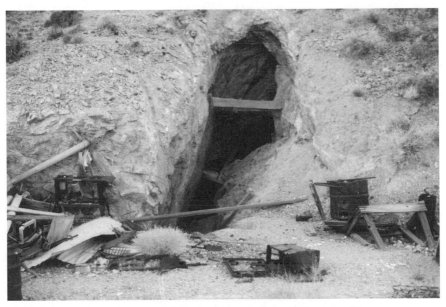

Mining camp and shaft adit at the Desert Hound Mine

The Desert Hound Mine. Located near the crest of the anticline separating Ashford and Scotty's canyons, this mine is one of the most isolated in the park. All approaches require strenuous cross-country hiking over steep terrain. The Scotty's Canyon route involves several technical climbs and extensive bypasses. The Ashford Canyon route is shorter, steeper, but easier. The Virgin Spring Canyon routes, via either one of two long, eroded trails, are the easiest, but they are still no Sunday stroll.

The lower trail starts a little further than the mill foundations as a faint trace ascending the right slope of the side canyon. For the first 2 miles or so, it climbs up to, then essentially follows, the sharp ridge separating this side canyon from the next one north. The trail then crosses the head of three drainages. Segments are missing here and there, mostly around the wash crossings. It resumes about 0.6 mile before the junction with the upper trail, marked by a small cairn on the left side. The rest of the trail to the old camp is in better shape and nearly level.

Built to access the Desert Hound, this trail has been rarely used since the 1930s, so don't expect a highway. More like a dim track, it has been taken out at many places by small slides and is overgrown by thorny bushes. By the time you are through walking it, your legs will look as if a cat used them as scratching posts. The lower part of the trail is quite steep, hard on your lungs going up, and hard on your knees coming down. However run down it is, it does a good job at minimizing elevation changes and distances, and it's far easier than the steep, slick slopes it crosses. The main problem is that the trail is easy to lose. If this happens, chances are that by climbing to higher ground you will run into it again. Knowing its general direction helps. Take along an enlarged copy of the 15' map and frequently check your location.

The upper trail starts in the west fork of Virgin Spring Canyon. Once known as the Desert Hound Trail, it climbs along a steep drainage and joins the lower trail 0.8 mile before the mine, crossing vast exposures of the Virgin Spring phase along the way. I have not hiked it yet. My guess is it's probably in better shape than the lower trail.

It is strenuous, but it's a small price to pay for glorious views of the desert, and the thrill of exploring a legendary location no one has visited in a long time. The Desert Hound Mine overlooks spectacular upper Scotty's Canyon, a wild panorama of deep canyons and chiseled mountain slopes. The mining camp is built on a leveled terrace right by the trail. One of the two main mine workings, a steep shaft still stoped with original timber, gapes in the hillside just behind the camp. The second tunnel is around the next bend in the trail. A long tailing, littered with rusted cans and trash, spills down the slope. The large rusted carcass stranded part way down is probably the furnace used in 1908.

From here the trail winds for half a mile before ending at a narrow divide. This is the site of the 1906-1908 mining camp. It is marked by a few tent sites, some of them well-preserved rock platforms, and the larger ruin of a rock shelter, constructed partly in the hillside just before

Virgin Spring Canyon		
	Dist.(mi)	Elev.(ft)
End of road/trailhead	0.0	1,580
Mouth	0.4	1,660
Side canyon to lower trail	2.0	2,250
Virgin Spring	(0.4)	2,410
Jct with Desert Hound Trail	(3.6)	3,970
Desert Hound Mine	(4.4)	~3,990
Old camp	(4.9)	~4,010
Rock house ruins	2.3	2,540
Fork	3.1	2,600
Desert Hound Trail	(1.5)	3,120
Jct with lower trail	(4.1)	3,970
4WD road	6.3	3,660
Head	7.2	3,790
Greenwater Valley Road	(5.6)	2,615

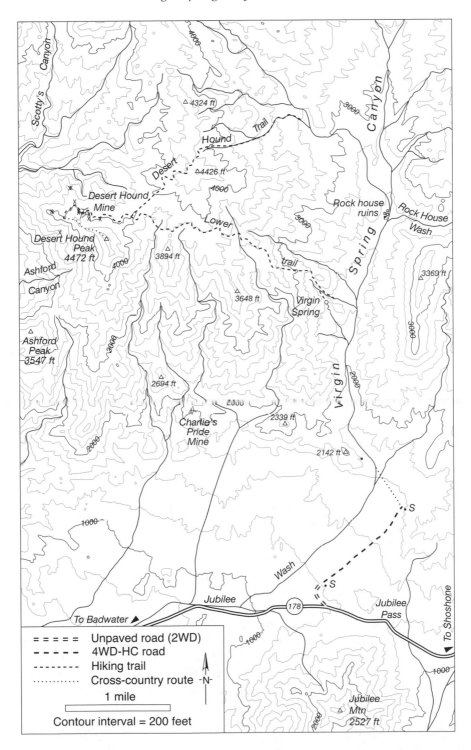

Scotty's Canyon

△ 4324 ft

Hound   Trail

Desert

△4426 ft

4000

Desert Hound Mine

Lower

Rock house ruins

Rock House Wash

Desert Hound Peak 4472 ft

△ 3894 ft

trail

3369 ft

Ashford Canyon

△ 3648 ft

Virgin Spring

△ Ashford Peak 3547 ft

Virgin Spring

△ 2694 ft

2000

2339 ft △

Charlie's Pride Mine

2142 ft △

Wash

S

To Badwater ▲

Jubilee

178

Jubilee Pass

Jubilee Mtn 2527 ft

To Shoshone ▲

===== Unpaved road (2WD)
- - - - 4WD-HC road
- - - - - Hiking trail
.... Cross-country route   -N-

1 mile

Contour interval = 200 feet

the end of the trail. These modest remains are completely eclipsed by the awesome views from the divide. Standing on the brink of Ashford Canyon, you will look straight down the sweeping curvature of a great wall, all the way to the small camp of the Ashford Mine more than 1,800 feet below. Far beyond sprawls the pristine southern end of Death Valley, framed by the Owlshead and Panamint mountains, with the Sierra Nevada peeking over them. Since you came this far, and you are probably late anyway, you might as well climb nearby Desert Hound Peak. The views are even more spectacular, especially at sunset.

The Desert Hound was no winner, and its remains are not the most plentiful. But because of its remoteness and mysterious connection with Death Valley Scotty, it will hold a special place in the heart of the few Death Valley lovers who trudge this far just to check it out. It's an adventure. I was here on a bright crisp winter day, left the highway at 11 a.m., spent most of the day chasing the erratic lower trail, did not reach the mine until 3 p.m. Much too late. Returning in twilight, I lost the trail twice, didn't reach the main canyon until dark, and hiked the rest of the way by flashlight. Come here preferably when the days are long enough, and get an early start. Bring a flashlight, or make sure the moon is on your side.

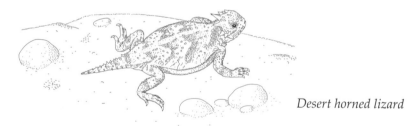

Desert horned lizard

The upper canyon. For the seasoned hiker, upper Virgin Spring Canyon provides a seldom-traveled backpacking route across the Black Mountains, up its east fork to its head and down a broad unnamed wash into the southern end of the Greenwater Valley. The upper canyon forks many times, and each fork splits over and over again. Unless you are particularly unlucky, no one will be around to share this vast piece of real estate with you. You will need to carefully check your whereabouts on the 7.5' map, or you may not come out of this maze where and when you intended. The second half of this route, from shortly before the head of the canyon, follows an old jeep road that eventually connects with the Greenwater Valley Road. I don't know the condition of this road. It may be possible to use it the other way, at least part way, to access this canyon from the Greenwater Valley.

∎

IBEX SPRING

This isolated area in the southeastern corner of the park was the site of small talc mining operations starting in the mid-1930s. Its ghost town, lush spring, and nearby mines make an interesting destination for a short day of exploring.

General Information

Road status: Easy access from primitive road (HC)
Shortest hike: Short strolls / easy
Longest hike: 4.9 mi, 1,800 ft one way (or more) / moderate
Main attractions: Mining camp, Ibex Spring, talc mines
USGS 15' topo map: Avawatz Pass
USGS 7.5' topo maps: Ibex Spring*, Ibex Pass
Maps: pp. 231*, 159

Location and Access

Ibex Spring is located in the Ibex Hills, near the southern end of the Black Mountains. Drive Highway 127 south from Shoshone (at Highway 178) for 16.3 miles (1.8 miles south of Ibex Pass) to an unmarked dirt road on the west side. This is the Ibex Spring Road. Drive it 5.3 miles to the first junction below the spring. The right fork goes to the Monarch-Pleasanton Mines, betrayed from quite a distance back by their white tailings. The main road forks again 500 feet further. The right fork goes up to the camp and spring. The main road continues straight to the Moorehouse Mine, hidden behind the hills.

Although its old pavement is mostly gone, the Ibex Spring Road has held up pretty well so far, except for a major washout 3.2 miles from the highway where it dips steeply in and out of a deep wash. If you are driving a standard-clearance vehicle, you will probably want to quit here while you are ahead, and walk the rest of the way.

History: Talc Mining

Talc mining around Ibex Spring took place around the same time and followed much the same pattern as near Saratoga Spring, a few miles to the south. The original instigator was John Moorehouse, who located 16 claims in the hills north of Ibex Spring in the mid-1930s. The Monarch deposit, half a mile to the east, was located around 1938 by Ralph Morris. Both men worked their mines for a few years, extracting relatively small amounts of talc. Large scale operations started only in the mid-1940s, when the Sierra Talc Company leased both properties, as well as the nearby Pleasanton Mine, first opened in 1942. Over the next few years, the company developed all three mines extensively, involving a sizeable crew who lived in a camp by the spring. It was not the rip-roaring camp typical of earlier decades, but a relatively modern, almost comfortable place. At its height there were a dozen wooden buildings, including sheds, living areas, and a bathhouse, with electricity and propane appliances in several of them. The spring had a concrete spring-house, which pumped and distributed water throughout the camp.

None of the three mines produced as much as their neighbor the Superior Mine (see *Saratoga Spring*), but they all paid out a nice little return. The Moorehouse yielded nearly 62,000 tons before it played out in 1959. The Monarch produced 46,000 tons until 1950, and remained inactive for several years. The production of the Pleasanton was more modest—16,000 tons—until it was shut down in 1947. In 1956, the Southern California Minerals Company, which was already busy mining talc a few miles south, leased the Monarch and the Pleasanton from Sierra Talc. The new operator connected the workings between the two mines and squeezed out another 7,500 tons of talc over the next three years. By then the deposits were largely depleted, and other than minor exploratory work up until the late 1960s the properties have been idle.

Geology

As elsewhere in the region, talc occurs exclusively in the Crystal Spring Formation. This formation is exposed irregularly along a belt stretching from Galena Canyon to the Kingston Range—a belt traced neatly on the map by the talc mines of the past. Talc was formed when diabase sills intruded the formation's carbonate member. Around the contact zone between the diabase and the carbonate, a complex process called contact metamorphism took place. It substituted large quantities of the calcium and carbon oxides of the original carbonate with magne-sium and silicon oxides (which is called silication), thus transforming the carbonate rock into talc. While browsing through the mines, look for the wide variety of talcose rocks. They range from chalky to porcelain-like, pure white to green, dull to shiny. The very dark rock scattered around the mines is diabase. Diabase sills are visible as the wide dark strata across the Ibex Hills just north of the camp.

Route Description

If the washout on the access road stops you, you may actually be getting the best end of the deal. The Ibex Spring Road is a scenic and easy place to walk, in full view of the Ibex and Saddle Peak Hills, and the gentle slope of the open desert will repeatedly lead your eyes south-ward to the Saratoga Hills and the striking Ibex Dunes. With a high-clearance vehicle you can drive it instead, but you may miss part of the scenery. If you do drive through, try to park at the junction below the camp and walk from there. It's healthy for the soul, good for the land, and a lot better for your body.

Ibex Spring.   The luxuriant spring nestled at the foot of the Ibex Hills was the core of this small mining area. With its tall palm trees tow-ering over a thick grove of mesquites and arrowweed, it has a striking oasis quality, unexpected in this barren desert. Birds don't exactly abound, but there are a few—I even saw a couple of owls nesting in the trees. The ghost camp below it still has about ten standing structures. Most of them will probably remain for many more years if visitors just leave them alone. Signs of vandalism are ubiquitous, ranging from torn sidings to punched-in sheetrock walls and bullet-ridden artifacts. One should obviously not let people drive all the way out here. But what is left is still a lot of fun to explore. Several large cabins are scattered under healthy saltcedars. Look for the disjointed network of water pipes run-ning through the camp, and for the concrete-floored bathhouse. Although the galvanized tank at the spring is empty (the bullet holes didn't help), there is a little surface water among the nearby cane, and the low wooden shack near the tank is full of water. At the foot of the

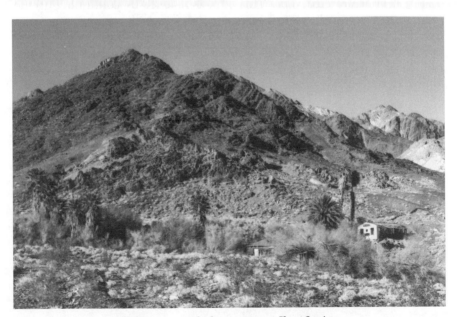

Palm trees and ghost camp at Ibex Spring

hills to the west are a nameless grave and the ruins of two stone houses, dating back to the Bullfrog boom of the early 1900s.

The Monarch-Pleasanton Mine. These mines are reached via the road that branches north below the camp. Again you can drive it, but portions of it are in poor shape and you may prefer to walk. The Pleasanton Mine is the closest one. The lower level has a large loading dock with a nice wooden ore chute. On the wide cleared area just above it there is a small shelter and the short rail spur that delivered the talc to the ore chute. From the far end of the tracks a short trail leads up to the main mines, which include an inclined shaft with its wooden headframe, and a long wall of talc above it, now fenced off for safety reasons.

The Monarch Mine is just a little further north, its lower level lined up with the ruins of three ore chutes. It worked the same long talc body as the Pleasanton Mine, and the two mines are connected by a 950-foot tunnel that follows this body most of its length. The main workings are higher on the hillside. Most of this area has caved in, leaving behind dazzling white talc walls. At the highest level, where the contact between the diabase wall and the talc body is exposed, notice how the talc grade deteriorates away from the wall. The small cabin and the few collapsed shacks below the mine are the homestead of Tom Wilson, an employee of the Southern California Minerals Company who lived here to avoid paying rent at the company-owned spring camp.

The Moorehouse Mine. This mine is reached by continuing up the main road westward to a fork. The left fork heads down and peters out in a deep wash. The right fork goes on to the mine loading area, where it is washed out. With its extensive complex of well-preserved ore chutes, rail tracks, ore bins, tunnels, and open cuts, this is the most interesting

Ibex Spring		
	Dist.(mi)	Elev.(ft)
Dip in road	0.0	1,090
Jct to Monarch Mine	2.2	1,025
Pleasanton Mine (headframe)	(0.9)	1,510
Monarch Mine (upper mine)	(1.0)	1,575
Jct to Ibex Spring	2.25	1,030
Ibex Spring camp	(0.15)	~1,100
Ibex Spring	(0.3)	~1,150
Moorehouse Mine (lower)	3.2	1,510
Moorehouse Mine (upper)	3.5	1,840

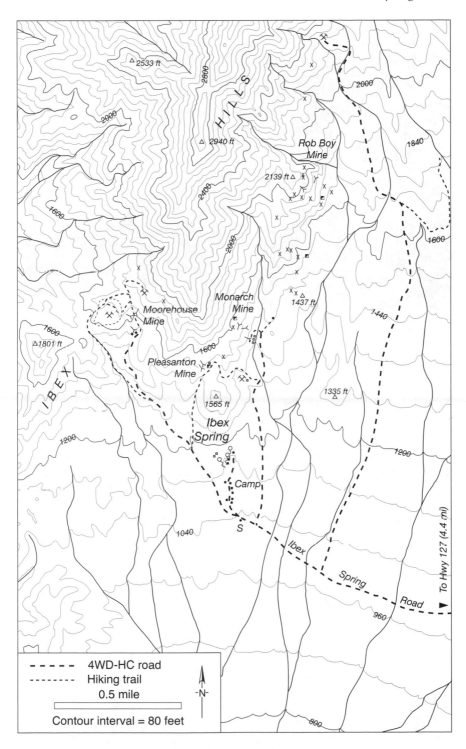

△ 2533 ft

2800

H I L L S

2000

2000

△ 2940 ft

Rob Boy
Mine

2139 ft △

2400

1840

2000

1600

1840

1600

Monarch
Mine

× × △
1437 ft

Moorehouse
Mine

1440

1600

1600

△1801 ft

Pleasanton
Mine

I B E X

1335 ft

△
1565 ft

*Ibex
Spring*

1200

1200

Camp

1040

S

Ibex

Spring

1200

To Hwy 127 (4.4 mi)

Road

960

800

– – – – 4WD-HC road
– – – – – Hiking trail

-N-

0.5 mile

Contour interval = 80 feet

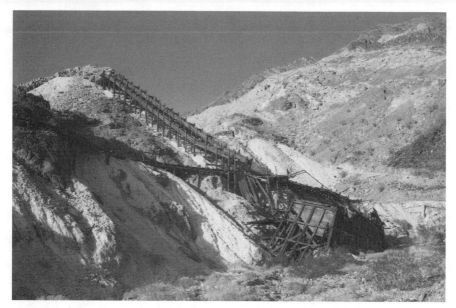

Ore bins and loading structures at the Moorehouse Mine

mine around. Walk up the steep washed-out road to the leveled area above for a closer look at the unusual twin ore chutes. Rocks from the nearby tunnels, and later on from the open cuts higher up, were railed on short tracks to the top of the chutes. The overburden was discarded on the dump. The talc rock was tossed down the chutes, stockpiled in the bins, then loaded into trucks and hauled away.

The road climbs on to the top of the hill, which was essentially beheaded by strip-mining. It created an eerie landscape of blinding white cliffs and terraces. Climb to the end of the road for spectacular views of the wide wash to the northwest, encroached in pockets of sand, and the Avawatz Mountains and Ibex Dunes to the south.

■

PART V

VALLEY FLOOR AND ALLUVIAL FANS

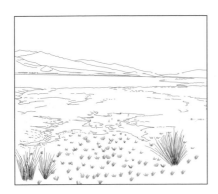

THE FLOOR AND FANS of Death Valley, bounded on both sides by high ranges, form the core of the park. This area is huge—about 140 miles long by 4 to 15 miles wide (see general maps on pp. 67, 103, 159, 289, and 393). The uplift of the Salt Creek Hills east of Tucki Mountain, roughly in the middle of the valley, divides it geographically into two parts, north and south. Although they both lie partly below sea level, the south valley is deeper over a much larger area. More than 200 square miles of it are covered by a salt pan. A good part of Death Valley is easily accessible. Paved roads run along most of its east side, and a graded road, the West Side Road, follows part of its west side. The Big Pine Road (graded) and the Harry Wade Road (primitive) explore the northern and southern reaches of the valley, respectively. Highway 190 and the Daylight Pass Road cross the valley generally east-west around its midpoint.

Hydrology

Death Valley has little to do with water, yet because it is such a huge closed basin it manages to collect more water than one would expect. For example, just a few feet under bone-dry Mesquite Flat, at the south end of the north valley, lies a huge underground lake. The water comes mostly from rain collected in the surrounding mountains, which percolates underground and collects behind the uplift of the Salt Creek Hills. The southern half of Death Valley gets its moisture from other sources as well. At its north end, seeps from the Mesquite Flat aquifer, including Salt Creek, flow south into Cottonball Basin, which empties—mostly underground—into the Middle Basin. The water then flows into the Badwater Basin, the last and lowest of all three basins. On its east side, the south valley receives water from several large springs near the mouth of Furnace Creek (Travertine, Nevares, and Texas springs), which originate from the Pahrump Valley aquifer in Nevada. Water also comes from smaller springs along the west side of the Badwater Basin, fed by precipitation in the high Panamints. The last intake is the small under-flow from the Amargosa River, at the south end of the valley. Since Death Valley has no outlet to the sea, water can escape only through evaporation. Most of it is locked just under the salt deposits of the pan, evaporating as fast as it is replenished. Very little of it is usually in the form of surface water. Every few years, however, the winter is wet enough that parts of the valley, especially Badwater Basin, get flooded under a lake 2 to 3 feet deep that often survives until summer.

Geology

Death Valley is not a valley but a graben: the primary forces that created it were tectonic in nature, not erosional. Tectonic forces supplied the energy that pulled apart the Amargosa and Panamint ranges. In the process, both ranges were tilted down eastward along an approximately north-south axis. As the east side of the Panamint Range slowly dipped towards the deepening graben, the Amargosa Range rose abruptly on the other side. The general eastward tilt of the ranges is reflected in the fans' physiography. At many places on the west side of the valley the fans extend more than 5 miles and reach up to 1,200 feet above the val-ley floor. The fans of adjacent canyons have essentially merged into each other. On the other hand, as the Black Mountains were being uplifted their fans sunk and became largely buried, which explains the small size of the fans on the east side of the valley. Many of them, like the first few fans south of Badwater, exhibit the conical shape typical of fresh piles of sand. At places, adjacent fans don't even overlap.

Perhaps the main geological curiosity on the valley floor is the salt pan. Drill holes at Badwater and Cottonball basins show that the salt layer is not very thick, and that beneath it alternating layers of mud and salt reach at least 1,000 feet down. It suggests that the area was flooded for a long time, with muds deposited in wetter periods and salts in drier periods. Today's salt pan is the most recent of many such playas of evaporites, this one left by Lake Manly when it dried up at the end of the Pleistocene. Because of the asymmetry of the valley, when the lake filled the valley it was much closer to the east side than to the west side. As a result, the salt pan is strongly offset in the same direction. At places it even comes right up to the base of the Black Mountains. As the lake slowly dried up, the least soluble salts—the carbonates—were first to precipitate. They cover the largest area, usually forming vast expanses of

Suggested Hikes on the Valley Floor and Alluvial Fans					
Route/Destination	Dist. (mi)	Elev. change	Mean elev.	Access road	Pages
Short hikes (under 5 miles round trip)					
Borax Haystacks	~1.5	50'	-245'	Graded	261-262
Harmony Borax Works	0.4	50'	-230'	Paved	261
Ibex Dunes loop*	2.8	1,280'	500'	P/1.0 mi	278
Kit Fox Canyon (lower loop*)	3.4	860'	290'	Paved	243-246
Midway-Surveyor's wells	1.2	50'	55'	Paved	238-240
Palm Spring-Triangle Spring	1.4	30'	20'	Paved	238
Saratoga Mine	1.7	350'	240'	P/9.9 mi	276-277
Saratoga Spring	0.5	30'	195'	P/9.9 mi	275-276
Shoreline Butte	1.6	500'	0'	Graded	266-268
Death Valley dunes (highest)	1.1	100'	~40'	Paved	249-252
Superior Mine	0.7	210'	620'	P/10.7 mi	278
Intermediate hikes (5-12 miles round trip)					
Badwater to lowest point	3.3	~10'	-280'	Paved	270
Cottonwd Cyn to Niter Beds	4.8	620'	410'	P/8.6 mi	240
Devil's Golf Course Road to					
Badwater	4.7	~10'	-277'	Graded	268-270
Salt Creek at West Side Rd	4.9	10'	275'	Graded	268-270
lowest point	3.3	~10'	-280'	Graded	268-270
Kit Fox Canyon (to head)	3.9	870'	505'	Paved	243-246
Mesquite Flat springs loop*	~7.4	150'	~40'	Paved	238-240
Nevares Springs	5.3	1,630'	1,420'	Paved	256-258
Pongo Mine	3.8	340'	250'	P/9.9 mi	278
Rhyolite-Skidoo Road	6.0	1,400'	770'	Paved	246
Stov. W. Campgr. to Stov. W.	6.6	~400'	~-20'	Paved	249-252
Long hikes (over 12 miles round trip)					
Badwater to Tule Spring	6.9	25'	-265'	Paved	270
Death Valley Sand Dunes,					
Palm Spr. to Stovepipe W.	11.0	~200'	-30'	Paved	249-252
Nevares Peak	7.9	3,650'	2,770'	Paved	256-258
Palm Spring to Niter Beds	6.4	60'	40'	Paved	240
Saratoga Hills talc mines*	9.3	1,000'	330'	P/9.9 mi	275-278
Overnight hikes (over 2 days)					
Death Valley trek					
Cucomungo C.-Mesq. Spr.	37.5	4,550'	3,230'	Graded	279-281
Mesq. Spr.-Stovepipe W.	36.0	1,850'	500'	Paved	281

Route/Destination	Dist. (mi)	Elev. change	Mean elev.	Access road	Pages
Overnight hikes (over 2 days) (Cont'd)					
Stovepipe W.-W. Side Rd	33.5	450'	-150'	Paved	281-282
West Side Rd-Ashford Jct	33.0	200'	-240'	Graded	282
Ashford Jct-Hwy 127	35.0	800'	110'	Paved	283-284
Mesquite Flat, Palm Spr. to					
Cottonwood Canyon Rd	13.4	720'	180'	P/8.6 mi	240

Key: P=Primitive (2WD)
* =Total distance and elevation change (ups + downs) for loops

fine silt mixed with salts on the outer edge of the pan. On top of them precipitated the second least soluble salts, the sulfates. At that point the lake was smaller, so that the sulfates cover a smaller area than the carbonates. The last minerals that precipitated were the most soluble salts—the chlorides. They cover an even smaller area, confined to the center of the salt pan. Although this distribution is not always this clear cut, sequential precipitation can be observed at many places in the evolution of both the minerals—dozens of evaporites have been identified—and the ground patterns from the edge towards the center of the playa.

Hiking

The floor and fans of Death Valley cover well over 1,000 square miles—a tremendous hiking playground. The three major terrains to look forward to are salt flats, sand dunes, and fans. Several hikes covering the first two terrains are described further on. Although no specific fan hike is suggested, you'll get to cover miles of fan to reach many of the canyons described in this book. If you like rocks, fans are also great destinations in themselves. The greatest variety of rocks is found at the foot of the longest canyons in the mountains that have the most varied formations. Fans hold many other treasures—desert pavement, ventifacts, water-worn cobbles, fault scarps, and many kinds of plants.

In a park notorious for its demanding cross-country hiking, the valley floor offers relatively easy hiking. It is also the warmest place in the park for winter hiking, and in early spring the fans offer the most stunning displays of wild flowers. The hikes suggested in this part of the book represent only a fraction of the valley floor potential. For lack of space, several interesting areas were not included, such as the Salt Creek boardwalk, or Ubehebe Crater, where trails lead down into the crater or to nearby Little Hebe Crater, amidst a dark-gray field of volcanic ash.

■

MESQUITE FLAT

> *With an approximate area of 50 square miles, Mesquite Flat has room enough to roam. This low desert offers a surprising variety of terrains, from sand hills to mud playas, salt-coated flats, and uncommon desert plants. Sample it with a short loop hike to small springs and wells, or take a long day hike or overnight trip clear across to the Niter Beds.*

General Information

Road status: Roadless; easy access from paved or graded road
Shortest hike: 0.4 mi, 25 ft one way / very easy
Longest hike: ~6.4 mi, ~65 ft one way (or more) / moderate
Main attractions: Open valley floor, low-desert plants, dunes, springs
USGS 15' topo maps: Stovepipe Wells*, Marble Canyon
USGS 7.5' topo maps: Mesquite Flat, E. of Sand Flat, Stovepipe Wells NE
Maps: pp. 239*, 67

Location and Access

Mesquite Flat is the vast stretch of open valley floor north of Stovepipe Wells. It is easily accessed from anywhere along the southern half of the Scotty's Castle Road, or from the Cottonwood Canyon Road. Refer to individual hikes for exact starting points.

Plant Ecology

A few feet under the dry surface of Mesquite Flat lies a huge lake, fed by underground discharge and precipitations occurring over the huge drainage of northern Death Valley. The water is impounded by the impermeable uplift of the Salt Creek Hills, which separates Mesquite Flat from the southern valley. This aquifer creates a unique environment that supports extensive stands of phreatophytes, plants that must have their roots in, or just above, perennial ground water. Over large areas, Mesquite Flat's soil contains a relatively high concentration of salts. Phreatophytes are picky about the amount of salt they can tolerate. Accordingly, their distributions are largely dictated by the soil salinity. The boundary between these distributions can be quite abrupt, reflecting sudden changes in ground chemistry. Mesquite trees and sacaton grass fare well in sandy soil, and are common around dunes and relatively salt-free mud flats. As the salinity increases, they are replaced by arrowweed, inkweed, and salt grass. In the saltiest soils, streaked with white swirls of salt, even they can't survive, and they leave the stage to rush and pickleweed. These plants are normally restricted to much more limited areas. Take your Ferris guidebook along, since identifying them is a good part of the fun of a random walk on Mesquite Flat.

Route Description

The springs loop. This circuit is a good, easy sampler of Mesquite Flat. Start from the Scotty's Castle Road 7.3 miles north of Highway 190. This is near the middle of a long S curve in the road; Palm Spring's tallest palm tree is visible to the northwest. Hike towards it, staying on the gravel fan at the foot of the mud hills (to avoid damaging these soft hills, do not climb on them). At the spring you'll find a cluster of palm trees, a few mesquites, an unmarked grave, and small white stone basins filled with lukewarm water. Not much of it, as usual. At one time, however, this spring was important enough to deposit the thick travertine beds exposed at the foot of the hills.

To go on to Triangle Spring, follow the foot of the hills north for about a mile (the faint track along the way is the old Scotty's Castle Road). You'll pass by a smaller spring where a little water trickles down salt-coated travertine. Triangle Spring is marked by a tall thicket of common cane and a mesquite grove. Although this spring had plenty of water until the 1940s, it is mostly dry today. Its namesake is a triangular concrete pool, once a popular stop along the road to Scotty's Castle where visitors could enjoy a bath and shade. You will find its remains, now partly buried under a fallen tree, in the middle of the grove.

To see Midway Well, you can either hike on from Triangle Spring in the same direction (about 1.6 miles), or go back and drive

		Mesquite Flat	
	Dist.(mi)	Elev.(ft)
Springs loop		
Scotty's Castle Road	0.0	~45
Palm Spring	~0.4	20
Triangle Spring	1.4	30
Midway Well	3.0	62
Surveyor's Well	3.9	45
Niter Beds		
Cottonwood Canyon Road	0.0	720
Niter Beds (west end)	4.8	100
Niter Beds (east end)	7.0	60
Scotty's Castle Road	13.4	~45

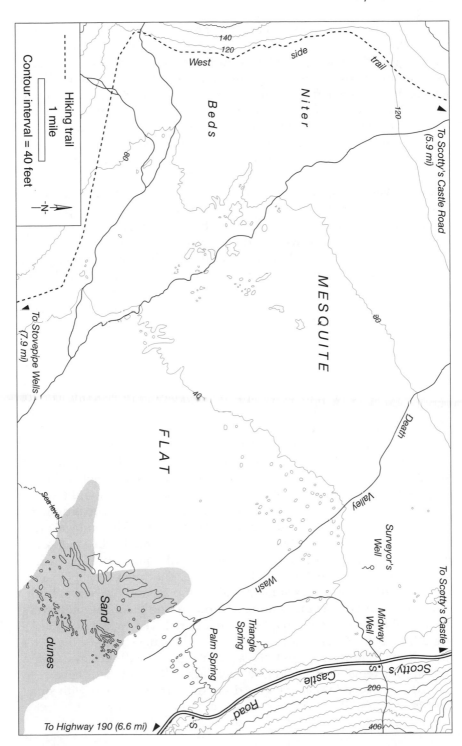

about 2.6 miles further north. Look for the well's white casing 0.25 mile west of the road, in front of the mesquite grove. Midway Well used to be a campground. Although the well water was too salty to drink, campers used it for cooking and washing. The campground was closed in 1972 to let the area recover from overuse. The pump stood on the concrete pedestal across the narrow wash from the casing. The campsites were scattered on either side of the wash down through the mesquite grove.

The next stop is Surveyor's Well. It has a tall dead cottonwood tree, which you can use as a beacon if you have good eyesight or binoculars. Otherwise just head due west from the west end of the grove at Midway Well. Along the way you will cross mostly salt-encrusted mud flats covered with salt grass. Surveyor's Well is a three-foot deep hole in the ground. It is said to have been dug by hand by an early surveying party in the 1850s. However, this spring was well known to the Shoshone, who called it *Oh yea hur* and had a village here named *Oiyo*. They may have dug the well long before that. Today, there is only wet mud in the well, but out of it grows a large mesquite and a young cottonwood. Underground water supports a long stand of common cane. Until the 1930s it was a water stop on the road to Scotty's Castle. A bleached road sign still stands near the well.

The Niter Beds.   To hike to the Niter Beds, on the west side of Mesquite Flat, start from either Surveyor's Well and head west, or drive to the mouth of Cottonwood Canyon (see *Lower Marble Canyon*). The Niter Beds are the grayish area down in the valley, about 5 miles almost due north. Much of this scenic approach is over the rough canyon fan. Either way is a pure desert hike, across sandy flats dotted with mesquite trees, small sand hills, silt playas, salt-laced ground, and extensive stands of phreatophytes. The sense of freedom and sheer isolation inspired by Mesquite Flat's oceanic vastness is truly exhilarating. Wildlife likes it here. Over the years, I have encountered roadrunners, coyotes, a kit fox, and a large, thickly-furred badger. The strangest feature, though, is the sand stacks. These isolated pyramids of sand, some over 40 feet high, dominate large portions of Mesquite Flat. Their angle of repose is so steep that they look manmade. They are probably magnified versions of the small sand pedestals found around the base of bushes in sandy deserts. As the wind piles sand around them, mesquite trees are forced to grow higher to avoid a fatal burial. The largest hummocks are a little before the Niter Beds. Unlike their name suggests, the latter are not made of nitrates, but of clay and mud mixed with evaporites, perhaps the remains of an old lake. Over time, these soft beds have been carved by erosion into a strangely dissected terrain covered with small turrets and mounds, a miniature landscape from another planet.

∎

THE KIT FOX HILLS

Although not the most spectacular, the colorful Kit Fox Hills are a good source of easy hikes along short, often tortuous gulches—ideal if you are new to the desert. For a longer outing, hike the historical Rhyolite-Skidoo Road from the Death Valley Buttes down through Kit Fox Canyon to the valley floor, over acres of surreal desert pavement.

General Information

Road status: Roadless; within easy walking distance of paved road
Shortest hike: 1.5 mi, 430 ft one way/easy
Longest hike: 6.0 mi, 1,400 ft one way/moderate
Main attractions: Rhyolite-Skidoo Road and telephone line, easy scenic
　　　　hikes in badlands, desert pavement
USGS 15' topo maps: Stovepipe Wells*, Chloride Cliff
USGS 7.5' topo maps: Stovepipe Wells*, Chloride City
Maps: pp. 245*, 67

Location and Access

The Kit Fox Hills are the low hills parallel to, and just east of, the Scotty's Castle Road and Highway 190, a few miles north and south of the Daylight Pass Road. These hills were formed by residual vertical movement along the Furnace Creek Fault Zone, which parallels their steep western slope. They are dissected by many short gulches, generally too small to qualify as canyons. The main hike suggested here is in Kit Fox Canyon, first named by Chuck Gebhardt in his book *Backpacking Death Valley*. The easiest approach to this canyon is from the Scotty's Castle Road. Park at the marked turnoff to the sand dunes, 3 miles north of Highway 190. The canyon mouth is 0.35 mile up the fan, in a direction opposite to the Historic Stovepipe Well Road. The second option is to start at the head of Kit Fox Canyon. Drive the Daylight Pass Road 3.1 miles from the Scotty's Castle Road to the emergency water tank at the upper end of Mud Canyon and park. Kit Fox Canyon and the Rhyolite-Skidoo Road are reached by walking across the fan northwest about 0.9 mile, staying on the uphill side of the hills to avoid minor washes.

To hike the Rhyolite-Skidoo Road downhill, start where it branches off the Daylight Pass Road, 4.8 miles east of the Scotty's Castle Road, at the lower end of the first major bend past Mud Canyon. The old road is to the west, and visible most of the way there. It is washed out at the bend; look for it about 0.2 mile downhill from that point.

Geology: Desert Pavement and Rock Varnish

The crest of the Kit Fox Hills and the fan east of them are coated with peculiar arrangements of close-packed stones. The ground looks as if it has been sprinkled with pebbles and pressed into a smooth cover. This is called desert pavement. In the Sahara, it is known as *reg* and covers hundreds of square miles of desert completely devoid of vegetation. In Death Valley, where it is fairly common although far less extensive, desert pavement manages to support a few plants, but it is still quite barren. If you lift a pavement pebble (and put it back), you'll find sand or silt underneath it. Desert pavement is believed to be formed by wind erosion in areas where the original ground was made of a mixture of silt and small stones. Wind preferentially blew away finer particles, leaving behind only heavier rock fragments.

Most of the pebbles are darker on their upper side than their underside. The dark top coating is rock varnish, a layer that develops on rock surfaces of all sizes, from gravel to cliffs, after prolonged exposure to sun and moisture. Rock varnish is very thin, typically less than five thousands of an inch. It is composed mostly of iron and manganese oxides, clay minerals, and traces of organic matter. Thanks to the latter, this benign coating can be accurately dated by C^{14} and used as a tool to study the recent past. It tells us, for example, that in the last few thousand years, the local climate has gone through several dry and "less dry" cycles. Like rocks, petroglyphs and stone artifacts often get coated with varnish over time. Their age, which is generally difficult to pin down, may be dated by this process in the future. In general, the older the varnish, the darker it gets. If you look at a distant fan, you should be able to tell its older from its younger areas by their relative darkness. Around Death Valley the lightest detectable varnish is at least a few centuries old. The darkest varnishes show that some of the fans have been mostly undisturbed for some 28,000 years.

History: The Rhyolite-Skidoo Road and Telephone Line

In the heyday of Death Valley a road connected the distant mining towns of Rhyolite, near Beatty, Nevada, and Skidoo, on the far side of Tucki Mountain (see *Telephone Canyon*). Known as the Rhyolite-Skidoo Road, it followed Boundary Canyon, passed along the eastern foot of the Death Valley Buttes, and dropped through Kit Fox Canyon to Stovepipe Well. It then crossed the valley to the foot of Tucki Mountain and climbed to Skidoo, along Emigrant Canyon in earlier years, later on along Telephone Canyon. The telephone line, completed in 1907, followed much the same route. On the eastern edge of the valley floor, a way station called Stovepipe Well offered the only water, brackish as it was, for miles around. In the early 1900s a settler built a one-room cabin here, with walls of mud and beer bottles. After 1905, when the Rhyolite-Skidoo Road was traveled by stage coach, this awkward dwelling was supplemented by a canvas store, a tent lodge, and even a tent saloon.

Route Description

Kit Fox Canyon. From the Historic Stovepipe Well Road it's an easy walk up to and through the canyon. No dramatic gorge here, but a serene landscape of rolling hills sliced by the wide open canyon. The rock exposed along the way, and throughout the Kit Fox Hills, is Funeral Formation fanglomerate. Its rocky chunks are bits of the Grapevine Mountains torn away by erosion during the Pliocene. The best times to be here are around sunrise and sundown, when the wrinkled hills fill up

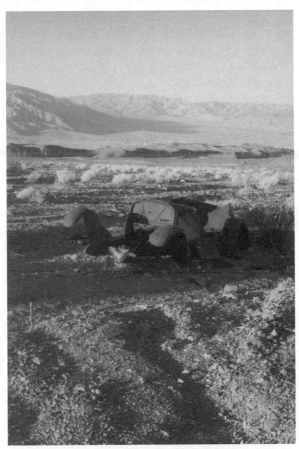

Rusted car body along the Rhyolite-Skidoo Road,
looking down at the Kit Fox Hills (middle distance)

with rich colors and intriguing shadows. This is a good area to see desert flowers in the spring, when wild displays of golden evening primrose, desertgold, gold poppy, and eriogonum brighten the fan and washes. In this barren landscape, they can be so abundant as to seem out of place.

At the main fork you can take the left branch for fast access to the crest of the hills and good desert pavement. If you continue up the main canyon (the right fork) instead, watch for the telephone line around 0.3 mile past the fork, on the hill to the right, then off and on further up canyon. The lower end of the Rhyolite-Skidoo Road is about 0.9 mile further, on the right side.

The telephone line. Another alternative is to return via the next canyon south, which makes an interesting short loop. To get to it, take the narrow ravine on the right, 50-100 yards before the main fork. It will take you shortly to a low divide overlooking the next canyon south. Along the way, look in the wash for a low, 5-foot wide boulder with a well-preserved patch of orange slickenside—another piece of the Grapevine Mountains. From the divide, climb to the prominent cairn on the hilltop to the east (elev. ~680') for good views of the Rhyolite-Skidoo Road and telephone line, marked by an alignment of standing wooden posts. The road used to follow Kit Fox Canyon all the way through, but just northeast of here the telephone line took a shortcut. You can still see where it climbs out of the canyon, up the hill you are on, then descends into the canyon south of Kit Fox Canyon. This narrower canyon is a good way to return. A few posts still line its steep south side. From its mouth, it's a short walk down the fan to the Scotty's Castle Road at the "Wagon Wheel History" sign, just 0.4 mile south of where you parked. The sign points out old tracks on the west side of the road, lined up with the canyon you came down and clearly visible from its mouth. This is

The Kit Fox Hills		
	Dist.(mi)	Elev.(ft)
Scotty's Castle Road	0.0	70
Mouth	0.35	220
Fork	1.5	500
Telephone line	~1.8	570
Lower end of R-S Road	~2.7	720
Head	3.9	940
Daylight Pass Road	(0.9)	~980
Upper end of R-S Road	6.0	1,470

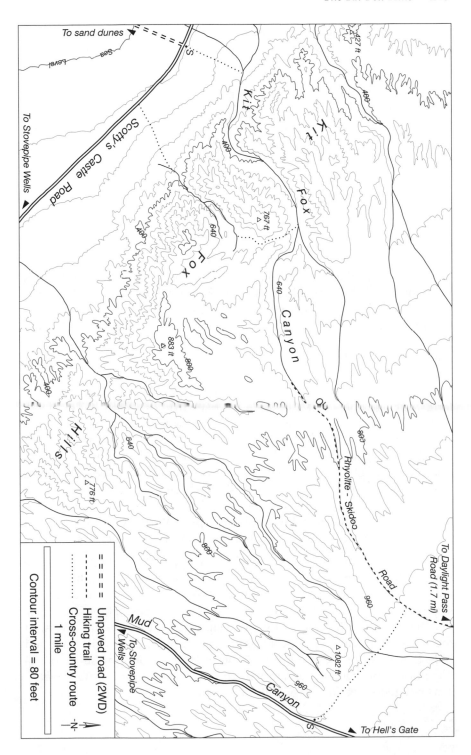

To sand dunes

Sea Level

Scotty's Castle Road

To Stovepipe Wells ▶

Kit

Fox

Kit

Fox

Canyon

Hills

Canyon

Mud

427 ft

400

400

400

640

767 ft

640

800

883 ft

400

400

640

776 ft

800

800

880

960

960

960

1082 ft

Rhyolite - Skidoo

Road

To Stovepipe Wells

To Daylight Pass Road (1.7 mi) ▶

To Hell's Gate ▶

====== Unpaved road (2WD)
- - - - - Hiking trail
·········· Cross-country route

1 mile

Contour interval = 80 feet

-N-

not the Rhyolite-Skidoo Road, as inaccurately claimed by the sign, but probably a road used to build and maintain the telephone line.

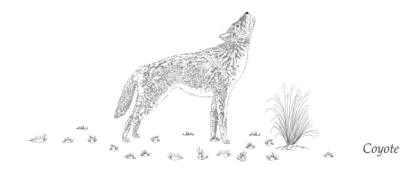

Coyote

The Rhyolite-Skidoo Road. This slightly longer, scenic hike will take you along the remaining stretch of historical Rhyolite-Skidoo Road (now a foot trail), from its upper end at the Daylight Pass Road down through Kit Fox Canyon to the valley floor and the site of Stovepipe Well. The old road first rolls gently down the flat fan towards the Kit Fox Hills. Aside from a couple of gutted old cars stranded along the way, the highlights are the sweeping views and the desert pavement. With its scant, ghostly cover of desert holly, the fan composes a surreal landscape, reinforced by the dramatic backdrop of Death Valley. Here and in the Kit Fox Hills, you may come across forgotten Indian trails— pale and narrow paths worn into the dark pavement. Look also for rocks sliced by the heat or faceted by the wind (see *Stretched-Pebble Canyon*). The road goes all the way down to Kit Fox Canyon and about 1.2 miles into it. The remainder, except for a 40-yard segment below the canyon mouth, is gone. The site of Stovepipe Well is on the far side of the highway, 0.8 mile down the Historic Stovepipe Well Road. Today it is marked by a sealed well and a rusted pump on the edge of the sand.

Other hiking areas. Further north in the Kit Fox Hills there are many other interesting canyons, shorter but winding through colorful and scenic badlands. From the Historic Stovepipe Well Road drive the highway north and pick the area of your choice along the next 3 miles. Try the canyons with traces of white evaporites at their mouths. Most of them are short gulches winding into brown, pink, and white rounded hills. Some are sprinkled with small mesquite trees, offering small, oasis-like pockets of shade. After a rain there can even be a little surface water. This is a good area for a peaceful, easy stroll in the desert.

■

THE DEATH VALLEY SAND DUNES

> *A trip to Death Valley would not be complete without a visit to its beautiful sand dunes. There is something magical and primeval about these great expanses of sand that seems to touch everyone. Whether for a short stroll or a day-long hike, there is little need for a set goal. Your whim is your best guide.*

General Information

Road status: Roadless; easy access from paved or good graded road
Shortest hike: Strolls and short walks/easy
Longest hike: 6.6 mi, 300-500 ft one way (or more)/moderate
Main attractions: Sand dunes
USGS 15' topo map: Stovepipe Wells
USGS 7.5' topo maps: Grotto Canyon*, Stovepipe Wells, Stovepipe Wells NE, Mesquite Flat
Maps: pp. 252*, 239, 67

Location and Access

The Death Valley Sand Dunes cover a long crescent-shaped region bounded to the south by Highway 190, and to the east by the foot of the fan below Scotty's Castle Road. Although you can hike to them from just about anywhere along these roads, the most popular starting point is around the small interpretive sign on the north side of Highway 190, 2 miles east of Stovepipe Wells. Another popular, quieter starting point is the end of the Historic Stovepipe Well Road, which starts off Scotty's Castle Road 3 miles north of Highway 190.

Geology

Whereas most sediments are deposited by water, the main engineer of sand dunes is wind. Death Valley and the surrounding desert valleys, bounded by continuous alignments of high, parallel mountain ranges, rank amongst the world's greatest natural wind tunnels. Winds driven by high temperature gradients are funneled between these ranges, sometimes racing up the deep valleys between them at more than 80 miles per hour. Finer dust gets picked up and scattered over great distances, generating the great mushroom clouds that come with desert storms. The intermediate, sand-size particles that make up the dunes are displaced by a slightly more organized process called saltation: they bounce and skip along, only a few feet off the ground. This

247

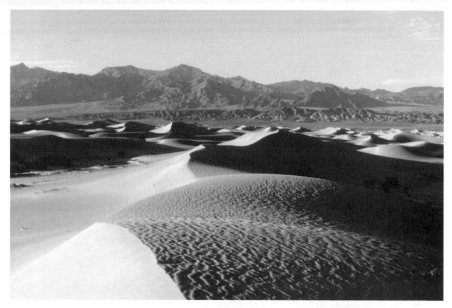

The Death Valley Sand Dunes in evening light

migration stops when the wind reaches an area where the local topography forces it to lose its velocity and to drop its burden of particles—over the same area, storm after storm, slowly building dunes.

Many first-time visitors to Death Valley, insisting on equating deserts with dunes, are surprised when they find out the entire valley is not buried in sand. By desert standards, Death Valley's sand dunes are quite modest, both in height and surface area. Several of the sandy deserts of the Sahara are larger than California. The main reason is not the lack of wind, as a single trip to Death Valley is likely to demonstrate, but the lack of an abundant source of loose sand particles. Although sand combines particles of vastly different compositions and origins, its primary building block is quartz, which resists weathering longer than any other mineral. There are plenty of quartz particles in Death Valley, but most of them are locked up in mud and salt on the valley floor, and by carbonates on the alluvial fans.

Nevertheless, there are several dune areas in and around Death Valley. The sand dunes near Stovepipe Wells cover by far the largest area. The quartz particles are thought to come from the fan of Marble Canyon and the Panamint Valley. The presence of dunes at this particular location has been explained by the abrupt widening of the valley north of Tucki Mountain. It causes local winds to spin off into eddies in the wind-shadow of the mountain. Eddies have lower velocities towards their center, where they drop their load of sand particles.

Dunes are differentiated by their shape, which tells something about their formation and migration patterns. The highest dune, composed of ridges rising to a peak, is a star dune. Barchan dunes, shaped like a crescent, are more common. They are formed when the wind blows constantly from the same direction, moving the sand on the edges of the dune faster than in its center. The two sharp ends of a barchan therefore point in the direction of the dominant wind. Another type of dune is the whaleback—a long, low cylinder of sand, produced at an angle to the prevailing wind. Parallel successions of whaleback dunes are also fairly common. Somehow, the complex process that continuously shapes these dunes is stable; the profile of the largest dunes changes little with time. On a human scale, they are as old as the hills. Yet they are clearly younger than the "hills" that are spawning them. On a geological scale, they are juveniles.

Route Description

The Death Valley Sand Dunes are one of the most popular hiking destinations in the park. Here as elsewhere, dunes provide a unique experience, stirring up emotions like few other landforms do. It has something to do with the simplicity of a landscape reduced to its most elemental components—sand and sky—with its harmonious forms and sensual rhythm. It can be a strange place, and its strangeness is pervasive. You may find yourself rolling in the sand, reverting to childhood games, crawling on hands and knees over fluid ground to stare at grains of sand inches away from your face. Out in the sand, while no one is watching, we all seem to become possessed by the same joyous spirits.

Although bare and simple, dunes have much to offer. Look for particularly unusual landforms—pristine stretches of sand, ripple patterns, simple sceneries oddly marred by one lone creosote. The vegetation is surprisingly varied (see *Mesquite Flat*). Inkweed, pickleweed, arrowweed, and mesquites grow on the sandy areas at the edge of the dunes, but only creosote and a few annuals manage to live in the higher sand. Look for circular arcs or even full circles surrounding isolated plants, inscribed in the sand by the tips of the plants as they are blown around by the wind.

Hardened playas of light-colored mud carpet the bottom of shallow sand troughs. Most of these troughs are miniature sinks, with no water outlet other than the thirst of the sand. Rainwater picks up silt from the sand and deposits it at the bottom of the sinks, where it accumulates as mud. The mud cracks upon drying, leaving behind a juxtaposition of nearly identical plates, as ornate as floor tiles.

Another fun thing to do is to try identifying animal tracks and burrows. Anything from beetles to lizards, snakes, birds, rodents, kit

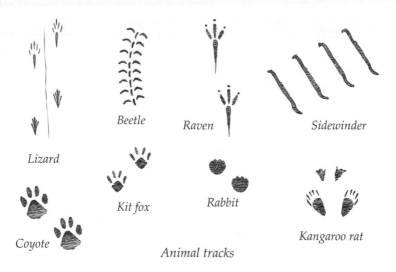

Animal tracks

foxes and rabbits leave marks in the sand. These cryptic messages are often the result of nocturnal activity and best preserved in the early morning. Among the greatest "finds" are the parallel stitches left by the sidewinder, the large imprints of road runners, the planned collision between a rabbit and a coyote. Keep an eye open for wildlife, especially in the early morning.

Dust and sand storms are relatively common in this area. They can be impressive, blotting out sunlight to a yellowish gloom, reducing visibility to just a few yards. During summer sand storms, the combination of heat and sand blasting can definitely be a negative experience. Yet if you do it right, a storm can also be a good opportunity to experience nature—and saltation—at work. Take plenty of water, a scarf, and light pants to protect your legs. In the worst gales, sit down facing away from the wind, wet your scarf, cover your mouth and nose with it, and wait it out. Or drive out towards Hell's Gate or Towne Pass to observe

The Death Valley Sand Dunes		
	Dist.(mi)	Elev.(ft)
Highway 190 at interpr. sign	0.0	0
Summit of tallest dune	1.1	~80
Stovepipe Wells Campground	0.0	-10
Summit of tallest dune	2.2	~80
Stovepipe Well	6.6	-50

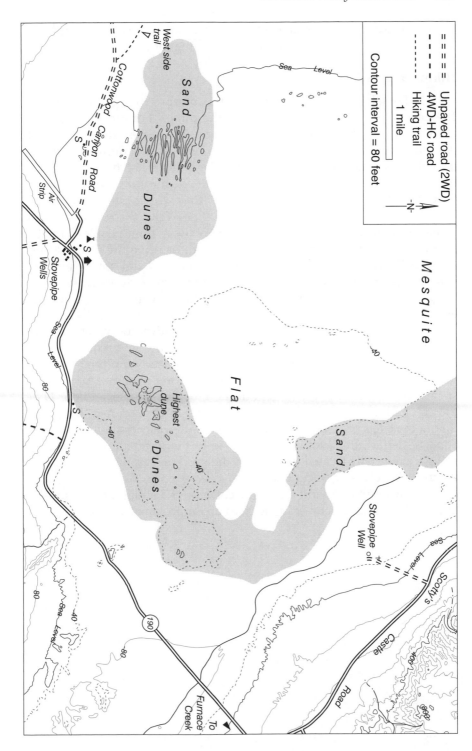

the storm from above. You'll see great plumes of dust reaching hundreds of feet up in the air, obscuring everything for miles.

Hiking Suggestions

For a leisurely walk, start from the interpretive sign on Highway 190 and take a random walk through the dunes. For a more vigorous workout, tackle the obvious local challenge—the highest dune. On a hot day it can be a frustrating climb, but the views are wonderful and you'll bring back a great crop of photographs. For another notch up in difficulty, do the same thing starting from the south end of the Historic Stovepipe Well Road off Scotty's Castle Road; this route is much less crowded. You can also continue to Stovepipe Wells; the round trip can be easily done in a day. If you want to stay away from people, hike the smaller dunes northeast of the campground, or drive the Cottonwood Canyon Road (see *Upper Marble Canyon*) about 1.7 miles and hike the small dunes north of the road. For a view of the main dunes from above and great zoom photography, try the Grotto Canyon Road. To see the entire sweep of dunes, start from Palm Spring (see *Mesquite Flat*) and follow the back side of the dunes all the way to Stovepipe Wells—a long day hike.

The best times to see the dunes are very early morning and just before sunset, when the deeper colors and long shadows produce a spectacular landscape. Try to get out there before sunrise; an hour later the colors and contrast are past their prime. In the summer, be aware that in the late afternoon the air can be scorching, especially if it's windy. Sand heals fast, but avoid walking close to the vegetation, where burrows are normally located. Also avoid the mud playas; they damage easily and take forever to recuperate.

Given that in sand dunes the concept of a straight line is murky at best, the distances shown in the chart are approximate.

■

NEVARES SPRINGS AND NEVARES PEAK

> *This hike will take you up a long alluvial fan to the old Cow Creek Ranch, where Dolph Nevares settled a homestead in 1900 and used the abundant spring water to support a small ranch. His wood cabin still stands next to the colorful springs, in full view of Death Valley. Dedicated hikers can ascend nearby Nevares Peak for spectacular views of the Furnace Creek area.*

General Information

Road access: Hiking from paved road
Shortest hike: 5.3 mi, 1,630 ft one way/moderate
Longest hike: 9.0 mi, 3,650 ft one way/difficult
Main attractions: Well-watered springs, Nevares Cabin, a peak climb
USGS 15' topo map: Chloride Cliff
USGS 7.5' topo maps: Beatty Junction, Nevares Peak*
Maps: pp. 257*, 103

Location and Access

Nevares Springs is at the western foot of Nevares Peak, in the central Funeral Mountains. The most direct route to it, via the Cow Creek Road and Nevares Springs Road, crosses the Park Service residential area and a firing range. Both areas are off limits. Do not drive or hike that way. Instead, start from Highway 190 1.7 miles north of the Cow Creek turnoff (or 6.0 miles south of Beatty Junction), which is due west of BM -254.4. The suggested route goes up the wash east of this point. Before going on this hike, you should contact the National Park Service to let them know you are planning to be out there. As a courtesy, it is a good idea to let the rangers and residents know you are coming.

History

Nevares Springs is at the heart of a historical homestead once known as Cow Creek Ranch. Central to its history is Adolph Nevares, known as "Dolph," a soft-spoken prospector, farmer and rancher who first came to the California desert in the late 1890s. Then in his mid-twenties, he worked for a few years as a driver and handyman out of Daggett for the borax companies. In his own words, Death Valley was then viewed as "a land to be shunned," but like many others he was eventually drawn to it. His first contact with Death Valley was in August 1900, when he participated in the much-publicized search for

253

Jim Dayton undertaken by the Pacific Coast Borax Company. Dayton was caretaker of the Greenland Ranch (now Furnace Creek Ranch), then run by the borax company. He had been missing for several days, and Nevares volunteered to help find him. Although the rescue was a failure—Dayton was found dead near Eagle Borax Works—upon his return from this heroic trip Nevares was offered Dayton's job by the borax company. Greenland Ranch then consisted of only a large adobe house, a barn, corral, and alfalfa field, so remote that the monthly mail stage was a local source of excitement. But Nevares loved the desert. He took the job, and stayed in Death Valley for the next 52 years.

During his long involvement here, Nevares lived at Cow Creek Ranch near the springs that now bear his name, a few miles from Greenland Ranch. He bought a cabin from a nearby mining town, carted it away and rebuilt it at its present location. For a few years after his new appointment, the ranch was co-owned by Nevares and M. M. "Old Man" Beatty, who periodically came here with his family. Even then the ranch was well known for its hot spring, fields of alfalfa, and well-irrigated garden. Nevares became sole owner of Cow Creek after Beatty's death around 1908, receiving title to the 320-acre property from the government as patented land.

For many years the springs on Nevares' homestead attracted ambitious entrepreneurs who coveted their abundant water for less organic purposes. Offers were made to use them to generate electricity for the Bullfrog mines, then to operate stamp mills for the Echo Canyon mines, but none of these plans came through. Right in the middle of Death Valley, Nevares enjoyed the luxury of tap water, a hot spring, and well-irrigated plots where he grew apricot and fig trees, beans, peppers, melons, and squash. He even had a small vineyard. His time was split between tending his ranch, his caretaker job, and indulging in prospecting when a new boom came along. Over the years he witnessed the gradual evolution of Greenland Ranch from a small rest area that supplied food to the mules and workers of the borax company, to a life-saving oasis that welcomed prospectors and miners, and ultimately to the tourist center now known as Furnace Creek Ranch. In 1942, at age 70, he was forced to retire by the borax company, lied about his age, and took a new job as gardener at Monument Headquarters. During his final years in Death Valley, Nevares negotiated the sale of Cow Creek with the Park Service, which planned to use the springs' water to support the burgeoning tourism industry. The homestead was purchased and added to Death Valley National Monument in 1949. Nevares retired three years later and returned to his birth place in San Bernardino. "Often I get mighty homesick of Death Valley," he reflected. "Wish I had time to relive every day of it."

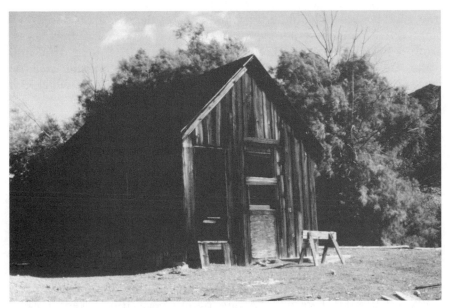

Nevares Cabin

Hydrology

With a combined flow around 330 gallons per minute (gpm), Nevares Springs are the second largest spring in Death Valley after Travertine Springs, located a few miles away near the mouth of Furnace Creek Wash. Its flow is about 2,000 gpm. Texas Spring, just east of Furnace Creek Ranch, ranks third with around 220 gpm. Considering the extreme aridity of the region, these rates are anomalously high. The reason is, of course, that the water is coming from elsewhere. Analysis of the springs' chemical composition suggests that the main source of water is Ash Meadows, 25 air miles east and 1,250 feet higher, which is thought to be replenished by the much larger aquifer under Pahrump Valley, another 25 miles to the southeast. Water travels along fractures to and through the permeable carbonate rocks of the southern Funerals until it is intercepted by high-angle faults in the Furnace Creek Fault Zone and channeled down the gravels of Furnace Creek Wash. There it flows over the impermeable layer of mudstones under the gravels, until this layer intersects the surface at the toe of the fan and forces the water to emerge in a line of springs.

Bedrock travel is slow. The water you see flowing out at Nevares or Travertine springs today may have started its journey several centuries ago. Along the way, it dissolved large amounts of carbonates, which precipitated over time near the springs to form huge travertine terraces. The underflow circulated at depths of 1,000 to 2,000 feet, which explains its temperature. Year-round, Nevares Springs is around 100°F. Despite its high fluorine content, it is good drinking water, and it has been used for years to supply the residential area. A few springs have been left untapped for the bighorn sheep, which do come here frequently, usually in the early morning.

Route Description

Nevares Springs. From the highway walk up to, then through, the wide gulch in the hills due east of you. The head of this short gulch is marked by a wind-carved sandstone ridge on the south side, and a green bluff across it (a good landmark when you return). From here, the shortest route is east-southeast to the western base of Nevares Peak, where Nevares Springs are located. However, this route is quite tedious because it crosses the fan diagonally and requires climbing in and out of many ravines. An easier route is eastward up the very wide wash for 2.5 miles (it angles southeast after 1.4 miles), then south across the fan to the springs (0.9 mile), betrayed by their palm trees. Honeysweet, desert holly, and creosote are common along this route, as well as desertgold, phacelias, gravelghost and desert five-spot in the spring.

The springs are scattered at the base of a wide travertine bench. Nevares' old wood cabin, a short distance below it, is shaded by a huge athel tamarisk. It is a good place to rest from the heat, as there is no shade on the way here. The small sunken wood structure next to it is a root cellar. The surrounding area shows numerous signs of past human activity, including the broad terrace below the cabin, which Nevares graded for his garden. In historical times, the original seeps and springs were consolidated by ditches into a small creek. This creek flows out into the narrow trench lined with vegetation just south of the cabin. The top of the travertine bench is densely covered with typical desert spring vegetation—salt grass, cane, mesquite trees—as well as a few alluring

Nevares Springs and Nevares Peak		
	Dist.(mi)	Elev.(ft)
Highway 190	0.0	-215
Leave wash and head south	4.2	1,130
Nevares Springs	(0.9)	~940
Nevares Cabin	(1.1)	850
Saddle	6.9	2,780
Nevares Peak	7.9	2,859

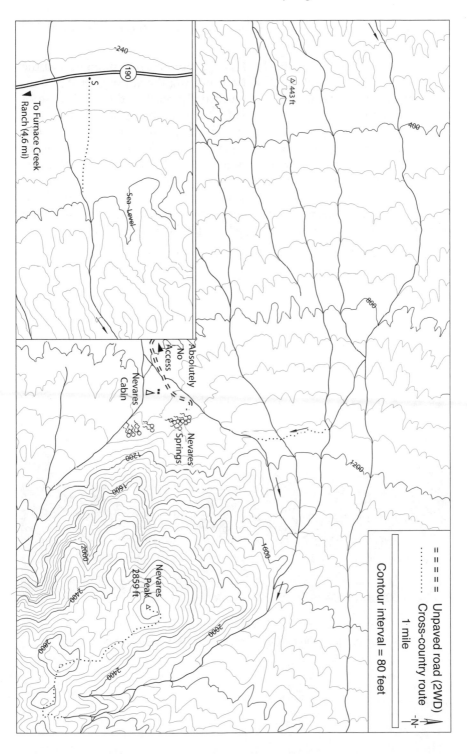

To Furnace Creek
Ranch (4.6 mi)

190

Sea Level

443 ft

400

800

No
Access

Absolutely

Nevares
Cabin

Nevares
Springs

1200

1200

1600

1200

2000

1600

2000

Nevares
Peak
2859 ft

2400

2800

2400

2000

=====   Unpaved road (2WD)
....   Cross-country route

1 mile

Contour interval = 80 feet

-N-

palm trees and other exotics. Avoid walking on the soft, salt-crusted ground or near the fragile plants.

Nevares Peak. Nevares Peak is the looming mountain east of the springs. If you want to climb it without visiting the springs, continue up the same wash (east-southeast). It eventually reaches the north base of the peak, circles around to its east side, then climbs up steeply to a saddle southeast of the peak. It is then a short scramble along the crest to the summit. If you start from the springs, hike northeast to the north base of the peak and follow the same route. The views from Nevares Peak are quite spectacular, encompassing Furnace Creek Wash and Ranch, the badlands below Zabriskie Point, and the shimmering salt flats of Cottonball Basin. Don't forget to bring binoculars. This is a long day hike, best tackled in the spring when the days are longer.

■

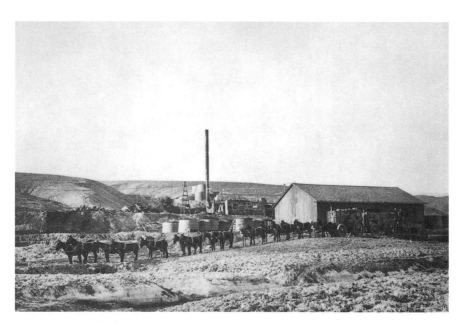

Twenty-mule team at Harmony Borax Works, circa 1885
(Courtesy of the National Park Service, Death Valley National Park)

HARMONY BORAX WORKS AND THE BORAX HAYSTACKS

> *These few hikes explore the area around Harmony Borax Works, one of the earliest borax industries in Death Valley. Take a short walk through the historical ruins of the small plant where the "white gold" of Death Valley was refined before being shipped out by 20-mule teams. Or go for a longer hike across the eerie salt flats to Cottonball Marsh, where the borax was harvested in neat rows of "haystacks," on the shore of the largest permanent lake in Death Valley.*

General Information

Road access: Hiking from paved or good graded road
Shortest hike: Short walks / very easy
Longest hike: 5.0 mi, 60 ft one way / easy-moderate
Main attractions: Harmony Borax Works, borax haystacks, salt pan
USGS 15' topo maps: Furnace Creek*, Chloride Cliff
USGS 7.5' topo maps: Furnace Creek*, West of Furnace Creek*, Beatty Jct
Maps: pp. 263*, 103

Location and Access

Harmony Borax Works is just off Highway 190, 1.4 miles north of the Visitor Center. You can also walk or bike to it from the Visitor Center on the paved trail along the west side of the highway. The borax haystacks are generally a couple of miles west on the valley floor.

History: Borax Mining and 20-Mule Teams

In spite of the excitement and glory surrounding gold and silver, the greatest wealth in the history of Death Valley mining was produced by a more prosaic mineral—borax. The first successful effort at mining, processing, and shipping this mineral took place in the 1880s. The original discovery was made in 1881 by Aaron and Rosie Winters. Aaron Winters was a miner with a background of unlucky finds, but this time he struck it rich. On the salt flats below Furnace Creek, he discovered boron ore, a combination of minerals now known as ulexite and probertite. The deposit looked so promising that he was soon bought out, reportedly for $20,000, by William Coleman, a prominent California industrialist who thus became one of the tycoons of Death Valley's "white gold."

In the winter of 1882, Coleman built a small refinery called Harmony Borax Works near the site of the discovery. Production started probably in 1883. Chinese laborers were hired to scrape the surface of the marsh, collect the ore into borax "haystacks," and haul it on sleds to wagons, then to the plant. The ore contained borax mixed with salts of little commercial value. Because markets were so far away, the operation could be profitable only if the ore was refined to reduce its weight and shipping costs. This was the purpose of Harmony. The plant had a large boiler fueled by mesquite wood from nearby groves, which heated water piped in from Texas Spring. The ore (sodium calcium borate) was mixed with sodium carbonate and dissolved in hot water tanks. After insoluble matter had settled and calcium carbonate precipitated, the solution was transferred to vats—the plant may have had as many as 57—with vertical crystallizing rods, where it was allowed to cool until borax (sodium borate) precipitated. At its apogee, the plant employed 40 men and produced 3 tons of crude borax daily. The process worked well, except that in the summer the temperature was so high the solution did not cool sufficiently for the borax to precipitate, and the plant had to shut down for the season. But Coleman was lucky. Another deposit was soon discovered at a higher location in the Amargosa Desert (along present-day Highway 127 near the junction to Tecopa Hot Springs). Coleman opened a second plant there, the Amargosa Borax Works, and summer operations were moved to that cooler location.

The greatest hurdle Coleman had to face was transportation. The nearest railroad was in Mojave, across 165 miles of largely waterless, roadless, and uninhabited desert. Initially, the ore was carried by 8-mule teams, until a 12-mule team was purchased and it was discovered that it could haul twice as much as eight mules. The concept of the 20-mule team emerged from this simple observation: hitched to two bulky wagons and a 1,200 gallon water tank, the 120-foot train was able to carry the capacity of half a railroad freight car. It is this awkward invention that spelled the success of Harmony. From the plant the train embarked on a 10-day trek across the salt flats to Eagle Borax Spring, out of Death Valley along Wingate Wash, then across the desert to Mojave. For five years, Harmony delivered about 20 million pounds of borax, a major portion of the country's supply. During this entire period the 20-mule teams did not experience a single failure, an accomplishment that has since been recognized as one of the world's most outstanding feats of transportation.

In 1888, because of fierce competition, a sharp drop in borax prices, and the collapse of Coleman's fortune, Harmony was forced to close down. Soon after, the property was acquired by Francis "Borax" Smith, but he owned richer deposits in the region and never reactivated Harmony.

Route Description

Harmony Borax Works. The ruins of Harmony Borax Works can be visited along a short paved foot trail. This little alchemist's den, with its rusted boiler, pipes, and crumbling adobe masonry, stands as a tribute to Coleman's ambitious enterprise. Just below the plant stood a large wooden barn and rows of cooling vats. On the flats below there was a small camp of wooden and adobe structures, including housing and a blacksmith's shed. The two adobe ruins by the road are all that remain. One of the original 20-mule team wagons is exhibited below the plant, still well-preserved after over a century of weathering.

If you want to see the type of terrain where the borax was mined, take the marked trail at the west end of the loop. In 0.3 mile it will take you to the edge of the salt pan. You can also continue along this trail around the hill behind the plant to Furnace Creek.

Borax haystacks and Cottonball Basin. The hike across the salt flats to the old borax workings is a Death Valley classic. To get to the starting point, drive the graded road 0.7 mile from Harmony to where it veers right into Mustard Canyon, and park.

Start in the wide wash below the canyon mouth, heading generally westward onto the vast depression ahead called Cottonball Basin. Along the first 50 yards, look for rocks imbedded in the gravel that have been neatly fractured into a stack of parallel slices, as if they had gone through a bread slicer. This is the work of salt. The likely mechanism is that salt dissolved in water infiltrates the rock. When the water evaporates, it leaves tiny crystals inside it. The heat of the sun expands the crystals, which induces small cracks and thus makes room for the salt to get in a little deeper the next time around. The process repeats itself, the cracks widening a little more each time until the rock breaks up. The cracks are parallel probably because they occur along weaker, parallel stress planes. These peculiar rocks are also quite common in the Coleman Hills, up canyon east of the highway.

The wash soon becomes completely covered with salt. It passes by a great assortment of weird, below-sea-level landforms, from fields of misshapen pinnacles to blistered salt crusts, salt flats covered with huge polygons, and buckled plates of salt and mud. Stay in the shallow washes to minimize damage.

The first borax workings are about 1.5 miles from the road. On a rainy year they may actually be flooded under the shallow lake that covers the bottom of the basin. This seasonal lake, with its scenic reflections of the mountains, is definitely a highlight. The borax mines are marked by small, geometric fields of haystacks, the small piles of mixed salts and mud that were raked from the surface. They were arranged either in parallel furrows, like small plowed fields, or in alignments of mounds, both typically 100 feet across. Some of them have been considerably worn down by flooding and rain, while others still stand a couple of feet high, carved into serrated pinnacles. The small, silky white clots lying on the ground are ulexite, the pay dirt mined in the past. Because of their appearance they are also known as cottonballs, the namesake of this area. Haystacks can be found at many locations all over the floodplain, for about 1 mile going either north or south.

Death Valley's borax haystacks are fragile historical remains. The soil around them is often quite muddy, and wherever you walk you will probably leave deep footprints that will take years, if not decades, to disappear. To minimize impact, please do not walk through the haystacks but stay a safe distance from them.

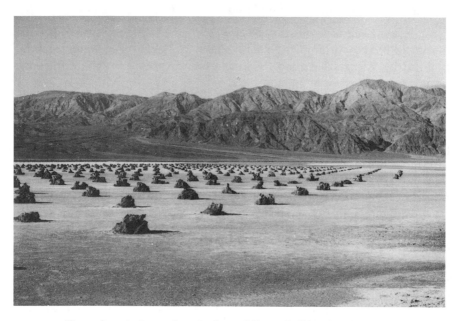

Borax haystacks on the salt flats of Cottonball Basin, circa 1960
(Courtesy of the National Park Service, Death Valley National Park)

If the temperature is right, this is an easy and delightful hike. Otherwise, get started very early in the morning and enjoy the bonus of a dramatic sunrise over the Panamints. Bring sunglasses (for the blinding salt) and binoculars (some haystacks can be spotted from a short distance into this hike). Keep an eye out for coyotes.

Mustard Canyon. After you return, take a short stroll along Mustard Canyon and the scenic mustard-colored hills it cuts through.

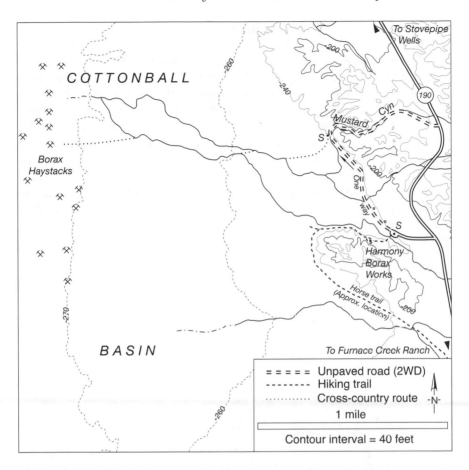

Harmony Borax Works and the Borax Haystacks

	Dist.(mi)	Elev.(ft)
Harmony Borax Works		
Parking area	0.0	-240
Harmony Borax Works	0.1	-220
Borax salt flats	0.4	~-250
Borax haystacks		
Mouth of Mustard Canyon	0.0	-220
Borax haystacks	~1.5	~-270

The rocks, probably from the Furnace Creek Formation, are fine-grained lake sediments deposited concurrently with evaporites. Evaporites actually permeate everything, and the land has been profoundly altered by these tiny crystals. The canyon walls contain so much rock-salt that they seem to be sprinkled with snow, and have developed ground features characteristic of salt flats. Throughout the canyon salt erosion has loosened the rocks and large portions of the walls have crashed in the wash. Erosion is in fact so active that you can actually hear it working. Even in the winter, walls exposed to the sun creak continuously as crystals buried within them heat up, expand and break. They produce unexpected sounds, like snapping twigs or light knocks on wood, loud enough to be heard from several yards away. In the middle of a hot summer day they can be strangely unsettling.

■

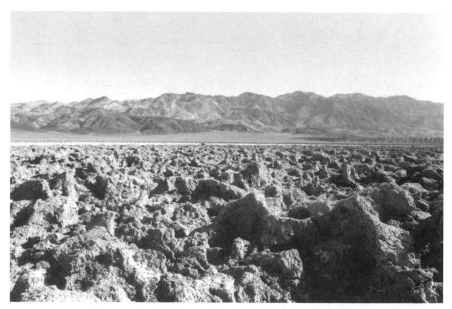

Salt pinnacles on the Devil's Golf Course

THE BADWATER BASIN

> *The Badwater Basin is the bottom of Death Valley, a blinding and barren desert of chemicals and mud left behind by a dying lake. It is an intriguing and magnetic place, and one of the weirdest hiking grounds anywhere. Somewhere out there you'll find small blue-green pools rimmed with shiny crystals, frozen rivers of salt, giant salt saucers, fields of sharp pinnacles creaking in the heat—landforms straight from the far side of Pluto.*

General Information

Road access: Easy access from paved or graded road
Shortest hike: Short strolls / easy
Longest hike: ~10 mi, 20 ft one way (or more) / moderate-difficult
Main attractions: Salt pan, salt formations, pools, springs
USGS 15' topo maps: Furnace Creek,* Bennetts Well,* Funeral Peak
USGS 7.5' topo maps: Devil's Speedway, Devil's Golf Course*, Hanaupah
       Canyon, Badwater*, Mormon Point, Gold Valley
Maps: pp. 269*, 393

Location and Access

      The Badwater Basin is Death Valley's lowest and largest basin. Its salt pan stretches roughly from the West Side Road south for about 17 miles, and the rest of the basin goes on for many more miles. One can hike into this vast area from anywhere along the West Side Road north of Johnson Canyon, or from the Badwater Road north of Mormon Point. The West Side Road is graded, and although it is a little rough at places, it is OK for all vehicles. Specific starting points are detailed below.

Plant Ecology

      Although the primary attraction of the Badwater Basin is its barrenness, one of its most interesting features is the unusual vegetation it supports on its periphery. Along the basin's west side, rainwater and snowmelt that have percolated down through the Panamints to the fan gravel encounter less pervious silt at the foot of the fan, which forces it to surface in a line of springs. Along good portions of the West Side Road, the water table is only 10 to 20 feet below the surface. The proximity of water and the presence of salt in the ground makes it a haven for phreatophytes (see *Mesquite Flat*), which cover extensive areas on the edge of the basin. Their distribution is dictated by the ground salinity, which increases towards the center of the valley (see *Geology* in *Valley Floor and Alluvial Fans*). Along the road, the most common plants are creosote, desert holly, and cattle spinach—plants that don't go all out for salt. Just east of the road, the dominant plants are mesquite trees, sometimes mixed with arrowweed and sacaton grass, which all tolerate a little salt. A little further east, where the soil is more alkaline, they are replaced by salt grass, tule, and rush. Pickleweed, the most salt tolerant plant, is the last one to give up. Along the entire west side of the basin it forms one huge pure stand, 0.2 to 2 miles wide, which coincides with the carbonate zone of the salt pan. The light brown ground just east of it, which is the sulfate zone, is completely barren.

The east side of the basin is considerably drier. Water surfaces only at a few small marshes and spring-fed pools like Badwater or Coyote Hole. Phreatophytes occur in limited numbers, mostly around these areas, except for pickleweed, which is fairly common.

Route Description

The West Side Road. This long, primitive road, which circumvents the west side of the Badwater Basin, offers a peaceful perspective of Death Valley, well worth the dusty, bumpy ride. Near its north end, where it crosses the salt pan, you can take a close look at the main types of terrain encountered on salt playas with minimal to no walking. It starts with large polygons of white rock salt delineated by fantastically shaped ridges, continues with the huge field of salt pinnacles known as the Devil's Golf Course, and finally crosses a featureless playa of compacted ground.

For many miles from here on south, the road parallels a long belt of mesquite trees, thickening to denser groves around four main springs: Tule Spring, Shorty's Well, Eagle Borax Spring and Bennetts Well. The springs have much in common: phreatophytes, at places small dunes and a little surface water. Eagle Borax Spring, with its green marsh of tule and rush covering over 40 acres and the small historic remains of Eagle Borax Works, is the most interesting. All along the road the striking contrast between the green vegetation, the empty basin, and the high mountain backdrop, produces spectacular scenery. The best way to see this area is to hike from Tule Spring to Bennetts Well, a route that encompasses the main springs. Or hike the salt pan from Tule Spring, where a track reaches out onto the sulfate zone for 0.6 mile—a longer, wilder approach than from the east side.

Shoreline Butte. Though not part of the basin, Shoreline Butte tells an interesting story about its evolution. For this short hike, start at the sharp bend near the south end of the West Side Road. Shoreline

Butte is the massive hill to the south. Walk on the old West Side Road (now closed to motor vehicles) about 1.2 miles to the foot of the butte. On your approach, notice how the butte's north face is conspicuously striated with long horizontal terraces. When Lake Manly began evaporating 11,000 years ago and slowly dried up over the next 1,000 years, it did so in stages, staying at a fixed level decades at a time. The terraces on the hillside are beach cliffs etched by waves lapping at the lakeshore. They mark the lake's successive stable levels. From the base of the butte, climb this giant stairway of about 25 terraces. The highest and most prominent shoreline is about 480 feet up—it was quite a deep lake! Similar shoreline sequences occur on the other side of the valley. Today, the west-side sequences are about 100 feet lower than the east-side sequences, showing that in just 10,000 years, downfaulting has deepened the valley by at least this much.

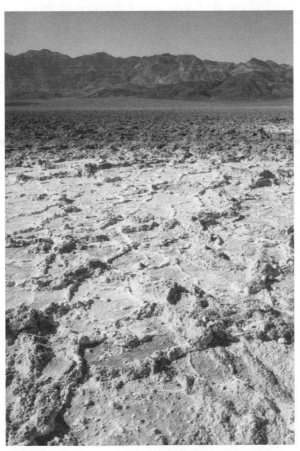

Polygonal salt patterns on the Devil's Golf Course

Shoreline Butte is an old volcano that erupted about 1.5 million years ago when basaltic lava crept up a fault (part of the Southern Death Valley Fault Zone) to the surface. Since then, lateral movements along it have slowly wrenched the butte apart, creating the steep-walled canyon on the butte's northwest side. A more dramatic effect of these tectonic motions can be seen at the much smaller volcano called Cinder Hill, about 0.8 mile north along the road. Since it erupted 700,000 years ago along the same fault, its eastern half has been transported some 600 feet southeast, and it is now neatly bisected into two hills. The gap between them is sitting right on top of the still active fault.

The Devil's Golf Course. With its fields of jagged pinnacles stretching out as far as the eye can see, the Devil's Golf Course is one of the most unusual landscapes around. Up to 2 feet high, the pinnacles are made of silty halite. What got them started is not fully understood, but what keeps them going is ground water that comes up through them by capillary action and leaves behind a little salt upon evaporation. Rain and wind prevent the pinnacles from growing too tall, trimming their tips to razor-sharp points.

The Devil's Golf Course extends in an irregular band from a little north of the West Side Road to several miles south of it. The two easiest points to start hiking into it are the northern part of the West Side Road and the Devil's Golf Course Road. Walking in this kind of terrain is awkward. The pinnacles are so densely packed there is not always enough room between them for a whole foot, and hobbling out there for more than a few minutes gets tedious. Salt crystallizes here in all kinds of pretty shapes—paper-thin tubes, clusters of cubic crystals, or delicate fibrous crystals growing inside small cavities. You may also find golf balls out there, the wrongdoing of occasional golfers who take the area's name a little too literally. If you head west far enough from the Devil's Golf Course Road, the pinnacles give way to a smooth playa covered

The Badwater Basin		
	Dist.(mi)	Elev.(ft)
Badwater	0.0	~-278
Lowest point in hemisphere	3.3	-282
Tule Spring	6.9	-253
Badwater	0.0	~-278
Devil's Golf Course Road	4.7	-277
Salt Creek at the West Side Rd	9.6	~-276

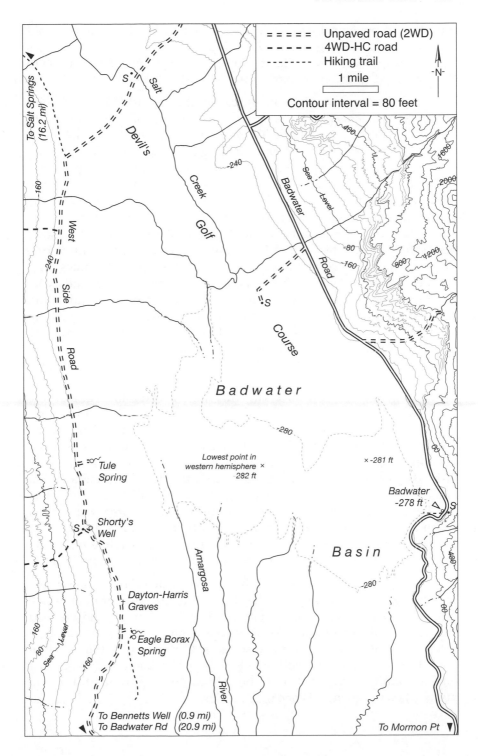

Unpaved road (2WD)
4WD-HC road
Hiking trail
1 mile
Contour interval = 80 feet

-N-

To Salt Springs
(16.2 mi)

S

Salt

Devil's

Creek

Golf

West

Side

Course

Road

Badwater

Road

Sea Level

240

160

240

80

160

Badwater

Lowest point in
western hemisphere ×
-282 ft

× -281 ft

Tule
Spring

Shorty's
Well

Badwater
-278 ft

S

Basin

Dayton-Harris
Graves

Amargosa

-280

Eagle Borax
Spring

160

Sea Level

80

160

River

To Bennetts Well   (0.9 mi)
To Badwater Rd   (20.9 mi)

To Mormon Pt

400

1600

2000

1200

800

400

with typical polygonal ridges. The ridges are just high enough to hold rainwater within the polygons, covering them with fresh salt crystals when it evaporates. If you like it here, try a longer hike, for example to Badwater, to the -282-foot point, or to the West Side Road.

Badwater. This place has character: it is almost the lowest point in the western hemisphere, the driest area in the nation, and, quite probably, the hottest spot on Earth. To experience what heat is all about try stepping out of your car here on a scalding July afternoon. The little salt pool is unfortunately a popular spot. In recent years, it has been considerably damaged by bus loads of visitors taking the obligatory stroll around it, which all but wiped out the poolside vegetation. Walk the short trail onto the salt pan instead, and stay away from the pool.

For a longer hike, try to reach the lowest point in the western hemisphere (-282'). It is located 3.3 air miles away, about 1° south of true magnetic west. The second lowest point (-281') is closer (1.6 miles, 341° magnetic bearing). The trouble is there are no landmarks to guide you. Unless you use a global positioning system, you are never quite sure when you get there, although with a pedometer and a compass you can get pretty close. From either low point you can continue towards the west side of the valley, possibly as far as Tule Spring.

Along this route, you'll first cross an immense smooth playa, then a chaotic field of salt "saucers" on the edge of the flood plain, a couple of miles out. Here the thick salt crust has buckled into large slabs up to 10 feet across, their edges curled up like saucers. Going further gets tricky. As unlikely as it seems, the main problem is water. Parts of the flood plain are always a little wet. In normal years, you will sink ankle deep in sticky mud-salt brine for up to a whole mile before hitting firm ground again. In wet years, you may run into a lake deep enough that you'll have to swim or use a canoe to get across! In *A Wolverine is Eating My Leg*, Tim Cahill relates a personal mishap in this area. For a good laugh and appropriate warning, read him first if you are dreaming of crossing to the far side. Wear shoes you aren't emotionally attached to, since they may be much the worse for wear by the time you are through.

A few words of caution. Much of the Badwater Basin has extremely fragile ground. Although it is hard to walk here without doing some kind of damage, take pride in minimizing it. Walk on ground the next rain is likely to smooth out. Avoid stepping on pinnacles or sharp salt ridges, as well as wet or crunchy surfaces. Camping is not allowed on the salt pan or along the West Side Road. This does not mean you can't take a midnight stroll out onto the salt pan on a glorious full moon night, when the eeriness is one notch eerier.

■

SARATOGA SPRING

Saratoga Spring, at the remote southern tip of Death Valley, is a nice little area to explore leisurely. The spring itself, with its cluster of ponds fringed with billowing fields of reed, is one of the prettiest in the park. Peaceful hikes along old mining roads will take you to the interesting remains of several historical talc mines in the nearby hills. For many visitors the area's highlight may well be the Ibex Dunes, strangely beautiful in their secluded setting.

General Information

Road access: Access via good graded road
Shortest hike: Short walks/easy
Longest hike: 9.3 mi, 1,000 ft loop (or more)/moderate
Main attractions: Saratoga Spring, talc mines, Ibex Dunes
USGS 15' topo map: Avawatz Pass
USGS 7.5' topo maps: Old Ibex Pass*, Saddle Peak Hills
Maps: pp. 277*, 159

Location and Access

Saratoga Spring is at the extreme southern tip of the Ibex Hills, near the southern boundary of the park. The easiest way to get to it is to drive Highway 127 from Shoshone south for 26.2 miles to the Harry Wade Road on the right. Continue on this mostly graded road 5.9 miles to the Saratoga Spring Road on the right. This road will take you in 2.7 miles to a junction (referred to, for convenience, as the Saratoga Junction). The Saratoga Spring Road goes left and ends at the spring in 1.3 miles. This route is well marked and easy with a standard-clearance vehicle (the only minor difficulty is the foot-high bank at the Amargosa River crossing). The other approach is from the other end of the Harry Wade Road, at the Badwater Road. It is then about 25.7 miles to the Saratoga Spring Road. Good clearance, if not 4-wheel drive, is needed for this route, especially at the river crossing about halfway through.

History: Mining Nitrates, Gold, and Talc

Although tucked away in a far corner of Death Valley, the Saratoga Spring area stimulated a lot of interest in its days, and over a period of some 80 years it acquired quite a colorful history. Before it got off to the right start, however, it witnessed two of the most pointless rushes Death Valley ever saw. The first one was the Amargosa niter rush. Although nitrates were first reported in the region as early as 1892, what touched it off was a 1902 report from the California State Mining Bureau identifying some 32,000 acres of rich niter beds. The choice grounds included low hills around Saratoga Spring, the Confidence Hills, and the Avawatz Mountains. By early October 1902, hundreds of people were on the scene or on their way to it. Many of those who made it there didn't even get a chance to stick a shovel in the ground. A week later the Geologic Survey denounced the futility of mining a cheap commodity like niter in such an inaccessible place. This announcement, combined with the bitter realization of the remoteness and low grade of the deposits, spelled out the end of the frenzy.

It still took 20 years before it completely died out. Over time, several skeptical government agencies and companies periodically came back to search for nitrates. In 1907 the Pacific Nitrate Syndicate and the American Niter Company were running tests in the area, rekindling grossly exaggerated reports from local newspapers. Two years later, the Pacific Nitrate had enough miners that a small camp was established at Saratoga Spring. Testing continued off and on until 1916, the main conclusion of each study being that further studies were needed. What finally put an end to it all was an authoritative report published in 1922 by the renowned geologist Levi Noble. He confirmed the presence of several large nitrate deposits in the region, but concluded that even "the richest is too scarce to be exploited commercially."

The second failed mining spree happened around 1907 and had to do with gold. Someone came up with the theory that since the Death Valley mountains appear to be full of gold, enormous amounts of gold must have been washed down to the valley floor by erosion. A sound concept, except for one detail: gold traveling downhill breaks down into fine particles and gets dispersed in enormous amounts of material. The only gold that could reasonably be expected in the valley fill was gold flour too diluted to mine. The primary advocate of this theory was a Rhyolite prospector named Clarence Eddy, also known as the poet-prospector. Another proponent was F. L. Gould, a prospector from Reno. In a local newspaper, Eddy claimed that it was to be the bonanza to end all bonanzas. There was enough gold beneath the desert floor that "all the world will be rich, and gaunt poverty will cease its weary journey in the land." Fueled by this appealing fallacy, prospectors started filing valley floor gold placers in early 1907. For a couple of years Eddy and Gould, sometimes allies, sometimes in vigorous competition, combed the southern end of Death Valley. Each party filed thousands of acres of claims, drilled test holes all over, and had hundreds of samples assayed. But even the best samples contained minimal gold and silver flour, worth at most 2 dollars per ton of dirt. Their find did not impress

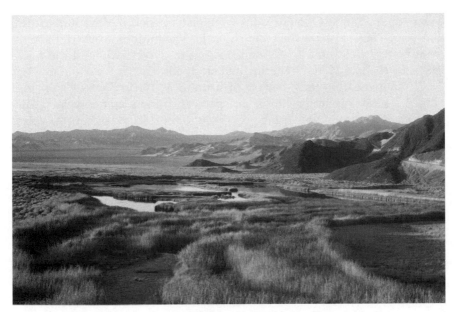

Saratoga Spring

anyone, least of all potential investors, and by the end of 1908 their dream had come to its predictable conclusion.

The irony of these two curious quests is that while a generation of prospectors was busily looking for imaginary niter and gold, the real bonanza—talc—was in full view all along, in the Ibex Hills. The presence of talc here was first recognized by Ernest Huhn in the mid-1930s, a few years after he and Louise Grantham discovered the huge talc lodes of Warm Spring Canyon. Huhn located a claim on the Pongo deposit, a few miles north of Saratoga Spring. Although he abandoned the property after sinking a shallow shaft in it, his find attracted others. In 1940 the Southern California Minerals Company opened the Superior Mine, a few miles south. It was the first of several mines the company would operate here over the next 20-odd years, but it turned out to be its bread and butter. The Superior deposit had the largest body of commercial-grade talc, and it produced up until the early 1960s. Between 1940 and 1959, its most productive years, it yielded 141,000 tons of talc, by far the largest production in southern Death Valley.

The other company mines did not fare quite as well. The Whitecap Mine, active between 1947 and 1951, yielded only 6,300 tons of talc. The Pongo Mine was put to work in 1948 and closed down seven years and nearly 13,000 tons of talc later. The last one, the Saratoga Mine, was developed in three stages. The northern group of mines, which had been worked for a year around 1944 by another company, was re-opened in 1949. New lodes were also opened in the south group that year. These also produced fairly little. The middle group did somewhat better, yielding a few thousand tons between 1955 and the mid-1960s. By the late 1960s all mining had stopped.

During this long period of human activity, Saratoga Spring played a vital role in the life of prospectors, miners and travelers. The first extensive use of the spring goes back to the 1880s. For several years the 20-mule-team wagons from the Amargosa Borax Works routinely stopped here for water and rest on their long journey to the Mojave Desert (see *Harmony Borax Works*). The springs were used again during the short-lived niter rush of 1902, in 1907-1908 by gold rush prospectors, then between 1909 and 1916 by parties exploring the Amargosa niter beds. At the time, a small town stood near the spring, consisting of a couple of stone houses, a large wood cabin, a springhouse, and several tents. Talc mining revamped the camp in the mid-1930s. During the entire life of the talc mines, water was trucked daily from the spring to the mines. Although the spring water was a little salty, it was drinkable, and it enabled a resourceful man to open a bottling business called the Saratoga Water Company. He also started a small tourist resort consisting of a few cabins, until war-time gas rationing killed both businesses. The area was abandoned in the late 1960s.

Geology

The central portion of the hills north of Saratoga Spring is essentially one massive tilted block made of a nearly complete sequence of three Middle Proterozoic formations collectively known as the Pahrump Group. Most of the west side is just one of them, the talc-bearing Crystal Spring Formation (see *Ibex Spring*). The local talc bodies are lenses located at the boundary of the conspicuous dark veins of diabase that intruded into the formation. All mining here was done by inclined shafts sunk into the tilted talc layers. Some distance down, lateral tunnels called drifts were excavated horizontally into the vein, generally in pairs, in opposite directions. When the drifts reached the edges of the talc zone, a second level of drifts was opened, deeper down the shaft, and so on until the shaft itself reached the end of the deposit.

Suggested Hikes

The easiest hike in the area is along the short trail on the east side of the spring, which provides close views of the ponds. There is also a small trail on the west side, but it dead-ends after a short distance. Please stay on the main trail to avoid trampling the sensitive spring soil and vegetation (and bugging the ducks).

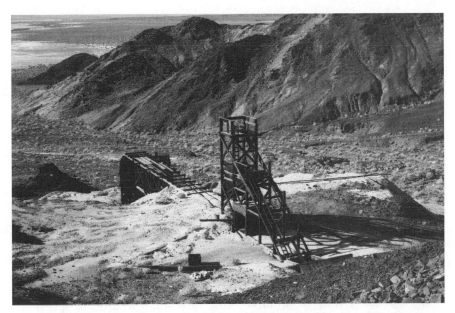

Headframe, loading dock, and ore bin at the Saratoga Mine (middle group)

There are several ways to visit the talc mines. None of them can be reached by car, although you can get fairly close by driving, even with standard clearance. The most interesting hike is up the road past the ponds to the Saratoga Mine; it's an easy half day. You can also continue on the same road to the Whitecap and Superior mines, and return via the road along the east side of the Ibex Hills. This loop takes a short day. An easier way to get to these two mines is to drive the east side road to the junction below the Superior Mine and walk up the old road from there (about two hours). For a very long day hike or an overnight hike, walk the long forgotten loop road around Old Ibex Pass (shown on the 15' map). It's about 17 miles, including side trips to all four mines.

Route Description

Saratoga Spring. This is one of the most amazing springs in Death Valley. With its large ponds and billowing fields of cane nestled on the edge of the immense valley floor, it is nothing short of a miracle. The water that feeds the spring rises along a fault at the foot of the hills and flows out along the strip of cane by the access road. It is impounded by the crescent of low sand hills visible on the north and west sides of the ponds. The ponds support a diverse wildlife. This area is known for its surprising variety of resident and migratory birds, including such unlikely critters as ducks, coots, and egrets. Bring binoculars, and approach the rise just west of the parking area quietly if you want to view the birds. You may also spot rabbits and coyotes, whose tracks abound. Pupfish (*Cyprinodont*) live in the ponds. They are similar to those found in Salt Creek, except that in 10,000 years they have evolved into a different species. To avoid disturbing wildlife, stay off the shores of the ponds (which are well guarded by thick vegetation anyway). The trail is lined with typical spring vegetation, in particular arrowweed, salt grass, and Cooper rush, which the Indians used for basketry.

The various camps that came to life here in the past were along the first 0.3 mile of the east side trail. Today, the ruins of two stone houses are all that remain. They were probably built in the 20-mule team days to serve as a saloon and a store. In 1909 the first one was used as a blacksmith shop by the Pacific Nitrate Syndicate.

The Saratoga Mine. The Saratoga has three groups of mines. The first mine north from the spring is the southern group. Its wooden chute and small tin shack are visible about 300 yards from the trail. The other groups are a little further, at the end of a right spur in the road (faint at first). Facing each other on either side of a small amphitheater, their well-preserved ruins are quite picturesque. The north group has an interesting two-chute ore bin. The disjointed metal ducts scattered around it were used to funnel the ore down from the workings directly above it. If you want to see talc, climb to them using the switchbacks past the ore bin. The talcose layer, around 300 feet long and as much as 10 feet thick, is exposed by a huge open cut and several shallow tunnels.

	Saratoga Spring	
	Dist.(mi)	Elev.(ft)
Road's end (Saratoga Spring)	0.0	220
Upper end of spring	~0.5	210
Junction (very faint)	0.9	190
Saratoga Mine (south group)	(~0.2)	310
Junction (faint)	1.2	180
Saratoga Mine (north group)	(~0.5)	490
Whitecap Mine junction	1.7	200
Pongo Mine	(2.1)	480
Whitecap Mine	2.7	310
Superior Mine	3.9	~720
Junction	4.6	510
Saratoga Junction	6.7	230
Road's end (Saratoga Spring)	8.0	220

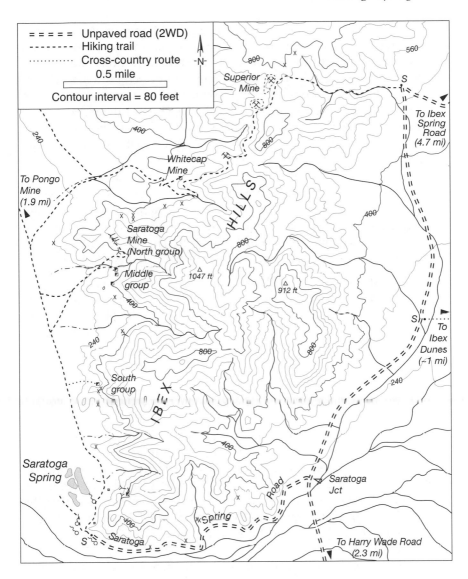

The middle group has the most interesting remains. Its tall wooden headframe was used to hoist the ore out of the 80-foot inclined shaft. The ore was dumped into the small ore bin beneath the hoist, and fed into a narrow-gauge ore car, which took it on the short set of tracks to the large ore bin at the tip of the tailing. The construction of this ore bin is unusual for Death Valley. Look for its X-shaped braces, and for the way it was unloaded into trucks that drove under it.

The Superior and the Whitecap Mines. The Superior Mine, scarred by last-ditch strip mining in the 1960s, has been cleaned up, filled in and graded, and no structures or adits remain. However, it has one impressive trench, maybe as much as 50 feet deep, cut directly into a thick talc layer. The old underground workings, which totalled more than 2 miles of tunnels, were located southeast of this trench, and extended underneath and well past the summit of the road. Perched at the crest of the Ibex Hills, this is still a scenic site, overlooking the vast salt-crusted delta of the Amargosa River. If you poke around you may find the rusted carcasses of old Southern California Minerals Company vehicles.

The Whitecap Mine, down the road from the Superior Mine, exploited a single talc lens, small and badly fractured, via a 200-foot inclined shaft with about 750 feet of drifts. The poorer northeastern end of the deposit was mined by shallow open pits. The most significant ruin here is a large wooden headframe, one of the best preserved around.

The Pongo Mine. The Pongo Mine, the most remote in this area, is nearly 4 miles up the east side trail from the spring—an easy walk. Most of its talc-bearing rock is of relatively low grade. The fairly small commercial-grade vein was mined by a 370-foot inclined shaft and about 600 feet of drifts. This site saw little development, and its ruins are minimal. The main attraction is certainly the lonesome hike to reach it, along colorful banded hills.

The Ibex Dunes. If you can, leave time to visit the Ibex Dunes. Isolated in a nearly enclosed valley, rising against the lunar scrags of the Saddle Peak Hills, they are truly beautiful, and hardly ever visited. Around sunset this whole area often turns to a dramatic fiery red.

For the shortest access, drive north from the Saratoga Junction until the road is closest to the dunes (1 to 1.5 miles), and hike from there. It is about 1.2 miles to the edge of the dunes. The loop connecting the three highest dunes and returning to this point is 2.5-3.0 miles. A longer (2.5 miles) approach is from the Harry Wade Road just west of the Saddle Peak Hills.

The Ibex Dunes sand comes mostly from local granitic and quartzite ledges and from the sandy wash of the Amargosa River. Because the dunes rest on a slope, they are very tall. From their western edge to the summit of the highest dune it is a 290-foot climb, more than twice as much as the Death Valley Sand Dunes. Some of the slopes are very steep, especially on the southernmost dune where at places they exceed 40°. It's a lot of slipping and sliding and fun, and you'll get a chance to take a peek at the two talc mines tucked behind the dunes.

■

DEATH VALLEY

This section describes a five-segment trek down the length of Death Valley. Each segment is short enough (30-40 miles) to make a great, 2 to 5-day backpacking adventure in the heart of Death Valley, with sumptuous views and plenty of solitude. Portions of these segments can also be singled out for day hikes. Much of this trek is nearly level, along dirt roads or old roads closed to vehicles, and fairly easy. In many ways this is the ultimate Death Valley experience: to meet the challenge of physical fitness and mental endurance it takes to cross one of the hottest places on Earth.

General Information

Road access: Hiking from paved, graded, or primitive roads
Shortest hike: ~33 mi, ~300 ft one way (or less)/moderate
Longest hike: 175 mi, 7,850 ft one way/difficult
Main attractions: Valley hiking and backpacking, grand views, solitude
USGS 7.5' topo maps: Last Chance Mtn, Tule Spring (Nev.), Sand Spring, Last Chance Range S.E., Ubehebe Crater, Tin Mtn, E. of Tin Mtn, Dry Bone Cyn, East of Sand Flat, Mesquite Flat, Stovepipe Wells, Grotto Canyon, Beatty Junction, East of Furnace Creek, Devils Speedway, Hanaupah Canyon, Badwater, Mormon Point, Anvil Spring Canyon East, Shore Line Butte, Confidence Hills W. & E., East of Owl Lake, Old Ibex Pass, Saddle Peak Hills
Maps: pp. 289, 67, 393, 159

Location and Access

The series of hikes suggested here covers the entire length of Death Valley, from its northern hydrologic boundary at the north end of the Last Chance Range to the southern tip of the Saddle Peak Hills. This very long route has been divided into five segments, each one starting and ending at a road that can be accessed with a standard-clearance vehicle. Remember that camping is not allowed on the valley floor from 2 miles north of Stovepipe Wells down to Ashford Mill.

Route Description

First segment: Cucomungo Canyon to Mesquite Spring. This segment begins at Cucomungo Canyon, at the north end of the Last Chance Range. Start hiking just before the sharp bend in the road past Willow Spring (usually reachable with a standard-clearance vehicle). Climb the

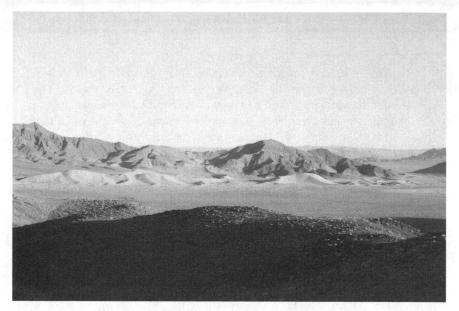

Ibex Dunes from the hills below the Superior Mine

old track south of the road to a low pass (elev. 6,070'), which is the very northern tip of Death Valley. On the far side, hike down into windy and desolate Last Chance Canyon to the upper end of the canyon road. For an interesting side trip, hike up the side canyon to the west (elev. 4,460') near here. In 1.8 miles it will take you to Last Chance Spring and its inviting cabin, a wonderful place to spend the night (see *Last Chance Mountain*). Otherwise hike down the road to the canyon mouth.

At the canyon mouth, leave the road and head across the open creosote desert southeast to Sand Spring (or hike the road to Crankshaft Junction, then the Big Pine Road, which not nearly as wild). Sand Spring has an open pool of water on the edge of small sand hills, but the water is contaminated by livestock and burros. Little Sand Spring, about 1.5 miles further, has a few mesquite trees but unreliable surface water.

From the road junction below Little Sand Spring, hike south on an old track, which is the north end of an abandoned segment of the Big Pine Road. It will take you to Death Valley Wash, which parallels the road less than a mile from it. After following the wash for about 7 miles, you will cross the road to Skookum, a small camp below the crest of the Last Chance Range that witnessed a short flurry of gold mining in 1926 and 1927. (For a long, out-of-the-way day hike or overnight trip, consider hiking this road from its start at the Big Pine Road to Skookum's old tunnels. It is 7.3 miles and 2,930 feet of elevation change one way.) Just beyond this road, you'll pick up the abandoned segment of the Big Pine

Road again. The next stretch is one of the highlights of this hike. The old road winds through rarely visited miniature badlands, a world of rounded hills and high walls eroded in whitish clay. This is the dry bed of Lake Rogers, a lake that filled this part of Death Valley in the Pleistocene. During this wetter era, mammals lived on the lakeshore, in particular horses and mastodons—the tusk of one of these elephant-like animals was recovered from these clay deposits.

The old road continues beyond the dry lakebed and ends near the Ubehebe Crater Road. The last leg of this journey is down Death Valley Wash to Mesquite Spring Campground.

Second segment: Mesquite Spring to Stovepipe Wells. Being the furthest from any road, this segment is by far the wildest. The first part of it is down the wide, silt and gravel bed of Death Valley Wash. Look for interesting animal tracks imprinted on the dry mud plates in the wash, especially in the weeks following a flood. At such times you may find small pools of water in the wash. The spectacular, high-reaching walls of the Cottonwood Mountains provide a scenic background all along this stretch. After 16.5 miles, below the wide mouth of Dry Bone Canyon, you will intersect the old west side trail. Follow this relatively well-defined trail south as it swings close to the foot of the Cottonwoods, then circles around the Niter Beds and the west side of Mesquite Flat. If time allows, explore one of the nameless canyons to the west. They are hardly ever visited, and some of them have great secrets in store. Much of what is to be seen along the trail is described in *Mesquite Flat*. At its south end the trail joins the Cottonwood Canyon Road 2.7 miles west of Stovepipe Wells. To avoid this road, leave the trail at the low sand dunes 1.5 miles before it and cross the dunes to Stovepipe Wells.

Third segment: Stovepipe Wells to West Side Road. Although this route partly follows the Stovepipe Wells-Furnace Creek transmission line, it is also quite wild, far from any road, and rarely hiked. From Stovepipe Wells, hike through the Death Valley Sand Dunes (to bypass Highway 190) and cross the highway at the foot of Little Bridge Canyon. To avoid the dense vegetation and critical pupfish habitat of Salt Creek, stay west of the Salt Creek Hills by following a contour line (~100 feet) around Tucki Mountain. South of the large fan of Trellis Canyon, descend to the edge of Cottonball Basin. The highlight of this segment is Salt Springs, at the easternmost foot of Tucki Mountain and just underneath the transmission line. These remote springs overlook Cottonball Marsh, which has a perennial lake. The field of salt pinnacles below the springs is the site of the West Side Borax Camp, also known as Shoveltown. Borax was mined here around the turn of the century. The site is marked by the weathered furrows of the borax works.

The rest of this route is along a trail that connects the Salt Creek Road to the West Side Road (no camping is allowed on the valley floor along this segment). It is faint and even missing at places. Use the transmission line as a guide, since it closely follows the trail, or cut across the fan of Tucki Wash to avoid it. This stretch is quite scenic, all below sea level and on the edge of the vast salt playa of Cottonball Basin. On a wet year, the shallow lake of the Cottonball Marsh can extend quite far south, and it adds unexpected reflections to this surreal landscape. About 7.4 miles south of the springs the transmission line angles sharply towards Furnace Creek. If you want to reach the ranch from here, remember that you'll need to cross Salt Creek. In the wet season the creek may have a few inches of water and be treacherous to ford.

The last part of this segment is along the Middle Basin. This area provides unusual views of the Black Mountains across the valley, including Red Cathedral and Manly Beacon. The trail remains at a nearly constant elevation of about -260 feet. Here as elsewhere, it is not always well-defined; just follow the foot of the fan. This segment ends at the sharp bend in the northern part of the West Side Road.

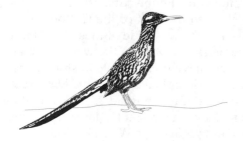

Roadrunners are prized encounters
in the low desert.

Fourth segment: West Side Road to Old Ashford Junction. This segment follows the West Side Road, and it is the least wild. Its main features, described in *Badwater Basin*, include the string of springs along the northern half of the road, and spectacular vistas of the salt pan and the Panamint and Black mountains. Along this entire route, camping is not allowed either on the valley floor or within 2 miles of the road. To visit the springs, you will need to hike down to them in the morning and hike back up the fan in the evening to camp. Consider camping part way up one of the canyon roads—they are easier to walk than the fans. South from Bennett's Well the springs are small and far apart, and it is best to stay away from the road. At the sharp left bend near the south end of the West Side Road, continue southeast along the abandoned southern extension of the road. You will pass by Shoreline Butte and its conspicuous lakeshore terraces, Ashford Mill, and finally join the Badwater Road at the old Ashford Junction (1.1 miles north of Ashford Junction).

Fifth segment: Old Ashford Junction to Highway 127. This south-ernmost segment parallels the Harry Wade Road, named after the Wade family, forty-niners who escaped Death Valley through here in 1849. Although this road is usually infrequently traveled, it is more interesting to hike along the Amargosa River, which remains close to it along this entire route. This beautiful hike will take you first through the Narrows, where the Amargosa River squeezes by the Confidence Hills. This long,

Death Valley		
	Dist.(mi)	Elev.(ft)
First segment		
Cucomungo Canyon	0.0	5,850
Last Chance Canyon Road	5.7	4,500
Sand Spring	15.0	3,160
Skookum Road	23.3	2,565
Lake Rogers (middle section)	26.7	~2,380
Ubehebe Crater Road	31.9	2,080
Mesquite Spring	37.3	1,780
Second segment		
Mesquite Spring	0.0	1,780
West side trail	16.5	230
Niter Beds (middle section)	21.5	110
Stovepipe Wells	36.2	5
Third segment		
Stovepipe Wells	0.0	5
Salt Springs/Shoveltown	15.0	-230
End of transmission line	22.4	-250
West Side Road	33.3	-260
Fourth segment		
West Side Road	0.0	-260
Tule Spring	5.6	-247
Bennett's Well	10.8	-255
Warm Spring Canyon Road	27.6	-244
Old Ashford Junction	33.1	-105
Fifth segment		
Old Ashford Junction	0.0	-105
Confidence Mill	9.5	-17
Road/river crossing	15.8	~30
Saratoga Spring	26.3	220
Highway 127 (via Ibex Dunes)	34.7	~475

eroded scarp, which reaches 700 feet above the river bed, was formed by tectonic movements along the Southern Death Valley Fault. Around the turn of the century famous mining failures occurred in this area, including the Amargosa niter rush (see *Saratoga Spring*) and the Confidence Mill. The mill was erected in late 1895 to treat gold-bearing quartz mined several miles up Confidence Wash to the north. The ore was so tough that little gold could be extracted, and operations were discontinued in early 1896. The mill site, in the bend in the road just past the Narrows, is dominated by the mill's concrete foundations.

Hiking the Amargosa River drainage is a unique desert experience. Remote and seldom traveled, it is a stunning area, alternatively crusted with salt and encroached in sand, surrounded by eerie mountains. The Amargosa River is one of the very few permanent valley streams in California's Basin and Range region. Incongruous in this parched land, it surfaces where bedrock is close to ground level and vanishes underground where gravel is deep. After heavy rains it turns to a muddy stream along good portions of its bed.

Towards the end of this segment, cut across to Saratoga Spring. Follow the road around the Ibex Hills, then hike cross-country to the southern part of the Ibex Dunes and over the dunes to the Saddle Peak Hills. At the talc mines an old road will take you across the hills to Highway 127—a spectacular conclusion to a majestic journey.

Logistics. A trip of this magnitude in Death Valley requires careful planning. Along this entire route the only reliable drinking water is at Mesquite Spring, Stovepipe Wells, and Furnace Creek Ranch. You will have to either carry or cache your own, or arrange for someone to drop off water and supplies (refer to *Water caching* in *Desert Hiking Tips*). The proximity of roads all along the valley makes caching relatively easy.

Choose your direction of travel carefully. Hiking downhill is easier and provides more spectacular views. However, remember that the prevailing winds come from the south. In the likely event of a wind storm, you will probably be forced to stop for several hours if you are headed south, but not if you are going north. In the winter, hiking south will keep you a little warmer. By hiking north you will not be staring towards the sun all day long, and in the summer your pack will provide some protection against the heat and light. The elevation is also an important selection parameter. With a mean elevation of 3,300 feet, the first segment is the best one for summer hiking, but in the winter it is noticeably colder than the other ones.

Much of this route crosses below-sea-level terrain where creosote bushes are the only source of what could pass for shade. The best time to do any portion of it is definitely fall to early spring.

PART VI

THE LAST CHANCE RANGE

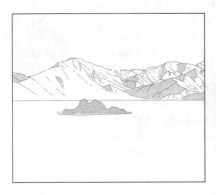

THE LAST CHANCE RANGE is the long and narrow range separating the extreme northern part of Death Valley from Eureka and Saline valleys to the west. It extends roughly north-south about 55 miles, from south of the Racetrack Valley to near the Nevada state line. With an elevation ranging from around 2,000 feet to above 8,500 feet, it is the third highest range in the park. Except towards its southern end, the elevation of the crest exceeds 6,000 feet along most of the range. The highest peaks are Dry Mountain (8,674'), Last Chance Mountain (8,459'), and Marble Peak (7,559').

Access and Backcountry Driving

The Last Chance Range is the least accessible range in the park. On its east side, the closest roads are the Racetrack Valley and Big Pine roads, both of which are unpaved and generally run several miles from the foot of the range. On its west side, it is paralleled by the Eureka Valley Road (graded) and its 4-wheel-drive southern extension along the Steel Pass corridor. The Last Chance Range is crossed at only two places, near its south end by the Lippincott Road, which connects the Racetrack and Saline valleys, and near its north end by the Big Pine Road. Although a little rough, in dry weather the Racetrack Valley Road can be driven with a normal clearance vehicle (see *The Racetrack Valley*). The Big Pine Road is graded, even partly paved, and a lot better. Only a few old mining roads give access to the interior of the range. The closest services and water, at Scotty's Castle and Big Pine, are nearly 80 miles apart. Come prepared. Bring plenty of water and food.

Mining History

Although the Last Chance Range was never heavily mined, the Racetrack Valley area, at the south end of the range, witnessed nearly a century of mining. The first metal discovered here was copper, in July 1875. Not much happened until the mid-1890s when several of the properties that had been claimed in the intervening years became increasingly active. The mines were mostly located on the slopes of Ubehebe Peak, on the low range between the Racetrack and Hidden valleys, and around the Dodd springs—places like the Ulida Mine, the Copper Knife, and the Blue Boy claims. For many years, their only access was a rough track through Saline Valley. The journey was so long and difficult that only the best ore could be shipped, and the rest of it had to be stockpiled. In spite of this hardship, by 1902 there were 80 copper, gold, and silver claims in the area, all within a 6-mile radius. Production probably remained minimal, although after 1904, when the price of copper started to increase, a few properties may have produced a little ore.

The era's most prominent figure was Jack Salsberry, who controlled some of the largest and richest claims. Salsberry had visionary plans. To open the area, he first completed a road from the Racetrack Valley up to the Montana railway station near Bonnie Claire, Nevada, via Tin Pass and Grapevine Canyon. In anticipation of a large production, he also negotiated with banking firms a 48-mile railroad extension from the Montana Station. The completion of the road in 1907 was probably the most significant contribution to the area's welfare. It provided improved access, sparked a new influx of miners, and allowed supplies to be teamed from Nevada. The other keystone in Salsberry's master plan was Salina City, a town just north of today's junction to the Ubehebe Mine, which would serve as the rail terminus and host the miners. A second site, Ubehebe City, was also targeted near the south end of the Racetrack, where Salsberry proposed to erect a smelter. The Ubehebe Mining District was created at the height of the copper boom, in the spring of 1907.

It is difficult not to admire the unwavering resolve—some might say foolish—of these early miners. Everyone took the venture very seriously. Surveyors were sent over to determine the best route for the railroad. At the site of Salina City, a 150-foot well was sunk in search of water, and arrangements were made for a hotel and other businesses. At one time the town had 20 tents, two saloons and a grocery store, and a post office was pending. By the fall of 1907, the area was so active that a coach service ran weekly between Bonnie Claire and Ubehebe City.

This heroic effort, as well as mining, continued feverishly until the middle of 1908, but Salsberry's dream never materialized. Soon after, perhaps as a result of the Panic of 1907, the investment banks interested in the area folded and the project died. In the following years, other rail-road propositions were discussed, in part to supply the large reduction plant in Ely, Nevada with the newly exposed lead and silver deposits of the Ubehebe Mine, but they never came through.

Over the next 50 years or so, with slowly improving transportation, intermittent work at the best mines did produce a little copper—an estimated 120,000 pounds. Yet it was lead and gold, not copper, that kept the district busy. The Ubehebe Mine, at the north end of the playa, began to show promising lead and silver veins around the peak of the copper era, and remained active, albeit sporadically, longer than any other mine in the district. Up until the 1960s, it produced about 1,300 tons of lead and 2,600 pounds of silver. The Lippincott Mine, at the south end of the valley, was active mostly between 1938 and 1952, and it became the third largest lead producer in Death Valley. The Lost Burro Mine, over in Hidden Valley, produced essentially all of the district's gold. These three mines were the district's only stars.

The area around Crater, in the northern Last Chance Range, boasts one of the largest sulfur deposits in the west. Discovered in 1917, it was mined from 1929 up until the 1940s and produced over 50,000 tons of nearly pure sulfur. Smaller-scale mining took place in the 1950s (with one notorious shutdown in 1953 after a mill was destroyed by a sulfur dust explosion) and continued sporadically until today. Mercury was also mined in the area, producing 115 pounds of quicksilver in 1968-1971. There is still quite a bit of both elements in the ground, which was the reason for the exclusion of the Crater area's patented claims from the park.

Geology

The vast majority of the Last Chance Range north of Ubehebe Peak is made of Paleozoic formations. Although most of this era is represented (Cambrian through Pennsylvanian), the most common exposures are from the Ordovician, Cambrian, and Devonian. Generally speaking, older formations (mostly Cambrian and Ordovician) dominate north of Marble Peak, and younger formations south of it. Although the stratigraphy is fairly complex, the formations are generally younger towards the west side of the range.

There are three main areas in the Last Chance Range where non-Paleozoic rocks are exposed. The first area, south from Ubehebe Peak, is composed largely of Jurassic granite from the Hunter Mountain Pluton. The second area is the southwestern tip of the range, where it juts into Saline Valley just east of the springs. This area is made of small exposures of granite and Pliocene basalt. Finally, Tertiary basalt and pyroclastic rocks are exposed on the east slope of the range facing Ubehebe

Suggested Hikes in the Last Chance Range				
Route/Destination	Dist. (mi)	Elev. change	Mean elev.	Access road	Pages
Short hikes (under 5 miles round trip)				
Big Dodd Spring	2.5	2,120'	~4,300'	Graded	325-326
Copper Bell Mine	0.6	230'	4,100'	P/21.9 mi	305
Corridor Cyn (first narrows)	1.5	460'	3,690'	P/22.6 mi	307-308
Grandstand	0.3	0'	3,710'	P/25.1 mi	312
Last Chance Spring loop*	0.8	480'	5,700'	P/3.5 mi	291-292
Lippincott Mine from					
Bonanza claim	2.5	1,230'	3,170'	P/4.4 mi	325
Homestake Dry Camp*	4.2	1,140'	3,870'	P/29.1 mi	328
Little Dodd Spring	2.1	1,580'	~4,400'	Graded	325-326
Racetrack moving rocks	<1.0	0'	3,710'	P/27.1 mi	313
Sally Ann Mine	1.6	390'	3,910'	P/27.1 mi	314-316
Ubehebe Mine and camp	<0.5	<100'	3,920'	P/22.6 mi	303-304
Ubehebe Mine (upper)	0.4	240'	4,040'	P/22.6 mi	304
Intermediate hikes (5-12 miles round trip)				
Copper Queen No. 1 Mine	3.1	1,290'	4,310'	P/25.1 mi	318-319
Copper Queen Mine	3.2	2,510'	4,280'	P/25.1 mi	318-320
Copper Giant No. 3 Mine	0.6	200'	3,830'	P/25.1 mi	314
Dry Mountain (to fossil area)	6.0	2,630'	4,910'	P/6.7 mi	295-297
Last Chance Mountain	2.6	2,900'	7,200'	P/3.5 mi	294
Racetrack to Blue Jay Mine	3.9	3,250'	4,080'	P/25.1 mi	318-322
The Corridor	3.8	1,050'	3,400'	P/22.6 mi	307-310
Ubehebe/Copper Bell mines*	2.6	~1,100'	4,000'	P/22.6 mi	305
Ubehebe Peak	2.8	2,020'	4,580'	P/25.1 mi	318-319
Long hikes (over 12 miles round trip)				
Corridor Canyon (mouth)	7.7	2,000'	2,920'	P/22.6 mi	307-310
Dodd Spring trail	6.8	3,940'	~4,200'	Graded	325-328
Dry Mountain to 80-ft fall	7.2	3,160'	5,200'	P/6.7 mi	295-297
Dry Mountain	10.5	5,100'	6,180'	P/6.7 mi	295-298
Skookum Mine	7.3	2,930'	3,860'	Graded	280
Overnight hikes (2 days or more)				
Dry Mountain	10.5	5,100'	6,150'	P/6.7 mi	295-298
Corridor Cyn-Saline Val. Rd	12.7	2,720'	2,560'	P/22.6 mi	307-310
Racetrack-Saline Valley Rd	9.9	4,660'	3,380'	P/25.1 mi	318-322

Key: P=Primitive (2WD) H=Primitive (HC)
* =Total distance and elevation change (ups + downs) for all loops

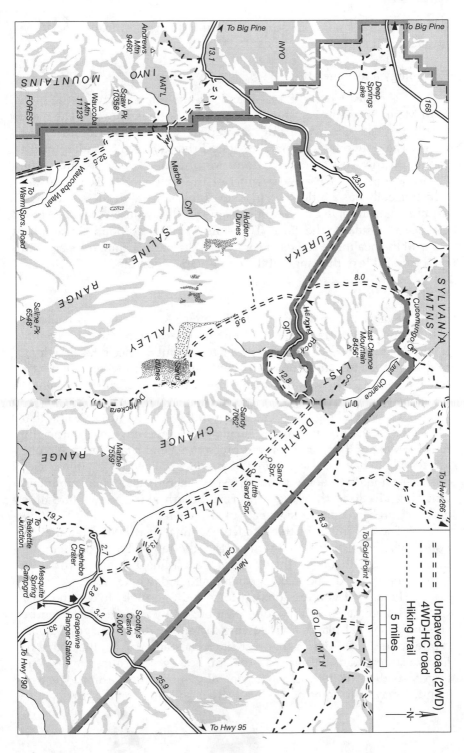

Crater. Several small exposures of similar Tertiary volcanic rocks are also found at a few locations near the foot of the range.

Hydrology and Vegetation

The Last Chance Range stands in the rain shadow of the high Inyo Mountains, and is generally fairly dry. Springs are rare. The main one is the Last Chance Spring, located near the northern end of the range. The only other springs are around the southern boundary of the range, on the west slope of Hunter Mountain—Big Dodd and Little Dodd springs, which are dry most of the time, and Jackass Spring, which usually has a little flow. In spite of this general dryness, the highest areas can receive quite a bit of snow in the winter, especially Last Chance Mountain to the north. This summit and Dry Mountain support some of the healthiest stands of conifers in the park. Joshua trees abound on the east side of the range, at the foot of Dry Mountain.

Hiking

Ever since I first saw the Last Chance Range, I have considered it to be a special attraction. This feeling comes in part from its largely unknown character, in part from its austere beauty. Since it takes so long to get to it, visitors are more infrequent here than elsewhere. Only at a few places did I see signs of passage, and I haven't yet run into a single hiker.

Canyon hiking takes on a different flavor here. Just consider that only four of the many canyons slicing this range have been officially named. Most of them are short but precipitous and challenging. No one knows when they were last visited. If you like isolated hiking, these simple facts should stimulate your curiosity. There is also good mountain climbing all along the range, offering breathtaking views of Saline and/or Eureka valleys from just about anywhere.

The old mines of the Ubehebe Mining District are definitely a bonus when hiking the southern part of the range. Some of them are easy to get to. Others, like the Copper Queen Mine, take hard work, are infrequently visited, and make great goals for a day hike.

Finally, if you are looking for good overnight hikes, the Last Chance Range has much in store. Its topography is such that it can be crossed at several places by following facing canyon drainages. Routes typically start from one of the west-side roads and end on the Saline or Eureka valley roads. Water is a problem, however. Because the range is largely roadless, water caching is generally out of the question. The best solution may be to come here when there is still snow on the crest.

∎

LAST CHANCE MOUNTAIN

> *The tin cabin, springs, and little mine at the foot of Last Chance Mountain, and the ascent of the forested mountain itself, make an excellent target for a short but strenuous hike in this remote corner of the park. In early spring the air is so clear that the views from this modest peak extend well over 100 miles.*

General Information

Road access: Long graded road and primitive road
Shortest hike: Short strolls / easy
Longest hike: 2.6 mi, ~2,900 ft one way (or more) / strenuous
Main attractions: A peak climb, woodland, springs, cabin and mine
USGS 15' topo maps: Madruger Mountain*, Last Chance Range
USGS 7.5' topo maps: Last Chance Mountain,* Hanging Rock Canyon
Maps: pp. 293*, 289

Location and Access

Last Chance Mountain is near the north end of the Last Chance Range, at the extreme northern tip of Death Valley. The starting point for this hike is the end of a primitive road that branches off the Big Pine Road. From the Ubehebe Crater Road, drive the Big Pine Road north 21 miles to Crankshaft Junction, marked by an old sign and a small cemetery of rusting crankshafts. Take the obviously less-traveled road to the right, then bear left 0.8 mile further onto an even less less-traveled road. Park 2.7 miles up this road, where it ends at the Last Chance Cabin.

The Big Pine Road is graded, and although it is a bad washboard at places, unless there have been recent washouts a standard-clearance vehicle is all you'll need to make it through. The road from Crankshaft Junction to the cabin is a little rough, but the crown is shallow and the rocks small, and I have had no problem getting through with a sub-compact car. Just drive slowly and carefully, especially the last 2 miles, which are steeper and a little worse.

Route Description

The Last Chance Cabin area. The little tin cabin at the end of the road is the heart of a small homestead and mining area, which were active from probably the 1930s until recent times. Although the cabin itself is not the most handsome, its peaceful, remote setting on the edge of timberline has received rave reviews from the occasional visitors who spent the night in it. Check with the Park Service whether overnight use is still allowed. The cabin is furnished with a small fireplace, a few chairs and a small table, and it has a wonderful old Far West flavor.

There are several springs in this area, all very different. One is in the ravine just below the cabin. A little water usually flows all of 200 feet along a narrow, algae-coated channel between rabbitbrush and cliffrose. The largest spring, betrayed by the wire fence surrounding it, is up on the wide bench across the ravine from the cabin. You can climb to it along a faint trail across the wash northwest of the cabin. It is locally known as Fan Spring, presumably for its shape, clearly visible from higher ground on the way up Last Chance Mountain. Hard to believe, but a couple of grazing easements are still active in the park, and this is one of them. As expected in a place as lush as Death Valley, overgrazing has essentially wiped out the native vegetation of this little spring.

Given the odds of finding a fortune right next to the only spring for miles, not much mining went on here. What little mining took place was done up the wash a short distance from the cabin. The workings consist of two deep shafts and a short tunnel. The shafts still have their access ladders, and a primitive hoist stands by the inclined shaft. The tailings are minimal, and so, probably, was the production.

The third spring, Last Chance Spring, is a short distance up the wash. Water seeps out from under a low tangle of mesquite trees and grapevine, feeding a grassy slope and a cluster of cottonwoods. Runoff from the spring collects in a large steel tub, which is always full. In the old days water was piped by gravity to the mine or the cabin—remnants of the pipeline are scattered below the spring. Please stay away from the grass area; use the stepping stones to get near the tub. Other living things, in particular burros and bighorn sheep, use this spring regularly. Don't camp within 200 yards of the spring. If you want to use its water, purify it first, as it probably contains giardia.

Last Chance Mountain		
	Dist.(mi)	Elev.(ft)
Last Chance Cabin	0.0	5,620
Mine shafts	0.05	5,660
Spring	0.2	5,780
18-ft fall	0.4	5,945
7,141-ft knoll	1.1	7,141
Saddle	2.0	~8,100
Last Chance Mountain	2.6	8,456

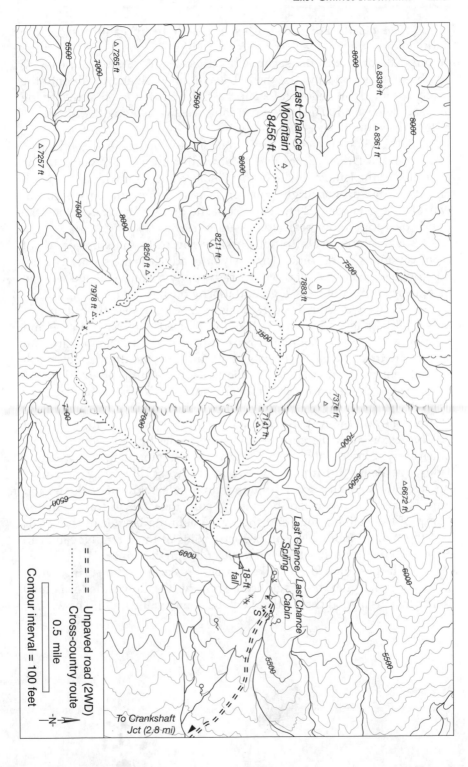

Last Chance
Mountain
8456 ft

△ 8338 ft

△ 8361 ft

△ 7265 ft

△ 7257 ft

△ 8211 ft

8250 ft △

7978 ft △

7883 ft △

731? ft △

7141 ft △

6672 ft △

Last Chance
Spring

Last Chance
Cabin

18-ft
fall

To Crankshaft
Jct (2.8 mi)

Contour interval = 100 feet

═ ═ ═ ═ ═   Unpaved road (2WD)
· · · · · · · · ·   Cross-country route

0.5 mile

-N-

The climb. For the shortest route, hike up canyon from the spring, bearing left at the first two forks (within 250 yards of the spring). About 120 yards into the second fork there is an 18-foot fall, easy to climb or bypass. Shortly past the fall, leave the wash and climb onto the ridge to your right. Follow it to, and past, the 7,141-ft knoll to the divide at a saddle near 8,100 feet, then continue westward along the divide 0.6 mile to the summit.

The route I prefer is about 1 mile longer, but it offers good views of the Eureka Dunes. From the 18-foot fall, continue 400 yards to the next fork on the left. Follow it a short distance and climb out of the wash onto the ridge on your right. Stay on it as it climbs and curves southward to a knoll near 7,720 ft, just east of the divide. Then hike along the divide over four minor peaks to the summit.

There are several other possible routes to the summit, all of them variations of the same theme. My only advice is the sooner you get on a ridge the better, as all canyon forks rapidly become clogged with an increasing number of trees, logs, and thorny bushes.

Either way, this is a great climb. The greenest summit in this range, Last Chance Mountain is heavily forested with pinyon pine and juniper, and it gives this hike a refreshing character. The density and size of the trees increase with elevation, until on the divide they reach magnificent proportions. Some of the trees are beautifully gnarled and varnished to a golden finish. From the summit the views are tremendous. You'll be able to look straight down the long shimmering sink of Death Valley all the way to the Black Mountains, with the high summit of Charleston Peak piercing the far edge of the horizon some 130 air miles away. Closer to the south rise Dry and Tin mountains, crowned by Telescope Peak. But it is the views to the west that steal the show. Pristine Eureka Valley sprawls more than a mile below, its golden sand dunes burning in the distance. On its far side, the valley is framed by the hump of the Saline Range and the overwhelming barrier of the Inyos and the White Mountains. Still beyond, miles of the Sierra Nevada can be seen on the horizon, white and immaculate in the winter.

The best time for this hike is probably early to mid spring, when snow adds charm to this magnificent scenery. The downside (or bonus) is that there is a good chance there will be some on the ground as well.

■

DRY MOUNTAIN

> *The highest summit in the Last Chance Range, 8,674-foot Dry Mountain makes a wonderful goal for a strenuous day hike or a more leisurely overnight trip. The route suggested here follows a tortuous and deep canyon to a secluded high valley at the foot of the mountain, then continues on to the summit, which commands stunning views of the Saline Valley area. A vigorous hike, long and tough, from pure desert to forested heights.*

General Information

Road status: Roadless; hiking from primitive road
Shortest hike: 6.0 mi, 2,720 ft one way / difficult
Longest hike: 10.5 mi, 5,100 ft one way / strenuous
Main attractions: A peak climb via a remote canyon, fossils, Joshua trees, woodland
USGS 15' and 7.5' topo maps: Tin Mountain, Dry Mountain*
Maps: pp. 299*, 333

Location and Access

Dry Mountain is about in the middle of the Last Chance Range, 10.5 miles southwest of Ubehebe Crater. There are several good routes to climb this prominent mountain. The one described here is not the most direct, but it is easier than most and quite varied, as it combines fan, canyon, and ridge hiking. The starting point is the Racetrack Valley Road about 6.7 miles from the Ubehebe Crater loop. This is half a mile or so before a group of low hills on the west side of the road. The ride is a little rough but easy to negotiate with a standard-clearance vehicle (see *The Racetrack Valley* for road conditions).

Route Description

The fan. The high peak towering to the southwest is not Dry Mountain but its unnamed and equally lofty 8,432-foot neighbor. Dry Mountain is about 2 air miles due west, separated from it by a 1,400-foot deep saddle. The route suggested here first goes nearly 4 miles up the long fan that sweeps into the mile-wide opening in the range to the west, then south up a nameless canyon to the saddle between the two peaks. From there it's a standard ridge climb to either summit.

From the road, cut a bee line towards the reddish hill at the northern foot of Dry Mountain (about 4 miles WNW). At first, try to stay

295

on the high parts of the fan. It is mostly even and well-compacted desert pavement with sparse vegetation, and it makes the walking easier. After about 2.6 miles, you'll reach the high north-facing bank of a large wash. If you traveled in a straight line, you should be at a low point in the bank, marked by the scattered relics of an abandoned camp. From here on, the fan is broken up into innumerable small, braided washes, and walking is more tedious. The easiest way is to stay in the main wash as it curves gently along the front of the mountain.

It's a long haul, and the scenery does not change very fast, but there are quite a few things along the way to keep you entertained, like the plants. You will find here all the common cacti of Death Valley—cottontop, beavertail, strawtop cholla, echinocereus—which are a floral treat in the late spring. On the upper fan a few Joshua trees will join you. The rocks will also catch your attention. The lower half of the fan could serve as a model of desert pavement. In this curious rock garden, most of the rocks are small, neatly arranged, and gauged, faceted, sliced, or grooved by wind and water erosion. Some of them also have another exciting feature, this one quite unusual. Once you notice it, it will likely keep your curiosity going, and even slow you down a little.

The canyon you want is the first one on the left. It's hard to miss: on the east side of its mouth there is a small arch at the base of the wall.

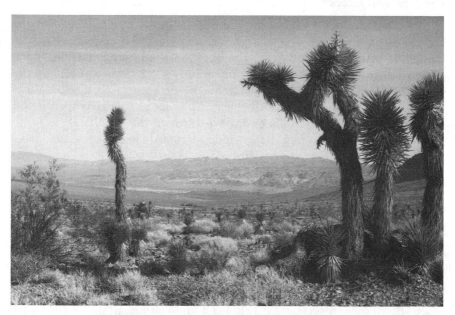

Looking back at the long alluvial fan that leads up
from the Racetrack Valley Road to Dry Mountain

The canyon. In more ways than one this canyon is atypical of Death Valley canyons. For one, it has Joshua trees—no giants, yet healthy specimens, some with multiple branches and over 10 feet high. These weird-looking plants will keep you company most of the way. Except for two short narrows, the canyon is never narrow. Rather, it cuts a deep, meandering swath through the mountain. Along the way you'll pass by all the formations from the Pogonip Group at the mouth to the Lost Burro Formation (from the saddle to the summit), thus time-traveling from the early Ordovician to the Devonian.

Above its mouth, the canyon slices through rocks deeply hollowed out by erosion. The many small caves that pockmark the east wall are tempting targets for inquisitive visitors—as well as sleeping lairs for bighorn sheep. After changing direction abruptly twice, the canyon narrows a little. Here and there sheer walls rise straight up from the gravel, on one side or the other. Check them out closely. Many beautiful Ordovician fossils are imbedded in them, especially just downhill from the first side canyon on the west side. Maclurites, a snail characteristic of the Ordovician, is the most common. Against the dark gray limestone (Pogonip Group), its shells produce strik-

ing white spirals, at places a few inches across. They can form more complex patterns, depending on the orientation of the cut. There are also large receptaculites, sponges called sunflower corals because they look like the pitted surface of a sunflower freed of its seeds. Further up canyon, dense carpets of rock spiraea and colorful lichen, both uncommon in this region, grow on a shady rock wall. A little past it there is a small seep at wash level, where water oozes out on a rocky ledge.

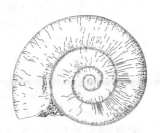

Maclurites, a snail that lived and died around 450 million years ago

Still further, the wash runs into a 12-foot fall, beneath a massive balanced rock. The fall is easy, the bypass a staircase, and the small trench in shattered quartzite above it is pleasantly cool.

The only serious obstruction is the 80-foot fall three quarters of the way through the canyon. It terminates a short stretch of deep narrows clogged with giant boulders. To go around it, walk back about 100 yards, to about 20 yards above an 8-ft fall, and scramble up the steep ravine on the west side. Gain about 100 feet of elevation, past the first large tree, to a roughly level ledge lined with a few trees on your left, and follow it to the lip of the fall. The fall can also be bypassed on the east side, but it takes more work.

Above the fall the canyon is different again. Rounded boulders litter the wash. Joshua trees run into timberline, and for a while you'll travel through a peculiar landscape where pinyon pines, junipers, and Joshuas thrive next to each other. A last high fall (about 20 feet) blocks the way just before the head of the canyon. To bypass it, retrace your steps 100-150 yards and climb out the side canyon on the east side. This will put you on the edge of the canyon's upper drainage, a lovely area covered with a welcoming pinyon pine forest, framed by the looming peaks of Dry Mountain and its facing neighbor. You can rest or camp here before assaulting the mountain, amidst large, beautifully gnarled pines and junipers.

The climb. Where the upper drainage opens up, the wash forks three ways. Half a mile up the middle fork, climb west over the low divide into a south-draining wash. From here you can climb the ridge directly east to the summit. For a longer but easier approach, you can also stay with the wash and climb it to the divide of the Last Chance Range, where you'll catch your first enthralling views of the other side— the Steel Pass corridor below and the Saline Range, the deep trough of Saline Valley beyond, and still further the high escarpment of the Inyo Mountains against the sawtooth peaks of the high Sierra. The final stretch—0.7 mile and 650 feet up—is southwest along the divide. There is snow here just about every winter, and even in the spring you are likely to find patches of snow lingering along this north-facing ridge.

Logistics. Most hikers confident enough to attempt this hike in a day will take close to 10 or 12 hours to complete it. That's a long day, and you'll need plenty of daylight hours. I was here a little too early in the season (early March), started a little too late in the day, and one hour

Dry Mountain		
	Dist.(mi)	Elev.(ft)
Racetrack Valley Road	0.0	3,620
Canyon mouth (arch)	3.9	5,350
Side canyon (fossil area)	6.0	6,190
12-ft fall & balanced rock	6.7	~6,450
80-ft fall	7.2	~6,720
20-ft fall	8.1	~7,100
Fork	8.2	7,170
Divide	9.8	8,020
Dry Mountain	10.5	8,674

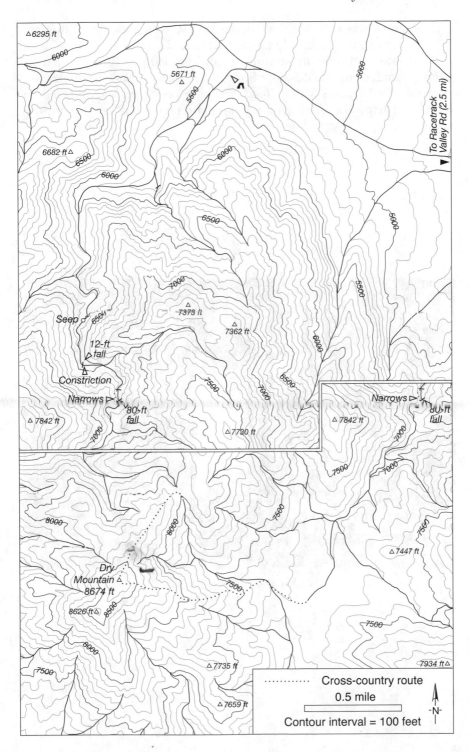

6295 ft

6000

5671 ft

To Racetrack
Valley Rd (2.5 mi)

6682 ft

6500

6000

6000

6500

5500

Seep

7373 ft

7362 ft

6000

12-ft
fall

6500

7500

7000

6500

Constriction

Narrows

Narrows

7842 ft

80-ft
fall

80-ft
fall

7730 ft

7500

7000

8000

8000

7500

7447 ft

Dry
Mountain
8674 ft

7500

8626 ft

8500

7500

8000

7934 ft

7500

7735 ft

·········· Cross-country route

0.5 mile

–N–

7659 ft

Contour interval = 100 feet

after sunset I was still dodging chollas on my way back down the fan. Mid to late spring is probably the best time to do it in a day. Since most of the route is in full sun, summer would be painful. To cut down on driving time, camp at Mesquite Spring Campground or at the starting point on the Racetrack Valley Road. For a slower-paced hike, make it an overnight trip. The open valley below the peaks has great camping spots.

■

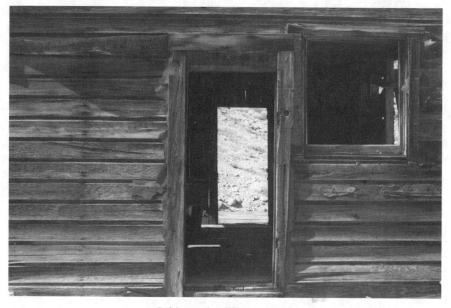

Cabin at the Ubehebe Mine

THE UBEHEBE MINE

While visiting the Racetrack, take a little time to explore the remains of historical Ubehebe Mine. Its small camp, ore tramway, and the scenic approach to its upper tunnels offer an interesting glimpse into the operation of a small-time lead and silver mine.

General Information

Road access: 22-mile primitive road
Shortest hike: Short strolls/very easy
Longest hike: 2.6 miles, ~1,100 feet one way (or more)/moderate
Main attractions: A historical lead and copper mine and camp
USGS 15' topo maps: Ubehebe Peak*, Dry Mountain
USGS 7.5' topo maps: Ubehebe Peak, Teakettle Junction
Maps: pp. 309*, 333

Location and Access

The Ubehebe Mine is near the head of a canyon draining the Last Chance Range from a low point in the Racetrack Valley divide. From the paved road at Ubehebe Crater, drive 19.7 miles to Teakettle Junction, then drive towards the Racetrack for 2.2 miles to the junction to the Ubehebe Mine, on the right. Standard-clearance vehicles can usually make it to this point (see *The Racetrack Valley* for road conditions), but the last 0.7-mile spur to the mine is narrow and rutted, and you may need to walk part of it.

History

Although the Ubehebe Mine was first a copper mine, probably on the nearby Copper Bell claims, it started to be operated as a lead-silver mine in late 1906 when one of the mine owners discovered a rich lead carbonate vein on the property. A little over a year later, several claims had been staked and assessment work had shown that the main vein was quite extensive. The mine already appeared as one of the most promising in the district. In March 1908, the owners, Smith and Watterson, two businessmen from Bishop, formed a partnership with Archibald Farrington, and incorporated the Ubehebe Lead Mines Company. By then the 25-ft mine tunnel and its two shafts showed 70% lead and a high silver content. In July it had reached 50 feet, still all in ore. That summer the mine was described optimistically as "easily the biggest undeveloped property of the kind in California."

Some ore was teamed that year on the newly completed road from the Racetrack Valley—which conveniently passed within a mile of the mine—to the Tonopah-Las Vegas railroad at Bonnie Claire, Nevada. By the end of 1908 the Ubehebe Mine had generated the first recorded production in the district—48 tons containing 491 ounces of silver. A trial shipment sent to a Salt Lake City smelter returned an average of $40 per ton. Although a decent figure by Death Valley standards, it was not enough to offset the high cost of animal-powered transportation to the railroad. Mining was also impeded by the lack of water. The nearest water supply was the scant flow from Quartz Spring, 7 miles away, which had to be piped to a storage tank below the spring and hauled to the mine. Perhaps because of this disappointing initial run, mostly assessment work was carried out during the following few years. The mine produced only a little high-grade ore again in 1913 and 1914.

In the fall of 1915, after lead prices shot up, Watterson and Farrington attempted to solve their transportation problem by hiring a contractor, Frank Campbell, to haul their ore with a ball-tread Yuba tractor. Although the round trip took a painstaking 52 hours, the tractor idea was a success. The 10-ton capacity tractor handled the rough, steep road far better, and the cost was down to $8 per ton. For several years, Campbell hauled out a good part of the combined ores of the district mines. His tractors were also busy with manganese ore in southern Death Valley. In 1916, with only three men employed, the Ubehebe production went up tenfold from that of 1914, to 250 tons of ore.

After a couple of years of inactivity, in the fall of 1920 some of the Farrington claims were sold to a Tonopah mining company for $125,000. The south workings mined so far had played out. A small crew was sent out to open the lower tunnel, which turned out to be the richest. The following year yielded nearly 284,000 pounds of lead and 500 pounds of silver. Shortly thereafter lead prices dropped again, the claims returned to the Farrington estate, and the mine was inactive for several years. But when the main tunnel was reopened by new lessees in 1927, it paid off again. That year 258 tons of high-grade ore were shipped. The following year, production reached an all-time record with over one million pounds of lead, nearly 1,000 pounds of silver, 1,500 pounds of copper, and a little gold. After paying $15 a ton in transportation, the lessees netted over $55,000 from 25 ore shipments to Salt Lake City. This was the highest annual production of lead and silver the district ever saw, and the mine's greatest output.

The Ubehebe Mine remained active off and on for nearly four decades, its production fluctuating in unison with the lead market. But in spite of improved roads, cheaper transportation by truck, and a more plentiful water supply trucked in from Goldbelt Spring or Scotty's

Castle, its annual production never reached one tenth of the 1928 figure. In 1929 and 1930, only small tonnages of mostly high-grade ore came out of the mine. A third area, the tramway stope, was opened around then, but it is said to have netted only around $5,000 of low-grade ore. In the late 1930s, Grant Snyder, who had been involved in the mine earlier, employed 10 men to mostly widen and clean out existing tunnels. Ore values still ran high, but there just was not much of it left, and only 1938 saw a little production. He came back in the late 1940s and early 1950s, working all five ore bodies and producing 100-400 tons of lower grade ore each year. A new lessee gave it another try in 1966, but the tunnels had already been gutted.

So it was that it ended with a whimper. But when it finally closed in 1968, it had left its mark as one of Death Valley's top lead producers, and the longest active mine in the district. Its total production has been estimated at 3,500 tons averaging an impressive 38% lead, 7% zinc, and 12 ounces of silver per ton, an enviable achievement considering its extreme isolation.

Geology

The formation exposed on the north canyon slope, up to the ridge and down the far side, is the Ely Springs Dolomite. In the mine area, it was greatly altered by contact metamorphism with a small pluton of quartz monzonite that intruded it about 400-800 feet to the northeast. The intrusion took place in the Mesozoic, probably around the same time as the much larger Hunter Mountain Pluton to the south (see *Ubehebe Peak*). The dark gray dolomite was recrystallized, bleached, and shattered, and bears little resemblance to the original rock. The metal deposits occur mostly in veins and in replacements of shattered rocks in the contact zone. The ore was mostly silver-bearing galena and cerussite (lead), hemimorphite (zinc), with traces of copper, gold, wulfenite (tungsten), arsenic, and vanadium minerals.

Route Description

The Ubehebe Mine camp. Nestled at the head of a wall-rimmed canyon, this little mining camp is the most picturesque around the Racetrack. The camp is now reduced to a single wood cabin, but at one time it also had a cook house, a three-room bunkhouse, and a two-bedroom cabin located near the main mine entrance. Look around for other remains—an old car carcass, thick stone walls, tent sites, a rusted stove, and scattered concrete foundations.

The mines. The Ubehebe Mine exploited three distinct areas. The timbered portal topped by a small tank near the canyon floor is the main adit. The mine about 45 feet higher is the south workings. The third area is the north (or tram) workings, on the far side of the ridge at the top of the tramway cable.

The south workings, mined mostly from 1906 to around 1916, are the oldest. They have a 60-foot tunnel, connected to the main mine by a vertical shaft. The main mine, which was opened next, was the largest producer. Its tunnel penetrates more than 700 feet nearly straight into the hill, sprouting six main drifts along the way, some of them a few hundred feet long. The narrow gauge rail used four mine cars to haul the ore out of the tunnel. The tracks still run part way along the loading ramp, which is made of overburden. At the end of the tracks stands the ore chute where the ore was downloaded from wagons onto trucks. Near the main adit stood a small compressor house, an air receiver, and a blacksmith shop (now resting sideways in the wash below the adit).

The smaller north workings were opened last, around 1930, although this deposit had been known for a long time. Never connected underground with the rest of the mine, it was serviced by the tramway that still spans the canyon wall from wash to ridge. It was a single-bucket tramway, powered by a 10-horsepower gas engine located on the ridge. Ore was delivered to it in wheelbarrows. To get there, look for the narrow trail about 200 yards up the road from the cable, to the left of a stone platform (perhaps an old tent site). The trail winds its way up to a saddle on the ridge, then continues a short distance to the tramway breakover tower. The tunnels are clustered just below it on the steep north slope. The tramway construction is interesting, and there are good views of the surrounding ridges and little camp below. This is also one of the few places where I have seen a bear poppy in bloom.

Not to put a damper on your fun, but do think twice before entering any of the mine tunnels. All three workings cut through shattered rock and have dangerous hidden shafts.

The Ubehebe Mine		
	Dist.(mi)	Elev.(ft)
Ubehebe Mine Junction	0.0	3,990
Copper Bell Mine	(0.6)	~4,220
Trail to north workings	0.6	~3,940
North workings (tramway)	(0.4)	~4,160
Ubehebe mining camp	0.7	3,920
Main mine	~0.75	3,920
Side canyon to prospects	1.2	3,765
Prospects	1.6	~4,120

The Copper Bell Mine. The Copper Bell Mine is high on the north canyon slope, about 1,500 feet east of the camp. The easiest way to reach it is to hike up the old mining road that starts at the junction between the Racetrack Valley Road and the Ubehebe Mine road. The mine is south of the last major switchback, below the road. The other way is from the north workings, hiking first along the ridge then cutting across to the mine, which takes a little scrambling.

The Copper Bell was worked on two unconnected tunnels, each about 150 feet long, and 20 vertical feet apart. Most of the copper came from the upper tunnel. These claims were held by the same owners as the Ubehebe claims, and mined concurrently. A good portion—a little over 15,000 pounds—of the Ubehebe Mine copper probably came from here. The rock exposed around the mine is limestone (Pogonip Group) metamorphosed into nearly white marble by the same pluton that altered the Ubehebe Mine area. The pluton (quartz monzonite), which is exposed all along the mining road, comes within only 25-50 feet of the Copper Bell tunnels. The Copper Bell minerals, found mostly in marble, include chalcopyrite, bornite, and malachite, with traces of pyrite and hematite.

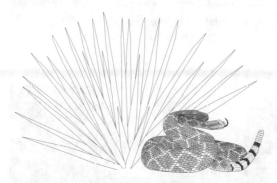

Mojave rattlesnake
(Crotalus scutulatus)

The prospects. There are a few prospects and mines on the next ridge north from the tramway, visible from the north workings of the Ubehebe Mine—a good excuse to take a little stroll around. For the easiest approach, hike down canyon from the camp. After a few turns along the narrowing wash, you'll get to an inconspicuous side canyon on the right. The workings are about 0.3 mile up this winding canyon, all lined up one on top of the other along a steep ridge on the north side. From the wash just below this ridge a narrow, worn-out trail climbs up a short distance to the highest adit.

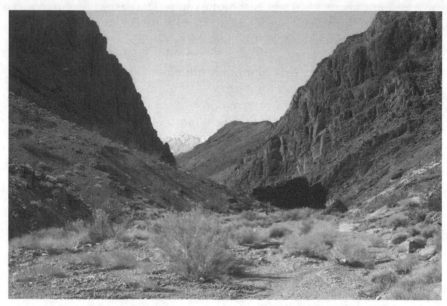

*High walls along the side canyon that leads from the Ubehebe Mine
to Corridor Canyon; snow-capped Inyo Mountains in the background*

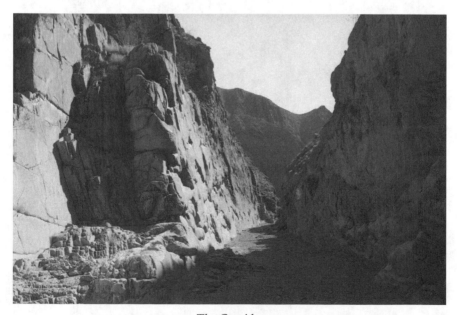

The Corridor

CORRIDOR CANYON

Corridor Canyon is a local name, probably coined by park rangers after the unusually straight narrows of the mid-canyon. Although these and other narrows are the main highlights, this long canyon and its numerous tributaries offer a variety of landscapes and little secrets waiting to be discovered.

General Information

Road access: Primitive road
Shortest hike: 1.7 mi, 520 ft one way / easy-moderate
Longest hike: 12.7 mi, 2,720 ft one way (or more) / difficult
Main attractions: Exceptional narrows, fossils, geology
USGS 15' topo maps: Ubehebe Peak*, Dry Mountain
USGS 7.5' topo maps: Ubehebe Peak,* Teakettle Jct, West of Ubehebe Pk
Maps: pp. 309*, 333, 477

Location and Access

Corridor Canyon drains the Last Chance Range from the northern Racetrack Valley to the south end of Saline Valley. The easiest starting point to hike to it is the small camp at the Ubehebe Mine. Refer to *The Ubehebe Mine* for directions and road conditions.

Route Description

The approach. The approach suggested here is only one of several possible routes into this extensive canyon system. From the Ubehebe mining camp, walk down the wash as it winds its way through the Last Chance Range. This is actually a side drainage, so you will not reach Corridor Canyon for some time. It's a nice little canyon, narrow at places, well-behaved and easy to walk. The rock formations get younger down canyon. The well-stratified high wall about 1 mile down is typical Lost Burro Formation. As all formations bear fossils, one of the fun things to do as you amble down canyon is to poke around for these small remains of long ago. They are not exactly all over, but locally fairly abundant. The most obvious ones are Mississippian crinoids and corals (see *Perdido Canyon*) left over from the time Death Valley was a tropical reef. They are quite striking, both for their quality and quantity. At places the rocks are literally crawling with fossils. The most scenic area is the short narrows just before the junction with the main canyon. Carved in light gray limestone, its exposed bedrock sculpted by erosion,

307

it is a pleasant place to rest in the shade in the summer months.

Down from the junction, the main canyon is quite broad at first. From a little below the junction down to near the canyon mouth, most of the exposed rocks belong to the Keeler Canyon Formation, Pennsylvanian in age. It is a beautiful, well-laminated formation, mostly made of limestone interbedded with calcareous siltstone. About another mile down, the canyon begins to narrow and meander in tighter curves. The transition into narrows is gradual, almost imperceptible: by the time you come to the brink of the first real fall you have already been immersed in them for some time. The fall, about 10 feet in height and not a great hurdle, is made of massive, polished limestone with good holds. Below it, the narrows tighten up. Several shallow potholes line the exposed bedrock. In the rainy months, they may hold the only water for miles. The best is kept for last: a deep and dark slot, no more than 4 feet wide. Curving gently beneath high-polished walls, its dark lime-stone crisscrossed with delicate white veins, this bare-rock passage is as smooth as a playground slide. A few more steps and you emerge into the Corridor.

The Corridor. In the vicinity of the Corridor, the Keeler Canyon Formation is upturned, so that its distinct strata stand almost vertically. Erosion has dug along a weaker plane in the stratification, leaving behind this long corridor trapped between vertical walls mostly less than 30 feet apart. At places the walls are so smooth that they seem to have been cleaved with a giant blade. Except for two small jogs, it is

	Corridor Canyon	
	Dist.(mi)	Elev.(ft)
Ubehebe Mine camp	0.0	3,920
Side canyon to prospects	0.5	3,765
First narrows	1.5	3,460
Junction with main canyon	1.7	3,400
Second narrows (start)	2.9	3,060
Fall	2.95	3,040
Slot	3.1	3,000
Junction with the Corridor	3.15	2,985
The Corridor (lower end)	3.8	2,870
Lower gorge (start)	5.9	2,320
Lower gorge (end)	6.3	2,250
Mouth	~7.7	~1,920
Saline Valley Road	12.7	1,206

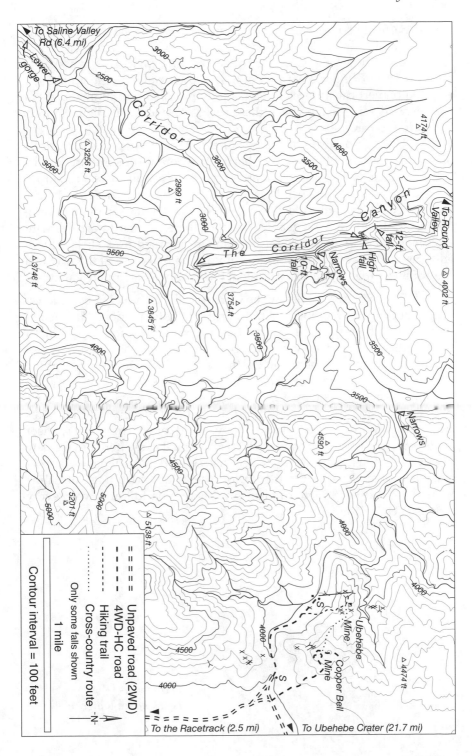

To Saline Valley
Rd (6.4 mi)

Lower gorge

Corridor

△ 3256 ft

2500

3000

3000

△ 2999 ft

3000

3500

The

Corridor

Canyon

△ 4174 ft

4000

3500

To Round Valley

12-ft fall

High fall

Narrows

0-ft fall

⊙ 4002 ft

△ 3748 ft

3500

4000

△ 3845 ft

△ 3754 ft

3500

3500

3500

Narrows

△ 4590 ft

4500

4500

4000

△ 5201 ft

5000

5000

△ 5138 ft

4000

4000

4500

4500

4000

4000

△ 4474 ft

Ubehebe Mine

Ubehebe Copper Bell Mine

S

S

To the Racetrack (2.5 mi)

To Ubehebe Crater (21.7 mi)

-N-

Unpaved road (2WD)
4WD-HC road
Hiking trail
Cross-country route
Only some falls shown

1 mile

Contour interval = 100 feet

almost perfectly straight for nearly 1 mile. The main canyon enters the Corridor at a right angle just below the jog. From this junction you can stare straight down the Corridor for over half a mile. This is a special place, worthy of a little extra attention. Down canyon, sea ripples are exposed on vertical surfaces 15 feet above the wash, frozen memories of the Pennsylvanian sea in which these rocks were formed. There is more. Look around carefully.

Hiking up canyon from the junction is equally spectacular. At its upper end the Corridor makes a sharp left where it runs into the undisturbed vertical strata of the formation. Its eastern wall soars straight up for nearly 70 feet. At the bend there is a high fall, which needs to be circumvented on its north side. It is not too difficult, but be extremely careful, as a fall here may be deadly. Beyond, there are short narrows with easy falls, then another straight corridor interrupted by a slick, 12-foot fall (low 5s). This pattern continues—if you can make it—all the way to a beautiful, completely enclosed alluvial basin known as Round Valley.

The lower canyon. Below the Corridor, the canyon offers a succession of short narrows, polished falls, and straighter sections. The geology is one of the highlights. At one place there is an impressive wall of thick vertical strata, deeply notched by differential erosion, rising several hundred feet above the wash. On the way to the lower gorge, near the bottom of the canyon, you'll pass by as many as seven side canyons. Some of them are less than a mile long. Others, far longer, form a complex web of side canyons splitting into more side canyons that takes many visits to just begin to know. They, too, have narrows, falls, sheer walls, winding passages, and fossils. Every time I come here I make new discoveries. You may find yourself so distracted that it will take you several visits to make it to the mouth, on the bright crisp edge of Saline Valley. But it doesn't matter much—in this canyon full of secrets, every step is a destination.

■

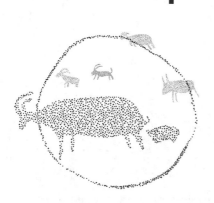

Petroglyphs,
Last Chance Range

THE RACETRACK VALLEY

> *This is a great place, remote, strange, and beautiful in ways only the desert can be. Just driving the rough road to it gives a wild flavor of desert exploring in pre-asphalt days. Take a stroll on the eerie dry lakebed called the Racetrack to check out its mysterious moving rocks, or hike clear across it to the ruins of a small copper mine.*

General Information

Road access: 25-mile primitive road
Shortest hike: 0.25 mi, level/very easy
Longest hike: 1.6 mi, 240 ft one way/moderate
Main attractions: A scenic, isolated dry lake, moving rocks, copper mines
USGS 15' and 7.5' topo maps: Ubehebe Peak
Maps: pp. 315*, 327, 333, 477

Location and Access

The Racetrack Valley is a long, north-south trending high desert valley between the Cottonwood Mountains and the Last Chance Range. The shortest route to it by car is the Racetrack Valley Road, which starts at the end of the Ubehebe Crater Road. From here it is 25.1 miles to the Grandstand turnout, near the north end of the Racetrack playa. To see the moving rocks, near its south end, drive 2 more miles and park by the interpretive sign.

A good part of this road is a bad washboard, and the lowest clearance passenger cars may not be able to make it, especially if the driver has little experience driving this kind of road. However, unless there has been a recent washout due to rain, most standard-clearance passenger cars can make it to the Lippincott Mine. Just roll up the windows and take it slowly. The other option is to drive in from the Saline Valley Road, which takes a high-clearance, 4-wheel-drive vehicle.

Camping along the Racetrack Valley Road south of Teakettle Junction is prohibited except at the marked camping area (Homestake Dry Camp) south of the Racetrack.

Route Description

The Racetrack Valley Road. If you've never ventured this far on a primitive road before, the ride to the Racetrack is likely to be an experience. You'll first drive through the dark ash field left by the explosion of Ubehebe Crater sometime in the last few thousand years, then climb a long, mountain-bounded alluvial fan bypassing the sheer face of the Cottonwoods on your way to Tin Pass, which is not even half way through. After a half hour of shaking and increasingly wild sceneries, you may well start feeling you are headed for the legendary "middle of nowhere." The Tin Pass area boasts thick stands of Joshua trees, a high density of chollas and other cacti, as well as bear poppy, an endemic plant that is striking when in bloom. South from the pass you'll start to descend into the Racetrack Valley, one of a series of high-elevation closed basins with no outlet to the sea. Teakettle Junction is the first sign of civilization in miles. The number of kettles attached to the sign varies greatly over time. There are almost always at least a few, and sometimes one can barely see the sign for the kettles. Along the Racetrack itself the road is a washboard, and it can be the roughest part of this ride.

The Racetrack. From just about any vantage point, the dry lakebed at the bottom of the Racetrack Valley is one of the eeriest sights in the park. Against the backdrop of rugged mountains surrounding it on both sides, this vast blinding expanse of dry mud seems strangely out of place. And the Grandstand, the island of rounded boulders sticking out of it, adds another incongruous element to this already outlandish scenery. The Racetrack is just about as flat as a natural surface can be over such a large area. Even a lake of similar size would be more wrinkled. You might think at first that it is manmade, or perhaps manufactured by space aliens for landing. Not such a bad thought: a few decades ago the Racetrack was used by drug smugglers as a landing field.

From the Grandstand turnout, take a short walk onto the playa to check out the lakebed and the Grandstand (0.25 mile). The playa mud cracked when it last dried, leaving behind a surface divided into millions of polygonal plates, each of them a few inches across, like a gargantuan tiled floor. If you are into photography, between the semi-infinite, fractal lake surface, the strange Grandstand rocks, and the alien-looking ranges all around, you are in for some pretty wild shots.

The Grandstand is a metamorphosed outcrop of porphyritic granite that intruded the area in the Mesozoic (see *Ubehebe Peak*). This granite contains very little quartz or mica, thus its unusual darkness and lack of sparkle, but many large crystals, which is the reason it is called porphyritic. Its long tabular crystals, commonly over 2 inches in length, are orthoclase. Each crystal is twinned, which means it is made of two crystals that grew within each other. If you look at one carefully in reflected light, you should see the difference in reflectivity between the two halves of the crystal, neatly dividing it down its length.

The Racetrack playa is vulnerable. Walking on it when it is muddy—which happens only after a good storm—can mar it with footprints for months. At such times, please stay away from it. Also, leave

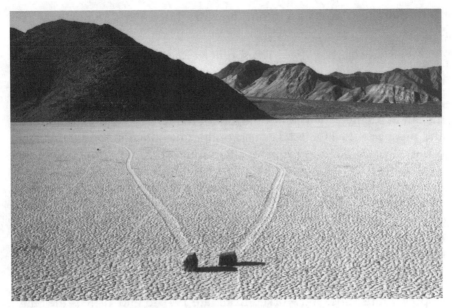

Moving rocks on the Racetrack

the rocks as you find them for others to enjoy. Wet or dry, the playa is off-limits to bicycles and, needless to say, all other vehicles.

The moving rocks. The Racetrack Valley is best known for its moving rocks. Rocks shed by the mountains southeast of the playa have been found stranded in the middle of the dry lake, each rock at the end of a faint trail. After a heavy rain, the normally dry playa develops a muddy surface layer slippery enough that the rocks can be herded across it by strong winds, imprinting a long track in the mud as they move. A usually good place to find moving rocks is the south end of the playa. Start your search from the interpretive sign 2 miles south of the Grandstand turnout, which gives more information about the moving rocks. My experience is that they can also be found at other places, even around the Grandstand. Bring binoculars to spot rocks from a distance. Most of the rock trails are straight, but if you are lucky you may find one making a sharp angle. They can be very faint. For best viewing, look for them under slanting sunlight. If heat is a problem, try evening when the lake is shaded by Ubehebe Peak. While exploring, note the 2-3 foot tall spiny brush common along the playa. It is called thornbush. In the early spring, it produces beautiful tubular, white-blue flowers. After the flower dies it turns a striking shiny red.

Moving rocks have been observed on several other dry lakes around Death Valley. If you can't make it here, check out for example

Little Bonnie Claire Lake along Nevada Highway 267 northeast of Scotty's Castle.

The Sally Ann Mine. The southern Racetrack Valley is surrounded by several mines and prospects (see map), most of them a short walk from the road. There is the Copper Giant No. 3 Mine, visible west of the road about 0.9 mile south of the moving rock sign. A foot trail crosses the fan in 0.6 mile, then climbs the foot of the range to its 100-foot tunnel and prospect. The Homestake, just south of the junction to Saline Valley, is the only talc claim in the area. The Lippincott Mine, at the end of the road, has by far the most interesting remains. But the most scenic mine here is certainly the Sally Ann, located up the mountainside at the southeast corner of the playa. To get to it you'll have to cross the lake bed starting from the "moving rocks" interpretive sign. Heading due east will take you just below the south group of mines, located between 350 and 500 feet above the playa. A short, very steep trail leads up to it. The north group, about 0.4 mile further north, is easier to reach.

These copper deposits were known as early as 1902 as the Copper Knife Mine, and worked from late 1947 to mid-1948 as the Sally Ann Mine. At the time, there was a small camp on the fan below the mines. Water was hauled from Goldbelt Spring. The two men who operated it then developed the main tunnel in the north group. They drove it 120 feet towards the mineralized zone to intercept a larger copper vein, apparently without success. The south group was even less developed; it has only a few trenches and shallow pits.

Although the workings are small, the geology is interesting. As elsewhere in this area, the copper deposits occur at the contact metamorphic zone between Paleozoic sedimentary rocks and an intrusive pluton

The Racetrack Valley		
	Dist.(mi)	Elev.(ft)
Ubehebe Crater Road	0.0	~2,510
Tin Pass	11.4	~4,940
Teakettle Junction	19.7	4,138
Ubehebe Mine turnoff	21.9	3,980
Grandstand turnout	25.1	3,710
The Grandstand (hike)	(0.25)	3,710
Moving Rocks Sign	27.1	3,710
Sally Ann Mine (hike)	(1.6)	~4,100
Lippincott Road	28.9	3,790
Homestake Dry Camp (end)	29.1	3,760

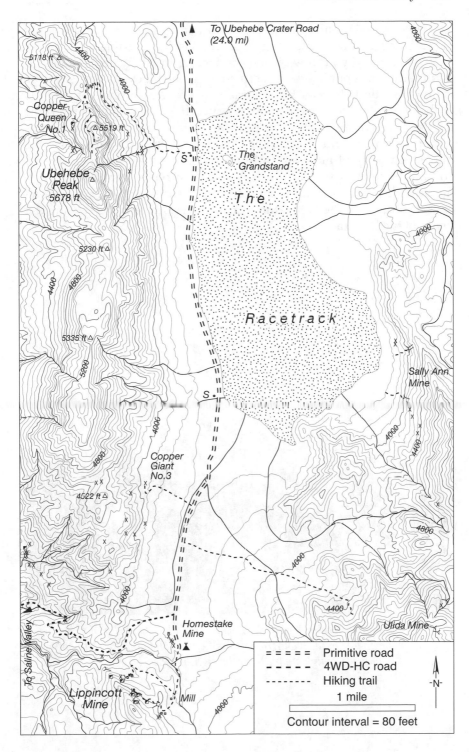

To Ubehebe Crater Road
(24.0 mi)

5118 ft △

4400

4000

Copper
Queen
No.1

△ 5519 ft

The
Grandstand

*Ubehebe
Peak*
5678 ft

T h e

5230 ft △

4400

4800

4000

R a c e t r a c k

5335 ft △

5200

Sally Ann
Mine

S

4000

4400

Copper
Giant
No.3

4800

4000

4522 ft △

4800

4000

4400

Ulida Mine

*Homestake
Mine*

4400

4000

To Saline Valley

*Lippincott
Mine*

Mill

4000

= = = = =	Primitive road
– – – – –	4WD-HC road
- - - - - - -	Hiking trail

1 mile

-N-

Contour interval = 80 feet

(see *Ubehebe Peak*). Almost all of the mountain west of the playa is made of plutonic rocks, with just a couple of small isolated sedimentary blocks along its base. If you draw a line connecting the Sally Ann workings, you pretty much outline the eastern edge of one block; its western edge is downhill, buried under fan material. As you walk uphill toward any of the workings you'll first come across nearly white marble (with some tactite and hornfel), then metal-bearing marble near the contact zone, and quartz monzonite (with some syenite and syenodiorite) above the mines. A variety of minerals are still exposed here—malachite, chryso-colla, a little azurite; the south group also has magnetite, garnet, hematite, serpentine, and a little scheelite (tungsten ore). But don't expect too much. The Sally Ann's greatest wealth remains its singular views of the Racetrack.

■

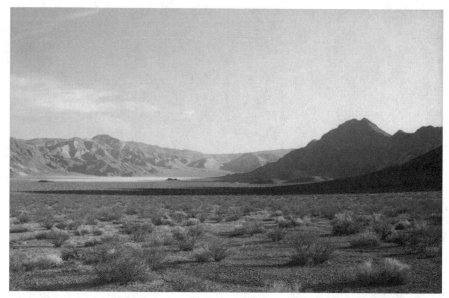

Approaching the Racetrack from the Racetrack Valley Road. The dark knoll near the middle of the photograph is the Grandstand, and the leftmost of the two high summits on the right is Ubehebe Peak.

UBEHEBE PEAK AND THE COPPER QUEEN MINES

> *From the edge of the Racetrack, climb an old mining trail to the colorful tailings of a forgotten copper mine, then to stark Ubehebe Peak for spectacular views of the deep sink of Saline Valley. A strenuous hike down the steep far side will take you into the winding granitic corridors of a rarely visited canyon to forgotten copper mines, and eventually down to the floor of Saline Valley.*

General Information

Road access: 25-mile primitive road
Shortest hike: 1.9 mi, 1,190 ft one way / moderate
Longest hike: 10.2 mi, ~5,500 ft one way / strenuous
Main attractions: A spectacular climb, copper mines in a remote canyon
USGS 15' topo map: Ubehebe Peak
USGS 7.5' topo maps: Ubehebe Peak*, West of Ubehebe Peak
Maps: pp. 321*, 315, 333, 477

Location and Access

Ubehebe Peak is the highest summit towering over the west side of the Racetrack playa, near the south end of the Last Chance Range. The copper mines described here are all on the west side of the peak. The trail to the peak starts at the Grandstand turnout, near the northwest corner of the Racetrack playa. Refer to *The Racetrack Valley* for directions and road conditions.

Geology

Sometime in the Mesozoic—late Jurassic, early Cretaceous, no one remembers anymore—a batholith of quartz monzonite intruded this area. Or, rather, what was to become this area, since way back then this was all deep down and somewhere else on Earth. Picture a huge bubble of hot magma slowly forcing its way up through the Earth's crust, shoving aside whatever formations happen to be in the way. The contact between the magma and the native rocks produced what is called a contact metamorphic zone, a region tens to hundreds of feet thick where rocks on both sides are metamorphosed—the native rocks from being heated and crystallized, the intrusive rocks from being cooled, and both from exchanging chemical constituents. Shales were transformed into hornfels, dolomite into marble and tactite, quartz monzonite into granite, diorite, gabbro, or syenite. Later on, rising metal-bearing solutions preferentially soaked up the weakened metamorphosed native rocks, slowly turning them into rich lodes.

Today, uplifting and erosion have exposed the pluton all over the southern Racetrack region. Ubehebe Peak, the mountain facing it across the playa, the north face of the Nelson Range, Hunter Mountain— they are all made mostly of quartz monzonite. Here and there, islands of the original sedimentary rocks are also exposed, and on their edges are the metal-rich contact zones that sparked the Ubehebe mining rush in the early 1900s. When miners searched for metals, unbeknownst to them, they were identifying contact metamorphic zones. On modern geology maps, their mines magically retrace the shattered outlines of the Mesozoic pluton.

Route Description: Ubehebe Peak

The lower trail to the divide. The Ubehebe Peak climb is one of the most spectacular hikes in this desert. For a change there is a trail, most of the way, probably built by miners to haul out their ore by mule. At the Grandstand turnout, the trailhead is identified by rocks lined up on both sides of it. The trail first heads west part way up the fan, then veers approximately northwest. It continues in this general direction for about 1 mile before climbing steeply to a low saddle north of Ubehebe Peak, on the divide of the Last Chance Range. This is quite a good little trail, with a total of 36 switchbacks nicely pacing the climb, and with increasingly fine views of the Racetrack Valley. In the summer it is best to tackle it in the late afternoon; this part of the trail is then in deep shade. Most of the rocks exposed along the way are essentially the same as what makes up the Grandstand—porphyritic granite with large crystals of orthoclase from the Mesozoic (see *The Racetrack Valley*).

Little can prepare you for the views when you top the divide and first look down the other side at Saline Valley, which is half a mile lower than the Racetrack. There is perhaps no better place to appreciate what a deep trough it is. The salt lake at the bottom of the valley, about 13 miles away and nearly 4,000 feet down, is dwarfed by the two-mile high wall of the Inyo Mountains. In the late afternoon, when it is obscured by the shadow of the mountains, the valley seems unfathomable.

If the climb to the divide left you breathless in more ways than one, this may be a good turning point. Do not feel too bad; the views do get better from here on up, but you have experienced most of the visual effect.

From the divide to the peak. At the divide the trail forks. The leftmost trail, lined with rocks and the most obvious of the two, goes to the peak. At first it climbs steeply along the ridge, offering at a couple of places dizzying views straight down the sheer east wall of the mountain. Then the trail circumvents the nameless peak north of Ubehebe Peak on its west side. In spite of a few switchbacks and rock stairs, this part is steeper and rougher than the lower mining trail. Near the saddle between the two peaks, the trail ends. The rest of the way is essentially cross-country. The best route is a little west of the ridge line; it is marked by a few cairns and faint trail segments. This is strenuous hiking. The average slope approaches 45%, there are plenty of loose rocks, and you may even forget to pay attention to the views. But you will not when you reach the narrow, wind-swept summit of Ubehebe Peak and are suddenly confronted with two very different worlds. On one side, you'll look, straight down it seems, at the pristine Racetrack playa and its tiny island of dark rounded rocks, with the high Cottonwood Mountains sprawling in the background. A 180° turn and you are on the brink of Saline Valley, with its small salt lake and dunes shining in the distance, completely isolated by high mountain ranges—the Nelson Range to the south, the Inyos to the west, the Saline Range to the north, and the Last Chance Range you are standing on. You may find, as I did, that two eyes are just not sufficient to take it all in.

Route Description: The Copper Queen Mines

The Copper Queen No. 1 Mine. This mine, the highest in the area, offers an easy side trip on your way to the peak. From the divide, take the rightmost of the two southbound trails, which is the old trail to the Copper Queen No. 1. It ends in about 0.2 mile, within sight of the mine openings. From here, head down to the tunnel with the yellowish tailing at the bottom of the ravine to the south (you may pick out the faint track of the original trail on your way there). Ore was first discovered here at the turn of the century, and the mine was worked episodically until the 1950s. It has a 35-foot shaft with remains of its primitive hoist, a tunnel and several exploratory trenches, and a few historical monument markers. The workings have a fair amount of copper ore, all in marble. Although brittle from decades of weathering, the ore is unusually colorful, and it varies greatly from site to site.

The approach to the other copper mines. The objective of this strenuous, full-day hike is the three copper mines located in the nameless canyon about 1.5 miles northwest of Ubehebe Peak. There are several routes to get into it, all of which start from the divide at the top of the lower trail. You can try hiking down the wash just west of the divide, which is the shortest route. Or you can follow the ridge north and try one of the next four washes, or the ridges between them. All routes are very steep and slow at places, some of them have falls, until around the 4,200-foot level where the grade eases up a little.

The canyon itself rapidly becomes the focus of this hike. All the way down to the Blue Jay Mine, it cuts through quartz monzonite. Fairly shallow in its upper reaches, the canyon deepens in the vicinity of the mines and remains on the narrow side most of the way. Though short, it has a surprising number of tributaries, with falls, narrower sections, and more abandoned mines. Wandering up and down this sinuous maze in search of forgotten vestiges certainly stimulated my curiosity. It is one of these totally isolated places where you could easily imagine that you are all alone on the planet—ignoring the occasional jet in the blue yonder. From the ridge down to the Blue Jay Mine, it's a 2,000-foot drop in just 2 miles. It's steep and physically demanding, but odds are no other human being will be sharing your canyon that day—maybe that year.

The Copper Queen Mines. The first mine, above the wash on the south side, is the Copper Queen No. 2. It has a 60-foot shaft, a short tunnel, and several trenches. The yellowish ore-bearing rock is tactite heavily stained with iron. The second mine, on the same side about 0.2 mile down canyon, is the Copper Queen. Faint trails lead up the very steep south canyon wall to a tunnel high above the wash. Like the Copper Queen No. 1, both mines are historically significant. They were probably part of the claims controlled around 1905-1908 by Jack Salsberry, a promoter who generated a lot of the original interest in the Ubehebe Mining District (see *Last Chance Range, Mining History*).

Ubehebe Peak and the Copper Queen Mines		
	Dist.(mi)	Elev.(ft)
Ubehebe Peak		
Grandstand turnout	0.0	3,710
Divide	1.9	~4,900
Saddle	2.5	~5,220
Ubehebe Peak	2.8	5,678
Copper Mines		
Divide	0.0	~4,900
Copper Queen No. 1	(0.3)	~4,910
Copper Queen No. 2	1.1	3,730
Copper Queen	1.3	3,580
Blue Jay Mine (lowest tunnel)	2.0	2,810
Canyon mouth	2.7	2,500
Saline Valley Road	7.4	1,430

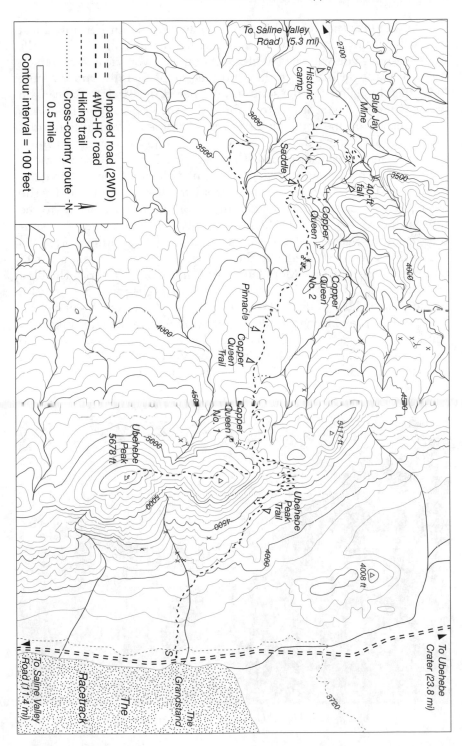

The Blue Jay Mine. This mine is only 0.7 mile further down, just below the narrows in the lower canyon. However, to avoid the high falls in the narrows you will need to hike out of the canyon via a faint trail on the south side, at a sharp right bend (see map). A little under a mile long, this trail climbs to the south ridge, then drops back to the canyon wash. The mine workings are a short distance up canyon from this point, mostly on the south slope and up the side canyon to the north. The largest working is the mineral-rich open cut just below the narrows, which is reached by a steep road. The deep-blue copper ore occurs mostly in tactite. This property is quite old; it had already been claimed and named by 1902. The owner, a man from Independence named Arlie Mairs, kept it for at least three decades, working it episodically, to the tune of the copper market. His property was then accessed by a spur road from the Saline Valley Road. Around 1914, Mairs transported his ore 12 miles across the valley to the salt tramway, which trammed it 13 more miles over the Inyo Mountains (see *Saline Valley, History*). The Blue Jay's only recorded production is 20 tons of high-grade ore in 1915, which yielded 4,000 pounds of copper and nearly 1,200 ounces of silver.

If you can arrange a ride, a great way to complete this hike is to continue down canyon to the old Blue Jay Mine Road (now closed to motor vehicles) and follow it to the Saline Valley Road. The long walk across the desolate floor of Saline Valley is a wild experience.

■

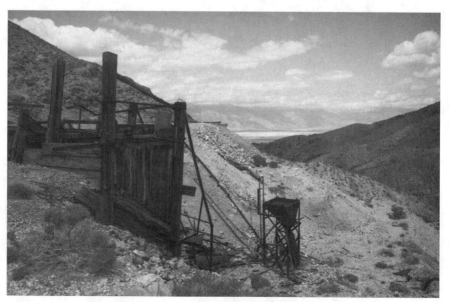

Tipple and ore bin at the Lippincott Mine (main group)

THE LIPPINCOTT MINE AND DODD SPRINGS

> *The main destination here is the Lippincott Mine, an interesting lead mine isolated at the south end of the Racetrack Valley. Besides the usual approach via the long Racetrack Valley Road, two alternative access routes are suggested—one a scenic climb along a primitive road from Saline Valley, the other a longer and more arduous hike on an old mining trail, past historical Little and Big Dodd Springs.*

General Information

Road access: Graded or primitive roads
Shortest hike: 1.1 mi, 200 ft one way / very easy
Longest hike: 8.1 mi, ~3,940 ft one way / difficult
Main attractions: A historic lead mine and trail, springs, wild flowers
USGS 15' topo map: Ubehebe Peak
USGS 7.5' topo maps: Ubehebe Peak*, Jackass Canyon
Maps: pp. 327*, 315, 333, 477

Location and Access

The Lippincott Mine is at the south end of the Racetrack Valley, near the head of a nameless canyon draining into Saline Valley. The first and most common way to get to it is to drive the Racetrack Valley Road. Park at the Homestake Dry Camp at the south end of the road (see *The Racetrack Valley* for directions and road conditions). The Lippincott Mine is on the hillside about half a mile to the south.

The second approach is the Lippincott Road. Starting from the Saline Valley Road 10.4 miles north of the Hunter Mountain Road, it heads east across the valley to the foot of the Last Chance Range, then crosses it to meet the Racetrack Valley Road just north of the Lippincott Mine. With a standard-clearance vehicle, you may be able to drive this road 4.4 miles to the roadside prospect a little past the Bonanza copper claims. This is the last spot wide enough to park before the road gets so rough as to make high clearance and four-wheel drive mandatory.

The third approach suggested here is the old Dodd Springs trail. To get to the trailhead, which is in Grapevine Canyon near the south end of the Saline Valley Road, drive this road 3.7 miles north from the junction with the Hunter Mountain Road. This will put you in the middle of a straight open section of road, about midpoint between two stretches of spring vegetation (across from BM 4412.3). Look for the trail climbing up the steep open hillside on the right side.

History

The earliest mining activity around the Lippincott Mine area was associated with the Wedding Stake, a group of seven claims discovered in December 1906, and the lead and silver Raven Mine, which was active from about 1917 through 1926. Little is known about their history, except that they were located on adjacent (or perhaps the same) ground, and they had partly common ownership. By 1926, the Raven Mine already had 2,000 feet of workings. The property then changed hands several times, being referred to in the 1930s as the Lead King Mine, then as the Southern Lead Mine, with some production of unknown value taking place at least from 1938 to 1941.

The area entered what was probably its most productive phase in early 1942, when George Lippincott, from Goldfield, Nevada, leased the property, then bought it two years later. With the help of his two sons, Lippincott began developing the property in May 1942, and over the next 10 years organized a nice little operation. The mine employed up to nine men, who first worked on the main tunnel (perhaps the original Raven Mine) then gradually opened other shafts and tunnels. There was a small camp near the mine, which was reached by plane in later years, using the Racetrack as a landing field. Water was a problem, as usual. Access to the closest water at Big Dodd Spring, less than 5 miles away, was difficult, and a pipeline was out of the question because of the danger of freezing in the winter. Water had to be trucked in from either Goldbelt Spring or Scotty's Castle, and the dream of an on-site mill never came through. The ore was trucked to Goldfield, which was a long, difficult route, and from there shipped by train to smelters in Utah. In the early years only the richest ore could be economically shipped out. The saving grace was that the mine had plenty of rich ore, assaying as much as 63% in lead and 35 ounces of silver per ton. Early on, the mine operators began constructing a new road to Keeler via the south end of Saline Valley to handle the lower grade ore, but it is not clear whether this road was ever used. Except for about a year during the war, when the area was under government control for aerial gunnery practice, the Lippincott Mine produced every year until 1952. During this period, it was the most active mine in the Racetrack area. It produced 2,000 tons of lead, silver and zinc valued at a modest $80,000, which still made it the third largest lead producer in Death Valley.

Geology

All the Lippincott ore deposits are found in sedimentary rocks of the Lost Burro Formation metamorphosed by contact with the Hunter Mountain batholith (see *Ubehebe Peak and the Copper Queen Mines*). The metamorphosed rock is mostly dolomite marble, light gray to white, often recrystallized. The main commercial ore was silver-bearing lead-zinc. It occurs in poorly defined veins along minor faults and in irregular replacement zones. Silver-bearing galena and cerussite, hemimorphite, wulfenite, a little pyrite, sphalerite, talc, and traces of chalcopyrite were found at the mine. During World War II, when the presence of silver in the ore had not yet been recognized, the ore went into the production of very expensive storage batteries!

Route Description

The Lippincott Road. This is probably the best way to discover the Lippincott Mine: it puts enough distance between your car and the mine to make you appreciate its isolation and surroundings. The walk from the Bonanza claim is straightforward, up the tight switchbacks of the steep road through a rugged canyon. In the spring, the roadside flower show is pretty good (look for spotted langloisia), and the rocks are interesting year-round—Paleozoic carbonates on the left, Mesozoic quartz-monzonite on the right, and Cenozoic olivine-basalt somewhere in the middle—but it is the views that will probably get you. The road offers good vistas of Saline Valley's salt flats and the towering Inyo Mountains, which get finer along the way.

You can stay on this road until it joins the Racetrack Valley Road (2.8 miles), then walk south 0.7 mile to the Lippincott Mine. You can also take the shortcut shown on the map and save 1 mile. About 2 miles into this walk, after the road has been level for a while, look for a prospect 100 yards down to the right, betrayed by two metal pipes dropping to it. Leave the road and head down to it (although it is called the Lead Giant Prospect, its two shallow pits show mostly copper ore). Continue down the ravine below the pits to the main wash. Another 220 yards up canyon and there is a fork; another 300 yards up the right fork and you'll see the ore bin of the Lippincott Mine just up to your right.

The Dodd Springs trail. This is the longest approach: about 6.8 miles and 3,530 feet of elevation change each way. It takes a whole day to get there and back, but the hike itself is as much of a reward as the final destination. The path you'll follow is the old Dodd Springs trail, which once connected Grapevine Canyon to the Racetrack Valley. From the trailhead, hike up the trail to the top of the first ridge. This part of the trail is well-defined because of cattle—this area has one of the park's few grazing easements. The rest of it is not nearly this good. At the first ridge the trail disappears, and you'll have to go some distance down the shallow ravine on the far side before finding it again, on the right side, a little before the first canyon crossing. There is a small seep here, usually dry, with dense thickets of willow and wild rose. The trail resumes near the upper end of the spring, heading north up to the next saddle. The rest of the way follows the same pattern: up and down.

Little Dodd Spring is beyond the third ridge. Trapped in a narrow canyon just up from the trail crossing, it has very thick vegetation. The mine on the next ridge is the Shirley Ann Mine, located in 1940. Its original discovery may date back to the 1900s, when a claim named Eureka was staked in this area. Both copper (mostly malachite) and lead (galena and cerussite) were exploited, probably in limited quantity given the remoteness of the site. It has several prospects, tunnels, and shafts, with colorful copper-stained walls. Big Dodd Spring, in the next drainage north, is impressively large and lush. Being in a more open canyon than its little brother, it is easier to visit. If it has surface water, it is well hidden in its dense grove of willow festooned with grapevine.

Like a giant roller coaster, the trail goes over another four main ridges before it finally reaches the Racetrack Valley, dropping after each ridge into a minor west-draining canyon, usually with a dry spring in it. Although the trail is not continuous, it is often present where it is most needed, on the steeper slopes. Elsewhere, it is faster to follow its approximate location than to look for it. To describe this route in detail would

The Lippincott Mine and Dodd Springs		
	Dist.(mi)	Elev.(ft)
Lippincott Road		
Bonanza claim prospect	0.0	2,580
Leave road	2.0	3,700
Lead Giant Prospect	2.05	3,590
Canyon wash	2.15	3,530
Main mine	2.5	3,760
Dodd Springs trail		
Saline Valley Road	0.0	4,410
Little Dodd Spring (wash)	2.1	3,910
Big Dodd Spring	2.5	3,830
Divide	5.0	4,660
Lippincott Mine (water truck)	6.8	3,870
Lippincott Mine		
Homestake Dry Camp	0.0	3,780
Water truck (junction)	0.4	3,870
Confidence No.2 (left fork)	(0.6)	4,020
Main mine (right fork)	1.1	3,760

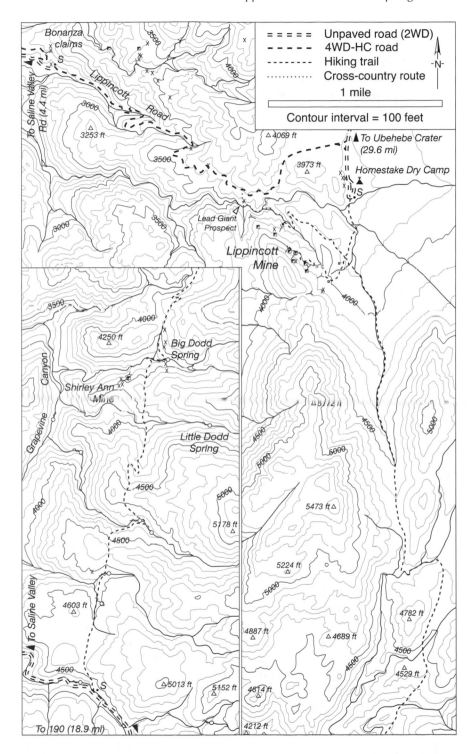

be tedious. If you are confident enough to hike it, you won't need it anyway.

This is a great hike, faithful to the desert spirit, spiced by the constant search for the almost imaginary trail. The hard outcrops of Hunter Mountain quartz monzonite mold much of the landscape, from exfoliating boulders in the washes to sheer walls in the Grapevine Canyon narrows to the west. The views are wild and the isolation exhilarating, but what got me was the wild flowers. In the spring of a particularly wet year, I saw more plants in bloom here than anywhere else in this desert, including less common species like desert mariposa and Parish larkspur. Dozens of species, in exuberant profusion, painted flamboyant canvasses all over the mountain slopes.

The Lippincott Mine. To get to the mine from the Homestake Dry Camp at the end of the Racetrack Valley Road, walk 0.4 mile down, then up the road to a fork, marked by a yellow water truck. The right fork goes to the main mine, offering good views of Saline Valley along the way. This area was worked in the early days of the mine and in Lippincott's era. It consists mostly of one tunnel, over 625 feet long, which splits into several shorter drifts. Both the large twin-chute ore bin just outside the tunnel and the metallic ore tipple below it were used to unload the ore, delivered from the tunnel by a narrow-gauge rail track. A couple of cabins once stood nearby, but only a concrete slab remains. From the slab a faint track climbs in switchbacks about 150 feet up the steep slope above the main tunnel to three impressively deep shafts.

The other road, straight ahead, continues up the hill. Just above the water truck it passes by several concrete foundations, including the signed slab of a mill. The main camp used to be just up the road, where it reaches a high point, but only the wooden floors of the cabins remain. The mines are a little further, past a low saddle in the road, strung along the south side. They were all developed after Lippincott acquired the property. The first one, about 400 feet past the saddle, is the Addison workings, the first to be opened after the main mine. A steep washed-out road leads up to its collapsed 120-foot inclined shaft and two tunnels, about 90 feet above the road. Its short tramway still spans the hillside. A little further down the road is the Inspiration Shaft, marked by its wooden framework. It was opened last, in 1951. The last two mining areas near the end of the road are the Confidence No. 1 and No. 2, opened after the Addison workings. The first one is the most extensive. It has a deep, nearly vertical shaft at its entrance (the Taylor Shaft) and a 250-foot tunnel (the Johnson Tunnel), a metallic headframe, and narrow gauge tracks. Good samples of the ore-bearing dolomite marble are exposed on the Confidence tailings.

■

PART VII

COTTONWOOD MOUNTAINS

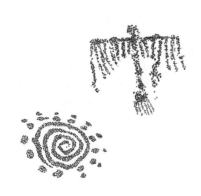

THE COTTONWOOD MOUNTAINS extend along the west side of northern Death Valley, from just north of Ubehebe Crater down to Towne Pass. To the northwest, they are separated from the Last Chance Range by a long and narrow alluvial corridor which climbs up, then down into the Racetrack Valley. To the southwest, they are bounded by Grapevine Canyon and Panamint Valley. About 45 miles long, they cover approximately 250 square miles. With a mean crest elevation over 5,000 feet, they are the second highest mountains in the park. From north to south they are dominated by Tin Mountain (8,953'), their highest summit, White Top Mountain (7,607'), Hunter Mountain (7,454'), and Panamint Butte (6,585'). Several unnamed peaks exceed 6,000'. The lowest point is near 200 feet along the middle section of their western flank.

The physiography of the Cottonwoods is as asymmetric as any mountain range in Death Valley. On their west side the mountainous area slopes 1,000 to 2,000 feet down into several high-desert valleys—Hidden Valley, the Racetrack Valley, Ulida Flat, and Sand Flat. Except for Ulida Flat they are all, like Death Valley, closed basins. In contrast, the eastern side drop precipitously towards Death Valley, especially in the northern part where the elevation change averages 6,000 feet over only 4 to 5 air miles. Some of the deepest and narrowest canyons are found along this steep eastern escarpment. The southwestern portion of the Cottonwoods, facing Panamint Valley, is also very steep and rugged.

Access and Backcountry Roads

The Cottonwood Mountains are generally poorly accessible, and together with the adjacent alluvial fan and valley floor, they contain one of the largest roadless areas in the park. Most of the eastern base of the mountains lies between 3 and 9 miles of paved roads (the Scotty's Castle Road and Highway 190). Only Marble, Cottonwood, and Lemoigne canyons have access roads. None of them are through roads, and they all require a high-clearance and/or 4-wheel-drive vehicle.

On their west side, the Cottonwood Mountains can be accessed by two long backcountry roads. The first one is the Racetrack Valley Road, which connects the end of the paved road at Ubehebe Crater to the Racetrack Valley. Although it is a gravelly washboard, this road can be negotiated with a standard-clearance vehicle, if you have experience in this kind of driving. This area can also be reached via the Lippincott Road, the rough track that connects the Saline Valley Road to the south end of the Racetrack Valley Road. The second main backcountry road is the Hunter Mountain Road. Starting from the Racetrack Valley Road at the north end of the Racetrack Valley, it skirts the west side of the Cottonwood Mountains and eventually meets the Saline Valley Road at the south end of the range. This road gives access to wonderfully remote high desert country, including Hidden Valley and the upper drainage of several isolated canyons. It is generally in good shape, and a standard-clearance vehicle can make it through, but given that it crosses some of the most remote regions in the park high clearance is advisable. The Hunter Mountain Road is often snowed-in and closed in the winter.

Geology

For the most part the Cottonwood Mountains are made of sedimentary and metasedimentary rocks of marine origin from the Paleozoic. With a few exceptions, these exposures stretch from around Mesquite Spring south to Goldbelt Spring, then resume south of Lemoigne Canyon. These formations are mostly limestone and dolomite, with ages ranging from Ordovician to Pennsylvanian. The stratigraphy of large portions of this region has not been mapped, so that both younger and older formations may also be present. The remaining central area, from Goldbelt Spring to Lemoigne Canyon, is a massive band of granitic rocks known as the Hunter Mountain Pluton (late Jurassic, early Cretaceous). They also outcrop around White Top Mountain and along the ridge separating the Racetrack Valley from Hidden Valley.

North from Mesquite Spring, mostly Tertiary nonmarine rocks and Cenozoic basalt flows are exposed, as well as quaternary volcanic rocks from the recent eruptions of Ubehebe Crater and smaller nearby craters. An extensive flow of Pleistocene basalt, several miles wide, also occurs at the southern end of the Cottonwoods, along the west side of Highway 190. Finally, a few nonmarine deposits, Plio-Pleistocene in age, are exposed along the east front of the range on both sides of

Cottonwood Canyon and west of Towne Pass. The high valleys on the east side of the mountains are made of Quaternary alluvium, lake deposits and other sedimentary rocks.

Hydrology and Vegetation

Because of their western location and high elevation, the Cottonwood Mountains receive the second highest amount of precipitation in the park, including snow just about every winter. This moisture feeds a relatively large number of widely scattered springs. From north to south the major ones are Burro, Quartz, and Rest springs east of White Top Mountain, and Goldbelt Spring. In the southern range, Cottonwood Creek is a rare desert stream that runs above ground along about half of a 5-mile stretch of canyon. It is the longest perennial creek in the mountains surrounding Death Valley.

The higher elevation and moisture create a favorable climate for pinyon pine-juniper communities, which thrive at several places in the high Cottonwoods. Tin Mountain and the central crest have scattered woodlands, but it is Hunter Mountain which has the best to offer—its slopes are covered with one of the thickest forests in the park. Several healthy Joshua tree forests can be found in the central Cottonwood Mountains, especially along the Tin Pass corridor and around Hidden Valley.

Hiking

As far as hiking is concerned, the best features of the Cottonwood Mountains are long isolated canyons, good narrows, challenging climbs, and a higher occurrence of rock art than anywhere else in the park. The main canyons—Bighorn Gorge, Dry Bone, Marble, Cottonwood, and Lemoigne, and many other unnamed ones—cut deeply into the abrupt eastern escarpment of the mountains, and they stand out for their magnificence. Only Cottonwood and Marble canyons have roads in them. The Lemoigne Canyon Road only reaches as far as the canyon mouth, and the canyon itself is roadless. For all other canyons, access is gained by either hiking to the canyon mouth from Highway 190 or Scotty's Castle Road, or hiking to the canyon head from one of the west-side backcountry roads. Although the latter approach usually minimizes leg work, both approaches require extensive hiking even just to get to the canyon itself. The canyons are also generally fairly long, Marble and Cottonwood canyons being two of the longest in the park. They often branch out into extensive networks of side canyons, some of which are comparable in length to the main canyons. These features, combined with their remoteness, low visitation, higher elevations,

Suggested Hikes in the Cottonwood Mountains					
Route/Destination	Dist. (mi)	Elev. change	Mean elev.	Access road	Pages
Short hikes (under 5 miles round trip)					
Burro Spring	1.6	900'	6,900'	P/28.1 mi	350
Cottonwood Cyn Mid. Spr.	1.7	330'	3,000'	H/19.2 mi	371-374
Dry Bone Cyn upp. narrows	1.5	500'	5,890'	P/30.3 mi	342
Harris Hill	1.5	1,300'	5,070'	P/27.3 mi	366
Lemoigne Canyon narrows	0.6	240'	2,920'	F/5.5 mi	379
Lost Burro Mine	0.3	260'	5,450'	P/24 mi	354-356
Lost Burro Peak	1.8	1,550'	5,320'	P/21.2 mi	356
Marble Cyn (first narrows)	1.1	295'	1,960'	H/13.4 mi	359
Quackenbush Mine	0.7	190'	5,080'	P/27.1 mi	365
Rest Spring	0.4	200'	6,550'	P/28.1 mi	350
Silver Crown Mine	1.5	900'	7,290'	H/32.5 mi	340
Intermediate hikes (5-12 miles round trip)					
Bighorn Gorge (60-ft fall)	4.1	2,140'	5,870'	H/32.9 mi	336
Cottonwood Springs	4.0	800'	3,230'	H/19.2 mi	371-374
Dry Bone Cyn mid. narrows	3.5	2,020'	5,250'	H/30.0 mi	342-343
Lemoigne Canyon narrows from Emigrant R. S.	3.6	690'	2,360'	Paved	379-384
Lemoigne Canyon north fork-south fork*	9.1	5,760'	3,990'	F/5.5 mi	382
Lemoigne Mine	3.8	2,400'	3,930'	F/5.5 mi	379-382
Lost Burro Peak-Mine loop*	6.1	3,100'	5,210'	P/21.2 mi	356
Marble Canyon up to third narrows	4.2	1,085'	2,360'	H/13.4 mi	359-362
Goldbelt to largest spring	4.1	1,400'	4,240'	P/27.3 mi	366
Mule Tail Mine Road	4.1	1,140'	4,750'	P/27.9 mi	365-366
O'Brien Canyon loop*	7.4	3,720'	6,220'	H/32.9 mi	340
Perdido Canyon gorge	3.2	1,080'	5,540'	P/23.7 mi	348-349
to Burro Spring	5.4	2,400'	6,200'	P/23.7 mi	348-350
Rest Spring Gulch loop*	11.4	4,800'	6,200'	P/23.7 mi	348-350
Long hikes (over 12 miles round trip)					
Bighorn Gorge down to main side cyn	6.7	3,320'	5,280'	H/32.9 mi	336-338
road to road	14.2	5,690'	3,960'	H/32.9 mi	336-338
Cottonwood Canyon Road to Hunter Mountain Rd	14.6	3,550'	5,250'	H/19.2 mi	374

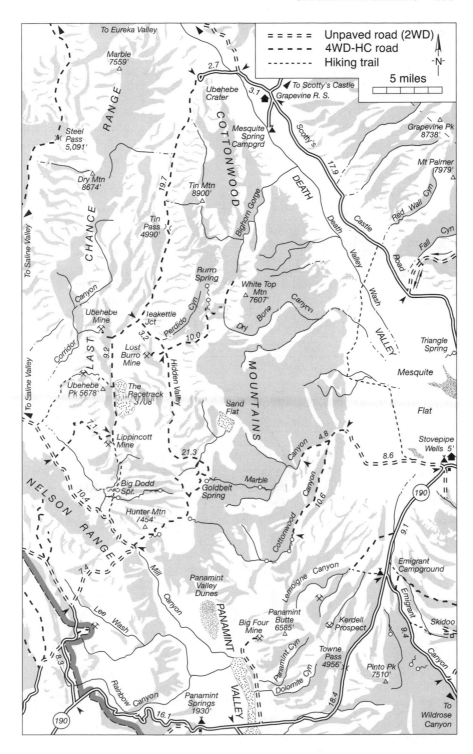

To Eureka Valley

Unpaved road (2WD)
4WD-HC road
Hiking trail

-N-

5 miles

Marble
7559'

To Scotty's Castle
Grapevine R. S.

2.7

Ubehebe
Crater

3.1

Grapevine Pk
8738'

Mesquite
Spring
Campgrd

Steel
Pass
5,091'

Mt Palmer
7979'

Scotty's

17.9

Red Wall Cyn

Dry Mtn
8674'

Tin Mtn
8900'

Fall Cyn

19.7

Bighorn Gorge

DEATH

Tin
Pass
4990'

Burro
Spring

White Top
Mtn
7607'

VALLEY

Triangle
Spring

Dry Bore Canyon

Castle

Wash

Death Valley

Road

Ubehebe
Mine

Teakettle
Jct

Perdido Cyn

10.0

9.2

3.2

Corridor

Canyon

Mesquite

Lost
Burro
Mine

Hidden Valley

Ubehebe
Pk 5678'

The
Racetrack
3708'

Sand
Flat

Flat

Stovepipe
Wells 5'

Lippincott
Mine

7.1

21.3

4.8

8.6

Big Dodd
Spr.

Goldbelt
Spring

Marble

Canyon

190

NELSON RANGE

Hunter Mtn
7454'

Cottonwood Canyon

10.6

9.1

Emigrant
Campground

10.4

LAST CHANCE RANGE

COTTONWOOD

MOUNTAINS

Mill Canyon

Panamint
Valley
Dunes

Lemoigne Canyon

Skidoo

7.4

Panamint
Butte
6585'

Kerdell
Prospect

9.4

Lee Wash

Big Four
Mine

PANAMINT

Towne
Pass
4956'

Pinto Pk
7510'

8.3

Panamint Cyn

Dolomite Cyn

18.4

Canyon

Emigrant

Rainbow Canyon

Panamint
Springs
1930'

VALLEY

To
Wildrose
Canyon

190

16.1

To Saline Valley

To Saline Valley

Route/Destination	Dist. (mi)	Elev. change	Mean elev.	Access road	Pages
Long hikes (over 12 miles round trip) (Cont'd)					
Dry Bone Canyon					
down to main side cyn	8.5	3,730'	4,340'	H/30.3 mi	342-344
Kerdell Prospect	7.9	3,700'	3,930'	Paved	384-386
Lemoigne Mine					
from Emigrant R. S.	6.8	2,850'	3,190'	Paved	380, 384
Marble Cyn third narrows					
from Goldbelt	6.7	2,080'	3,900'	P/27.3 mi	364-368
Marble Cyn (road to road)	10.7	3,130'	3,380'	H/13.4 mi	358-368
Overnight hikes (over 2 days)					
Dry Bone Canyon (rd to rd)	18.3	6,200'	3,190'	H/30.3 mi	342-346
Lemoigne Canyon Road					
to Cottonwood Cyn Road	17.1	4,890'	4,070'	H/19.2 mi	382
Marble-Cottonwood Cyn*	30.0	~8,000'	2,960'	H/10.8 mi	374

Key: P=Primitive (2WD)   H=Primitive (HC)   F=Primitive (4WD)
* =Total distance and elevation change (ups + downs) for all loops

and cooler temperatures, make the Cottonwood Mountains particularly appealing for extended backpacking trips. Marble Canyon and Cottonwood Canyon, in fact, have long been considered as Death Valley's classics.

The Cottonwood Mountains have been left comparatively untouched by prospectors and miners. The only significant mining areas are east of the Racetrack Valley, around Ulida Flat and Hidden Valley, and in Lemoigne Canyon. On the other hand, this area was highly prized by prehistoric cultures, as may be inferred from its relatively large number of rock art sites.

■

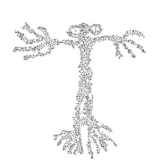

Petroglyph,
Cottonwood
Mountains

BIGHORN GORGE

Bighorn Gorge is a long, rugged, and isolated canyon with much to offer, from pine woodlands and Joshua trees to tight narrows, falls, and beautiful fossils. But it is one of the most remote canyons in the park, and the price to pay for these sights is a lot of walking. With a high-clearance vehicle you can drive fairly close and explore a good part of it in a day, but otherwise it will have to be an overnight trip. Either way, Bighorn is for serious hikers only.

General Information

Road status: Roadless; long, primitive road to canyon head (HC)
Shortest hike: 3.1 mi, 1,700 ft one way / moderate
Longest hike: 16.4 mi, 5,700 ft one way (or more) / strenuous
Main attractions: A remote canyon, several narrows with falls, fossils, woodlands, Joshua trees
USGS 15' topo map: Tin Mountain
USGS 7.5' topo maps: White Top Mountain*, Tin Mountain*, East of Tin Mountain
Maps: pp. 339*, 333

Location and Access

Bighorn Gorge is the northernmost major canyon in the Cottonwoods. To hike to its mouth, start from the Scotty's Castle Road 13.3 miles north of the Titus Canyon Road (or 3.9 miles south of the Grapevine Ranger Station), in the wide bend in the road. Bighorn Gorge is at the top of the broad, light-gray gravel wash coming straight down the fan to the southwest. You can also start from the Mesquite Spring Campground and hike down Death Valley Wash, then up the same way.

The head of Bighorn Gorge can be reached by driving to the White Top Mountain area. From the Ubehebe Crater Road, drive the Racetrack Valley Road 19.7 miles to Teakettle Junction. Turn left and drive 3.2 miles to the unmarked four-way junction just beyond Lost Burro Gap, at the pass into Hidden Valley. Take the White Top Mountain Road on the left, and follow it 10 miles to the divide overlooking Bighorn Gorge. At this point the road forks. The left spur goes to nearby O'Brien Canyon. Take the right spur and park at the small, pine-shaded turnout a short distance on the right. Bighorn Gorge is down the wide forested opening to the north. The White Top Mountain Road is usually passable with a standard-clearance passenger car up to the wash of Dry Bone Canyon. Just a little further on there is a rough spot, and the road is more rocky beyond; high clearance is needed for the last 2.7 miles. The drive from Ubehebe Crater takes at least one and a half hours.

Hiking Suggestions

If you have a high-clearance vehicle, drive to the head of the canyon for the shortest access by foot to the more interesting upper gorge. Hiking from here down to the main side canyon and back in one day is strenuous. Since the round-trip drive gobbles up several hours, it is best to camp at the head of the canyon and start hiking early the next day. To hike through the entire gorge to the road is about the same distance, but all downhill and easier. It's still a long day if you are in shape, purgatory otherwise, and you will need to arrange a ride.

If you have a passenger car, you can either hike up from Death Valley or drive as far as the wash of Dry Bone Canyon and hike the rest of the way (2.7 miles) to the head of Bighorn Gorge. Both routes are lengthy; the best way to explore this long canyon is overnight.

Route Description

The upper canyon. The upper drainage of Bighorn Gorge is a large basin where several broad, steep valleys converge from the crest of the Cottonwood Mountains down to the bottleneck of the gorge. This area is densely forested with pinyon pines and junipers, which is one of the delights of hiking in from this end. For the first 1.4 miles down to timberline, the canyon is a narrow, rock-strewn ravine crowded with large trees and occasional falls. From timberline down to the gorge, it broadens to a beautiful valley dotted with Joshua trees.

The upper gorge. The upper gorge, above the main side canyon, is deep and tortuous, and delightful for its solitude and unpredictability. At places the high walls display colorful strata, usually limestone and sandstone interbedded with dolomite. The wash squeezes through several smoothly polished narrows. Although short (0.1-0.3 mile), these beautiful, often very sinuous passages are the main attractions. Progress is impeded by a few falls and chockstones, although most of them are not serious obstacles.

The first narrows come as a surprise, in a tight bend in the canyon. They start as a dark crevasse plunging over a 60-foot drop-off, followed by a 15-foot fall just below it. This drop-off can be bypassed on the west side by scrambling down a steep talus of large square boulders. When you get to the bottom, walk back up into these short narrows. Rock climbers may want to take a close look at the majestic, wall-rimmed drop-off by climbing the 15-foot fall (about a 5.6).

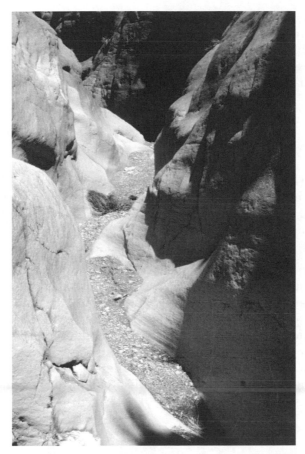

Polished bedrock in the third narrows of Bighorn Gorge

The second and fourth narrows start with the only falls that are slightly more difficult (especially going up), both about 7-feet high, slick and near vertical. The second narrows, somewhat wider, have high, vertical and jagged walls. The third narrows, finely polished up to 10 feet above the wash, are the windiest and tightest, narrow enough at places to brush both walls with your hands. The floor is scooped into small basins and hollows, sometimes filled with rain water.

Starting a little above the third narrows, beautiful fossils grace the canyon walls, an uncommon occurrence in Death Valley. The best and most numerous exposures I found are in the fourth narrows. The fossils are marine shells, probably from the early Paleozoic, distributed on several horizons in the thick deposit of limestone/dolomite. The polishing action of water has revealed these ancient fossils as pale, curly lines against the smooth, darker rock. They resemble the common shells found on today's beaches—bivalves, snails, and the slender, conical spirals of gastropods, smaller than an inch. The most striking are large fossils, probably ammonites, curling around several times, often 3 or 4 inches across. They are so finely preserved that some of them still show the inner chambers the animal filled with air for buoyancy.

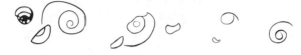

The lower gorge. The lower gorge, between the main side canyon and the mouth, is a broader canyon. I only saw its upper portion, which is wide and framed by high, rugged walls. I was told the rest of it does not have any major falls, but this is third hand news. If you decide to check it out, you may be favorably surprised.

The side canyons. The many side canyons of Bighorn Gorge can also be exciting destinations. There are in fact so many that if you are going up canyon on your first time here, you'll need a map to make the right turns, especially in the upper canyon where forks often look alike. The main side canyon, 2.9 miles above the mouth, is one of the longest (about 3.1 miles). I have not explored it, but the little I saw definitely made me want to go back. The map suggests several steep areas with potential high falls and narrows. It is likely more challenging than the main gorge, and equally interesting.

	Dist.(mi)	Elev.(ft)
Bighorn Gorge		
End of White Top Mtn Road	0.0	6,940
O'Brien Canyon	3.1	5,230
Head of the gorge	3.5	5,020
1st narrows (60-ft fall)	4.1	~4,800
2nd narrows	4.6	~4,650
3rd narrows	5.2	~4,180
4th narrows	5.6	~4,070
Main side canyon	6.7	3,620
Mouth	9.6	2,640
Mesquite Spring Campground	(6.8)	1,780
Death Valley Wash	12.9	1,470
Scotty's Castle Road	14.2	1,690

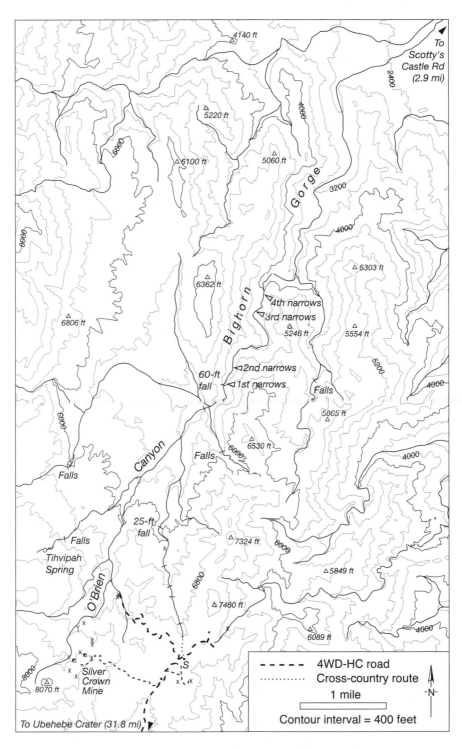

To
Scotty's
Castle Rd
(2.9 mi)

4140 ft

5220 ft

6100 ft

5060 ft

Gorge

3200

4000

2400

4000

5303 ft

6362 ft

Bighorn

4th narrows

3rd narrows

5246 ft

5554 ft

6806 ft

5200

60-ft
fall

2nd narrows

1st narrows

Falls

4000

5065 ft

Canyon

Falls

6530 ft

Falls

4000

25-ft
fall

7324 ft

6000

Falls

Tihvipah
Spring

5849 ft

O'Brien

6800

7460 ft

6089 ft

4000

S

Silver
Crown
Mine

8070 ft

To Ubehebe Crater (31.8 mi)

– – – –	4WD-HC road
··········	Cross-country route

1 mile

-N-

Contour interval = 400 feet

O'Brien Canyon, in the upper canyon, offers a nice alternative route to get in and out of Bighorn Gorge or to make a loop through the upper drainage. It is reachable from the main access road via one of two mining roads, which lead to its rim. The first one is the left fork near road's end. The other one starts near the picturesque wood cabin 0.4 mile further south. O'Brien Canyon was first prospected in 1912 for copper, which occurs in small silicate veins scattered in limestone. Prospects were located in 1917 as the Silver Crown group, then relocated and renamed several times and worked for years, but they were never exploited commercially. The most extensive prospects, at the top of the southernmost road, are two short, steeply inclined shafts. The narrow veins nearby contain small amounts of malachite, azurite and bornite, and small crystals of yellow-green or light purple fluorite. There are other prospects and cuts near copper-stained veins down canyon and near the end of the other road.

Bighorn sheep. Given its name and the abundant signs of sheep in nearby Dry Bone Canyon, I was surprised to find no traces of this graceful desert dweller in the upper gorge. The sheep of the Death Valley region are known to temporarily abandon certain areas for years at a time for no apparent reason, and this may be a case in point. They will likely return.

■

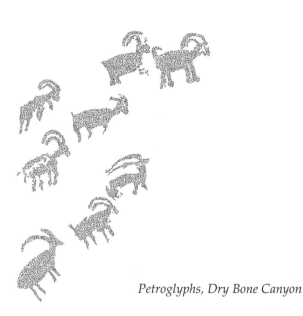

Petroglyphs, Dry Bone Canyon

DRY BONE CANYON

Dry Bone Canyon is hard to reach, rarely visited, and perfect for a long trek in the mountains. After the long backcountry drive to the upper canyon, a short walk down its broad wash, studded with Joshua trees, will take you to the spectacular upper narrows. Below this deep passage, the canyon floor drops 550 feet in a series of high falls. To see the rest of Dry Bone—a majestic canyon framed by sheer limestone walls—takes either a strenuous scramble around these falls or a long hike up from Death Valley.

General Information

Road status: Road in upper drainage; hiking from long primitive road
Shortest hike: 1.6 mi, 510 ft one way / easy
Longest hike: 19.3 mi, 6,230 ft one way (or more) / strenuous
Main attractions: Good narrows, high falls, grand sceneries, petroglyphs
USGS 15' topo maps: Tin Mountain, Marble Canyon, Grapevine Peak
USGS 7.5' topo maps: Sand Flat, White Top Mountain, Dry Bone Canyon
Maps: pp. 345*, 333

Location and Access

Dry Bone Canyon is located in the central Cottonwoods, south of Bighorn Gorge. The easiest access is to the upper canyon, although it requires a fair amount of driving on primitive roads. The directions are the same as for Bighorn Gorge, via the Racetrack Valley Road to Teakettle Junction (19.7 miles), then left through Lost Burro Gap and left again 3.2 miles further on at the White Top Mountain Road. Drive this last road 7.4 miles to the wash of Dry Bone Canyon (elev. 6,140') and park. This route usually does not require anything more fancy than a standard-clearance passenger car.

The other, far more demanding approach is to hike in from Death Valley. Start from the Scotty's Castle Road about 2.8 miles north of the Titus Canyon turnoff (or 15.1 miles south of the Grapevine Ranger Station). Dry Bone Canyon is the northernmost of the two canyons that converge at the apex of the fan, to the west-southwest.

Hiking Suggestions

From the upper drainage it is a short, two hour round-trip hike to the upper narrows, an easy walk even in the summer at this fairly high elevation. For a more challenging day hike, continue around the

341

drop-off to, and through, the second narrows. To make the Scotty's Castle Road takes a very long day. The other approach, up the long alluvial fan from the road, is a true Death Valley experience that requires at least two or three days.

Route Description

Joshua trees and leaning rocks. The walk down the funnel-shaped wash to the canyon is a little strange, through gentle terrain dotted with blackbrush and dwarf Joshua trees. In this remote location, these spiky trees stand like sentinels guarding the approach to a secret place. The entire landscape seems to be leaning towards the distant narrowing at the end of the wash, as if pulled to it by a mystical force, or to entice wanderers into the hidden canyon beyond. This canyon was in fact once referred to as Leaning Rock Canyon. The name is still attached today to the tilted ridge on the southern horizon.

The upper narrows. At the bottom of the funnel the wash narrows down and the true canyon begins. Around the first bend a 9-foot slanted fall, well polished and easy to climb, guards the entrance to the upper narrows. A short distance down, the canyon turns into a magnificent narrow corridor of polished gray dolomite walls, reminiscent of Grotto Canyon. Facing walls match each other's curves to create a contorted passage, filled with deep shadows. After about 100 yards the smooth gravel bed is abruptly interrupted by a 20-foot fall beneath a large boulder—the first of many back-to-back falls. In the next quarter of a mile the canyon floor drops about 600 feet along one of the tightest and most impregnable slot canyons in Death Valley.

The slot. To reach the canyon below, there is not really any option but to circumvent this major obstruction. The shortest and easiest route, such as it is, involves walking back through the narrows, up the slanted fall and around the bend to the small side canyon on the right. Go up its rocky wash (north-northeast) for about 250 yards, then climb the short bank on the right, east towards the prominent pyramid-shaped peak. This should take you to a 200-yard long, nearly level ridge within sight of Telescope Peak. The ravine on the east side of this ridge drops into Dry Bone Canyon below the slot. Go far enough north, up along the ridge, before climbing down into it, or you will get stranded at the top of high cliffs. It is then a slow, strenuous, 800-foot, 0.35-mile descent along this boulder-choked ravine to the canyon wash.

When you get to the bottom of the ravine, by all means walk up canyon into the narrows, dark and windy, encased in craggy summits. There are a couple of easy falls to climb, but the third one is a 20-foot wall—the bottom end of the slot. Climbing it is difficult and dangerous

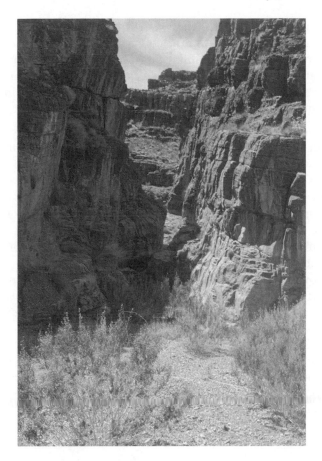

In the second narrows of Dry Bone Canyon

(especially using the crude and unsafe ladder of two by fours lying around) and should be attempted only by experienced climbers.

The middle narrows. Below the ravine the canyon opens up and meanders in wide loops beneath high limestone cliffs. This area and much of the rest of the canyon is reminiscent of side canyons of the Colorado River inside the Grand Canyon. High angular cliffs form giant stairways climbing in 100-foot steps to distant rims, stained with dark tapestries of desert varnish. About 0.8 mile below the ravine the canyon squeezes through the second narrows, a 0.3-mile gorge winding between vertical black-veined walls. At the lower end of these narrows the wash cuts through a 20-foot thick vertical strata of cream-colored conglomerate. Large angular boulders from this strata are stranded in the wash just down canyon. Rocks resting on top of them mark the high tide of past floods, as much as 10 feet above the wash!

Throughout this area, the wash is alive with many blooming plants in the spring, including brittlebush, stingbush, and penstemon. Small hanging gardens of Panamint phacelia thrive in wall fissures. At higher elevations the striking blossoms of cottontop, calico, and beavertail cacti brighten the rocky slopes. Sightings of solitary birds, in particular hawks and hummingbirds, are common.

The lower canyon. The lower part of Dry Bone Canyon is considerably wider than the upper canyon. Much like Titanothere Canyon, it is a far-away world of silence and grand panoramas, a perfect place for desert lovers. For about 1.7 miles past the second narrows, the landscape is shallower, with low rolling hills on both sides. Then the wash enters the third narrows as it swings into a pronounced S-shaped meander. Beyond, the canyon becomes more deeply entrenched again. The side canyon 1.3 miles above the mouth is a whole world in itself, forking several times into secret passages perhaps never fully explored.

Below its mouth the canyon opens onto a vast amphitheater, the common terminus of Dry Bone Canyon and the major, nameless canyon to the south. It is a great camping spot, far away from everything. Beyond the vast sweeping sea of gravel and creosote spilling out of the mountain, the jagged rampart of the Amargosa Range provides the backdrop for rare and spectacular views of Death Valley.

If you hike on from here to the road, you'll intersect the old west side trail about 5.5 miles below the canyon mouth. From this point you can continue cross-country (east-northeast) 3 miles to the road. You can

	Dist.(mi)	Elev.(ft)
Dry Bone Canyon		
White Top Mtn Road at wash	0.0	6,140
1st narrows (9-ft fall)	1.5	5,650
20-ft fall (edge of slot)	1.6	5,630
First narrows (end/bypass)	2.4	~5,020
Second narrows (start)	3.2	~4,570
Second narrows (end)	3.5	~4,360
Third narrows (at meander)	5.3	3,740
Main side canyon	8.5	2,510
Mouth	9.8	2,000
Trail	15.3	240
Scotty's Castle Road (via trail)	(4.0)	420
Scotty's Castle Road	~18.3	305

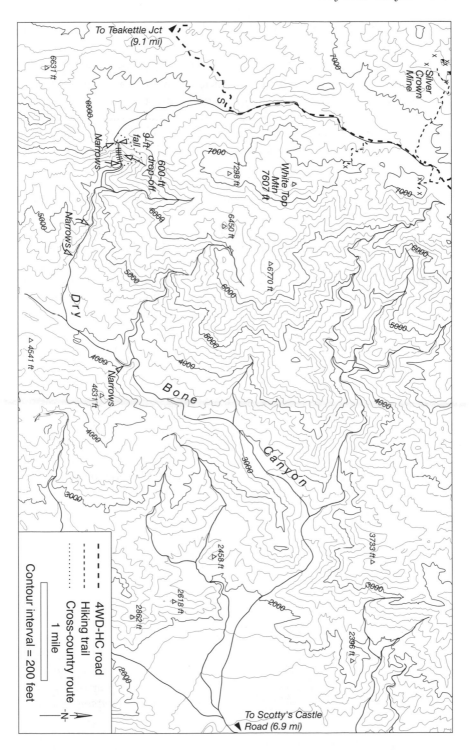

To Teakettle Jct
(9.1 mi)

Silver
Crown
Mine

6631 ft

6000

Narrows

9-ft
fall

600-ft drop-off

7000

7298 ft

White Top
Mtn
7607 ft

7000

7000

6000

Narrows

6450 ft

6770 ft

6000

5000

Dry

5000

6000

5000

5000

4541 ft

4000

4631 ft

Narrows

4000

Bone

4000

4000

3000

Canyon

3000

3733 ft

3000

2458 ft

2618 ft

2862 ft

2396 ft

2000

2000

2000

4WD-HC road

Hiking trail

Cross-country route

1 mile

Contour interval = 200 feet

-N-

To Scotty's Castle
Road (6.9 mi)

also follow this trail 4 miles until it joins the road about 2.5 miles further north, which is a little easier route.

The place where the bighorn come to die. There are petroglyphs in Dry Bone Canyon. Although they include many abstract compositions, human stick figures, and a horned snake, the most striking ones represent bighorn sheep. The sheep's horns are unusually long, their bodies depicted in numerous positions—resting, running, jumping, and even upside down. There is something magic about this site, born from its remoteness and unusual setting. It is a wonderful invitation to try, once again, to decipher these cryptic messages. Was this canyon the lair of a shaman or a hunter's blind? I always feel that if its walls could talk, they would tell a powerful secret.

Coincidentally, I saw here more signs of bighorn sheep than in any other desert bighorn habitat I have visited. The sheep bed along the wash, on protected gravel benches below canyon walls, in shallow depressions in the bedrock. Look for places where they have pawed the gravel to smooth it before lying down, and for telltale droppings. After a rainy summer night I found a small hole dug in the dry gravel of the second narrows, surrounded by sheep droppings. The bighorn taught me a lesson—at the bottom of the hole there was a little water.

The most exciting signs of bighorn sheep are the many bleached bones and skulls scattered along the wash. I saw here three ram skulls with almost fully curved horns, all six years old at the time of death. Considering the usual scarcity of bighorn skulls in the deserts of the Southwest, this abundance is a mystery. It made me wonder whether, like the legendary elephant cemetery of Africa, this is the secret place where bighorns come to die, whether it is the origin of the intriguing proliferation of sheep petroglyphs in this canyon. Maybe we are not the first ones to name this place Dry Bone.

■

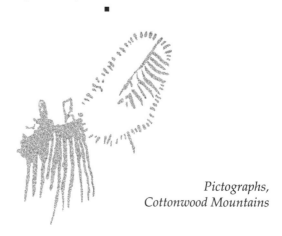

Pictographs,
Cottonwood Mountains

PERDIDO CANYON

> The main feature of Perdido Canyon is its wide gorge of dark cliffs
> bearing numerous fossils of Devonian goniatites, brachiopods, and
> corals nearly 400 million years old. If you like looking for fossils, you
> will enjoy browsing along its pleasant wash sprinkled with Joshua
> trees. This hike can be extended to include Burro Spring and the
> pretty narrows of Rest Spring Gulch.

General Information

Road status: Roadless; access by long primitive road
Shortest hike: 2.4 mi, 760 ft one way / easy
Longest hike: 5.7 mi, 2,350 ft one way / strenuous
Main attractions: A remote canyon, fossils, geology, Joshua trees
USGS 15' topo maps: Marble Canyon, Tin Mountain*
USGS 7.5' lopo maps: Sand Flat, White Top Mountain*
Maps: pp. 351*, 333

Location and Access

Perdido Canyon is at the north end of Hidden Valley, in the central Cottonwood Mountains. To get there, drive the Racetrack Valley
Road to Teakettle Junction and turn left towards Hidden Valley. After
3.2 miles, at the pass just past Lost Burro Gap, turn left at the White Top
Mountain Road. Drive about 0.8 mile and park. In normal weather you
can make it this far with a normal-clearance passenger car (see *The
Racetrack Valley* for road conditions). Perdido Canyon is 0.5 mile north of
the road, hidden behind the low hills at the end of the fan.

Geology: The Slow Braking of the Earth

Four formations are exposed along Perdido Canyon: the Lost
Burro Formation, Tin Mountain Limestone, Perdido Formation, and Rest
Spring Shale. They contain mostly dolomite, limestone, and shale. The
Devonian and Carboniferous seas in which they were deposited were
teeming with hundreds of plant and animal species: lungfish, clams and
brachiopods, crinoids, trilobites, goniatites and other ammonites, and a
wide variety of corals. Many of them were preserved as fossils, and they
provide us with a wealth of information about that era.

Few fossils have had a more amazing story to tell than horn
corals—a story about the past of our planet, but also about its distant
future. Horn corals are small animals that lived in a horn-shaped,

slightly curved shell a couple of inches long. The shell is made of lime secreted by the animal in unison with the seasons. Much like tree rings, it bears annual circular grooves that tell the age of the coral. In the early 1960s, American geologist John Wells discovered that each annual groove in a Devonian horn coral is subdivided into many smaller rings, each one marking one day in the life of the coral. He counted the diurnal rings and made a fascinating discovery: back in the Devonian, the year had 395 days! It was not that the year was longer. The Earth took just as long to travel around the sun then as it does today. But it was spinning faster, completing a revolution in 22 hours only, and there were more days in a year. Wells' discovery was a spectacular confirmation of predictions made by physicists: the spin of the Earth is continually slowing down because of the friction between the Earth's surface and the ocean tides caused by the moon. This force is very weak; in 400 million years it has increased the length of a day by only 2 hours. But given enough time it will bring our planet to a virtual standstill. The tiny corals give us a clue about our planet's ultimate fate. One hemisphere will freeze and the other will roast—if the sun is still around.

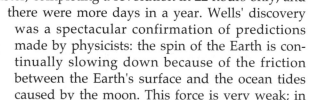

Horn coral

The formations exposed in Perdido Canyon contain some of the sea dwellers who lived in that distant era of 22-hour days. The Tin Mountain Limestone has abundant horn corals, tabulate (*Syringopora*) and honeycomb (*Favosites*) corals, and brachiopods (*Spirifer*). The Lost Burro Formation, named after nearby Lost Burro Gap which cuts right through it, contains several genera of brachiopod (including *Cyrtospirifer disjunctus* and *Atrypa*), corals, and crinoids, also known as sea lilies. Crinoids look like undersea flowers. They are made of a tall, slender stalk anchored to the sea floor and topped by a calyx. They formed extensive colonies in shallow Paleozoic seas, and several species still live today. The Perdido Formation has a beautiful goniatite called *Cravenoceras*. These tiny time capsules are the highlight of this canyon. You may not be able to find horn corals, but the magic of the past is there, silent messages frozen in the rocks, waiting to be deciphered.

Route Description

The lower canyon. It is an easy, nearly level walk from the White Top Mountain Road to the wide mouth of Perdido Canyon. Aim for the leftmost reddish talus (Rest Spring Shale) visible on the far side of the canyon, and look back for bearings to find your car when you return.

The most scenic part of Perdido Canyon is the wide gorge bounded by steep high walls a short distance above its mouth. It is by no means the most dramatic, but the Joshua trees scattered along the wash against the backdrop of dark walls produce an unusual landscape. Walls of cavernous dolomite host scores of small alcoves, undercuts, and a few odd-shaped windows. This area offers good face or slab climbing. Look in the wash for smooth, flat, discoidal rocks, grayish on the outside and a few inches across. These are septarian concretions, shed by the Rest Spring Shale. They are often broken clear across, exposing their colorful, radially veined core.

The fossils.   The gorge cuts through two formations. The Lost Burro Formation, mostly dolomite, is exposed for about 0.3 mile at the lower end of the gorge (along the first cavernous cliff on the east side), and 0.4 mile at its upper end. The rest of the gorge is Tin Mountain Limestone. The fossils you are most likely to spot are the corals and crinoid stems of this formation. Corals commonly look like a small circle, 5 millimeters across or larger, with many fine radial lines. They are often isolated, protrude a little, and being light tan in color they contrast sharply with the gray rock. Crinoid beds consist almost exclusively of broken stems; the calyces are far less frequently preserved. A stem fragment sliced perpendicular to its length looks like a tiny donut. On its side, it looks like a thin rectangle, typically 4-7 millimeters wide by a few centimeters long, with fine divisions across its width. Brachiopods are preserved as shell imprints, abundant only at a few places, and more difficult to find. Some of these bivalves are particularly attractive for their wing-shaped shells, especially *Cyrtospirifer disjunctus*, found in the very upper part of the Lost Burro Formation.

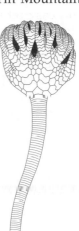

Crinoid

If you are new to fossil hunting, here are a few clues. Fossil sites are numerous, though only a few sites have abundant fossils. The foot of the walls and boulders on the edge of the wash are the easiest places to check, so start there. As with gold panning, if you find indications of fossils on a rock fragment, also look further uphill where they most likely came from. You may not be lucky at first but don't give up too soon; what made my day was a 45-foot fall of encrinal limestone—limestone made almost entirely of crinoid stems.

Shade is scant. Come here in the cooler season, or looking for fossils will be the last thing on your mind.

The upper canyon.   Past the gorge, Perdido Canyon opens up, then narrows to a steep ravine as it climbs a 200-foot escarpment. Most of the rock from the gorge up to and beyond the springs is Rest Spring

Shale, which has no well-preserved fossils. The exception is the escarpment. It cuts through the Perdido Formation, which is known to contain beautiful goniatites (*Cravenoceras*) and brachiopods (*Cyrtospirifers*). The rim of the escarpment is essentially the end of the canyon, and as far as most people will go. Others may want to continue along the steep gully beyond it all the way up to the head of the canyon, then cross over to Burro Spring, in the second drainage to the northeast.

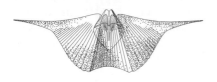

Cyrtospirifer disjunctus

Rest Spring Gulch. This little, out-of-the-way canyon offers a nice and easy return route from Burro Spring and upper Perdido Canyon. There used to be a road along it, but most of it is now roadless. The pipeline partially buried along the gulch was constructed, probably around 1917, to pipe water from Burro Spring to Lost Burro Mine (see *Lost Burro Mine*). Rest Spring is an area of yucca, Joshua trees and denser, greener vegetation in a beautiful setting of reddish rolling hills. The lower part of the gulch is crossed by the White Top Mountain Road. It has short, scenic narrows with steep walls made of thin interbedded layers of gray limestone and sandstone or siltstone—a pretty visual effect. This is the Perdido Formation. Look for *Cravenoceras* near the upper end of the narrows. The wider, lower end of the gulch is Tin Mountain Limestone.

■

Perdido Canyon		
	Dist.(mi)	Elev.(ft)
White Top Mountain Road	0.0	5,040
Mouth	0.7	5,040
Gorge (start)	1.7	5,400
Twin side canyons	2.4	5,760
Gorge (end)	3.2	6,080
Escarpment	3.8	6,400
Burro Spring	5.4	7,350
Rest Spring	6.6	6,650
Road	7.0	6,446
Back to starting point	11.4	5,040

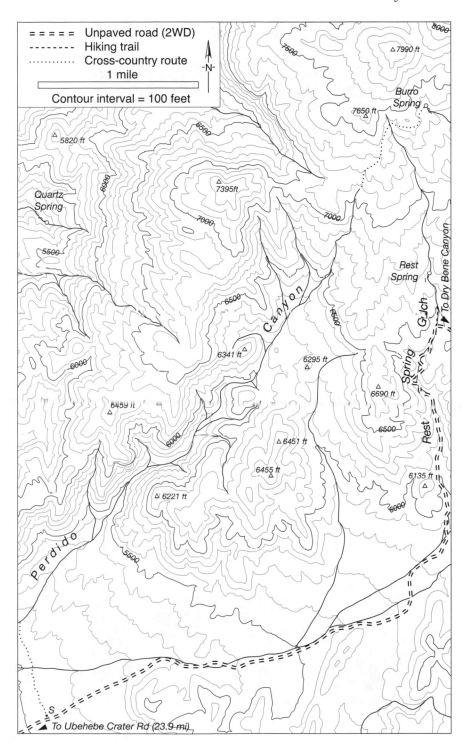

Unpaved road (2WD)
Hiking trail
Cross-country route
1 mile
Contour interval = 100 feet

-N-

To Dry Bone Canyon

To Ubehebe Crater Rd (23.9 mi)

Quartz Spring

Burro Spring

Rest Spring

Spring Gulch

Rest

Perdido

Canyon

5820 ft
7990 ft
7650 ft
7395ft
6341 ft
6295 ft
6690 ft
6451 ft
6455 ft
6135 ft
6221 ft
6459 ft

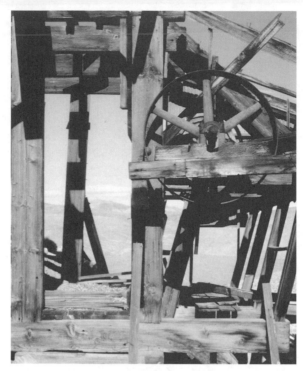

Detail of the mill at Lost Burro Mine

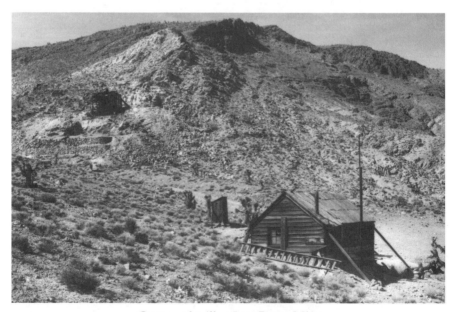

Camp and mill at Lost Burro Mine

LOST BURRO MINE

The remains of this little gold mine include a small camp and an impressive mill. Although it is usually reached by car, you may want to hike to it along a nameless canyon, which offers tight narrows, sweeping vistas from nearby Lost Burro Peak, and another little treat.

General Information

Road access: Access by long primitive road
Shortest hike: Short strolls / very easy
Longest hike: 2.5 mi, 2,100 ft one way (or more)/ difficult
Main attractions: Lost Burro Mine and camp, narrows, a peak climb
USGS 15' and 7.5' topo maps: Ubehebe Peak
Maps: pp. 355*, 333

Location and Access

To get to the Lost Burro Mine, drive the Racetrack Valley Road to Teakettle Junction (see *The Racetrack Valley*), then turn left and continue 3.2 miles, past Lost Burro Gap, to the four-way junction on the edge of Hidden Valley. The right spur ends at the mining camp in 1.1 miles. A standard-clearance vehicle can make it this far in normal weather, although some people may prefer to walk the last 1.1-mile stretch.

The other approach suggested here is to hike to the mine from Lost Burro Gap via a nameless canyon and Lost Burro Peak. The starting point is the canyon mouth, which is 1.5 miles from Teakettle Junction, or about 0.3 mile into the gap, on the south side.

History

Several natural features in this area—a peak, a gap, and a geologic formation—have been named Lost Burro, after a gold mine located in a small draw in the northwest corner of Hidden Valley. The original discovery was made in April 1907 by Bert Shively, a prospector who fortuitously stumbled upon it while rounding up his burros. The deposit looked promising, and Shively and a few partners immediately filed several claims in the area. Although assays indicated at an early stage that the deposit was valuable, the Lost Burro had a slow beginning. Over the next few years the owners bonded, leased, and attempted to sell their property to several parties. Each time the new operators developed the mine for a while, then soon called off the deal for one reason or another, and the property returned to the original owners, who eagerly

353

worked it themselves while waiting for another offer. At least they made a few thousand dollars in the process, and the property was worked fairly diligently. The workings exploited a vein up to 10 feet thick and assaying $15 to $18 per ton, as well as a smaller pocket that produced samples worth as much as $1,000 per ton. There was enough gold that by 1909 $30,000 worth of ore had been stockpiled at the mine.

The most glamorous era of the Lost Burro Mine started in 1915, when the Montana-Tonopah Company bonded the property and went ahead with ambitious plans. To cut down on transportation costs, the company decided to treat the ore on site and began constructing a five-stamp mill. With its 50-ton capacity, the mill was anticipated to recover up to 85% of the gold. It was to be powered by water piped all the way from Burro Spring, about 8 miles away north of Hidden Valley. The pipeline was eventually installed, but no records indicate whether the mill itself was completed. For some reason this flurry of activity stopped around 1917, and the mine remained idle for many years.

But the deposit was rich, and it eventually yielded a nice little return. From the late 1920s to 1938, Andy McCormick, who had been associated with the Lost Burro since its early days, worked here with a partner and recovered $85,000 in gold. Shorty Borden, always on the lookout for an abandoned mine to scavenge, relocated the claims in the 1940s with a partner, W. C. Thompson. After Shorty's death, Thompson worked the mine sporadically, keeping it alive up until the 1970s. All told, the Lost Burro Mine produced probably close to $100,000 of gold— it was definitely one of the richest in the Ubehebe Mining District.

Route Description

Lost Burro Mine. The small camp at the Lost Burro Mine, with its scattered wooden cabins and artifacts, is a picturesque site, although a little austere in its desolate valley sprinkled with stunted Joshua trees. On my last visit, it had a cabin, a dilapidated shelter and an outhouse. The cabin was still fairly well-preserved, furnished with odds and ends resting on dusty shelves, and parts of a stove. Yellowed newspaper and magazine clippings from a long-gone era served as wallpaper.

The most extensive structure is certainly the ruins of the mill, a short distance past the camp. Towering above several terraced levels on the hillside, it is an impressive sight. Its massive timber frame, darkened by decades of sunlight, still support its intricate machinery. The ore bin is more recent, and was probably constructed by Thompson.

The mines are up the small gulch beyond the mill, strung out mostly along the south side. There were essentially three mining areas. The first one is the east shaft, at the top of the first large dump and 30 feet above the wash. The second area is the main mine. One of its adits is

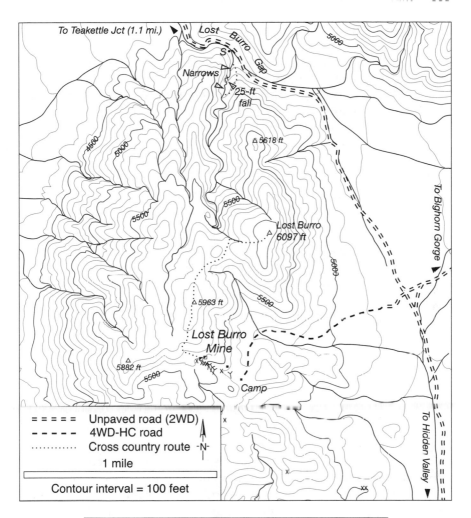

	Dist.(mi)	Elev.(ft)
Lost Burro Mine		
Lost Burro Gap (canyon mouth)	0.0	4,550
25-ft fall	0.1	~4,650
Wide U-turn (climb to saddle)	1.2	5,490
Saddle	1.4	~5,810
Lost Burro Peak	(0.4)	6,097
5,963-ft summit	1.8	5,963
Highest mines	2.2	5,580
Lost Burro camp	2.5	5,320
Lost Burro Gap (via road)	(2.8)	4,550

just before the next large dump; the other one is 50 feet up the slope. From here the tunnels run roughly parallel to the ravine for about 450 feet. A good part of the production came from here. The third mining area is the west shaft, near the end of the ravine, on the north side.

The gold occurs in a siliceous vein near the contact metamorphic zone between a small syenodiorite pluton and the native rock (see *Ubehebe Peak, Geology*). The pluton is exposed throughout the mines and along the wash. Some samples contain sizeable crystals of hornblende and biotite. The rock it intruded, Tin Mountain Limestone, is exposed higher up on the slope north of the wash. The contact zone, where the gray limestone was turned to nearly white marble, is between them. There are fine samples of marble below the tailings of the west shaft.

The hike via Lost Burro Peak. For this scenic alternative route to the mine, start at the side canyon in Lost Burro Gap. Hiking up canyon, at first you'll go through a narrow, windy passage framed by high walls. After a couple of bends there is a constriction and a 6-foot polished slant, then a 25-foot fall—vertical, slick, and impassable. Above the shiny lip of the fall, the canyon resumes as a narrow slot. To reach it, backtrack until you find a route on the east side where you feel comfortable to climb out of the wash. You'll need to scramble up a steep incline to the canyon rim, then drop to the canyon floor on the other side. This bypass is about 0.3 mile. Before continuing, walk down canyon to explore the hanging slot. Its tight, shaded narrows form a dark corridor of finely striated walls. At places it is almost enclosed overhead by the leaning walls, which are so tortuous your line of sight doesn't exceed 10 feet in any direction, until you get to the dizzying edge of the 25-foot fall.

Up canyon from the slot the scenery is less spectacular, but things soon pick up again. Follow the yucca-dotted wash, past a small arch, up to the middle of the wide U-turn (about 0.9 mile), and to scramble up to the saddle to the south. The going gets steep, but it's straightforward. This saddle sits between two high peaks. Besides the lower canyon, the highlight of this hike is definitely the spectacular views from the high spine of this small range, once known as the Dutton Mountains. From the saddle, climb along the ridge to the left (northeast-east) to Lost Burro Peak for the best views of Hidden Valley—a pristine canopy of shrubs surrounded by moon-like, barren hills. For equally impressive views of the Racetrack, climb the ridge the other way to the 5,963-foot peak, or better yet to the next one over (5,882'). To get to the Lost Burro Mine, climb down the south side of the 5,963-foot peak to the saddle, then southeast down the steep ravine to the workings and the camp below them. For a change of scenery and pace, you can return from the camp to your starting point via the road along Hidden Valley.

■

LOWER MARBLE CANYON

> *If you like narrows, rock art, or both, put Marble Canyon high on your list. Along the scenic canyon road and in the roadless canyon beyond it, you will go through several spectacular narrows. The petroglyphs adorning the canyon walls rank among the most elaborate and extensive in all of Death Valley.*

General Information

Road status: Rough road in lower canyon (HC); access by primitive road
Shortest hike: 1.1 mi, 300 ft one way/easy
Longest hike: 9.9 mi, 2,400 ft one way (or more)/difficult
Main attractions: A deep canyon, narrows, petroglyphs
USGS 15' topo map: Marble Canyon
USGS 7.5' topo maps: East of Sand Flat, Cottonwood Canyon
Maps: pp. 361*, 333

Location and Access

The lower part of Marble Canyon described here, located in the southwestern Cottonwood Mountains, is reached by a primitive road known as the Cottonwood Canyon Road. It starts in Stovepipe Wells, to the left of the campground entrance. Stay on it for 8.6 miles until it veers north, parallels the mountains, and eventually reaches a cleared area on the edge of the Cottonwood Canyon wash. This road is sandy at first, then a washboard for several miles, and it has a little soft gravel near the end, but a passenger car can make it this far. From here the road continues up the wash for 2.2 miles to the junction with Marble Canyon. This rougher stretch usually requires high clearance (although I saw good old VW vans make it apparently unscathed). The junction is easy to miss: look for the old "Marble Canyon" sign on the north side of the wash. The Marble Canyon Road is up to the right. It goes 2.6 miles to just inside the first narrows. This last stretch does require high clearance.

Rock Art and Historical Inscriptions

Many visitors come to Marble Canyon mostly for its petroglyphs. These prehistoric figures, pecked on smooth rock surfaces by aboriginals centuries ago, are fairly common in the deserts of the Southwest, but the sites found in Death Valley are generally smaller, perhaps a reflection of its harsher climate and lower prehistoric populations. Marble Canyon, however, was blessed with more petroglyph sites than any other canyon in the park. Often reminiscent of the style of rock art found in the Coso Range further west, Marble Canyon's petroglyphs 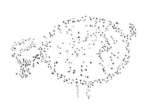 are extremely varied in subject matter, size, and level of detail. To anyone who enjoys searching every nook and cranny for rock art, this is a special place. There are beautiful figures to be found, from abstract drawings and pregnant bighorn sheep to lizards, desert foxes, human figures, and finely crafted birds. The antiquity of these figures covers many centuries. While many of them are quite prominent, others are faint and much older—and if you look closely you will find even fainter images, even older.

Pecked on a canyon wall there is also a very faint historical inscription of the date "1849" and initials "J.B." mixed with petroglyphs. It has been attributed to one of the men of the ill-fated Savage-Pinney party, a group of immigrants who split from the Jayhawkers and left Death Valley at the end of 1849 along this canyon (see *Jayhawker Canyon*). Of these 12 men, who were among the first immigrants to see Death Valley, only two are known to have reached the coast.

It is sad that much of Marble Canyon's rock art has suffered considerable degradation from modern graffiti, mostly in recent years. Unless something is done to slow down further damage, like closing Marble Canyon Road altogether, there will not be much left to look at in a few years—except for senseless graffiti. To help reduce the incidence of vandalism, I am not divulging the specific location of these sites. Remember that 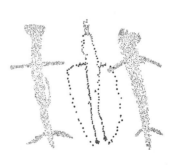 petroglyphs are part of a sacred cultural heritage. Do not touch them, or they will eventually darken and fade. Do not climb on walls near rock art. If you are upset by the graffiti, here or elsewhere, please share your concerns with a ranger or the superintendent.

Route Description

The canyon road. The Marble Canyon Road goes up the wide open wash on the right. The next 2.4 miles are over coarse alluvia, a long stretch if you are walking, but it's well worth the effort. Eventually the road enters the first narrows, and ends a short distance in. Park and hike from here.

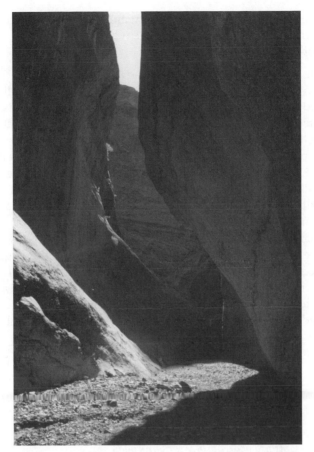

High walls in the second narrows of Marble Canyon

The first narrows. For the next mile or so, you'll be walking through a colorful corridor framed by sheer high walls that rival Titus Canyon for majesty. Along the way there is an interesting side canyon with falls, thick limestone beds loaded with black chert nodules, and overhangs with welcome shade. You will be craning your neck to gaze up massive strata that shoot at awkward angles to the distant rim. The first narrows end at a giant quartz monzonite chockstone wedged between the canyon walls—a piece of Hunter Mountain carried all the way down here by running water.

The second narrows. The second narrows of Marble Canyon are among the most impressive in the park. They begin shortly above the chockstone as a narrow passage in gray dolomite. They gradually deepen, open up for a short distance, then tighten again. The leaning walls, polished high above the wash, fold and unfold into a smooth contorted passage. For hundreds of feet you will wander through a dim, cool and naked world, closed and mysterious, where the light continuously changes with the time of day.

The mid-canyon and the third narrows. The middle section of Marble Canyon is scenic for its high, rugged and colored walls of thickly-stratified limestone and dolomite. Although most of it is an open, brush-dotted wash, it is sprinkled with surprises—constrictions, side canyons, a few slickensides (see *Red Wall Canyon*). Not far above the second narrows there are a few good exposures of fossil shells, mostly fragments of crinoids and gastropods—particularly on the polished, slanted walls of dark dolomite on the south side. The first side canyon on the north side above the second narrows has unusual walls packed with large nodules, scattered fossils of large gastropods, and eventually some amazing narrows.

The third narrows, less spectacular than the others, go through high black and white banded walls. This area contains finely polished displays of marble, white grading into gray—a rock that is also exposed around Goldbelt Spring and perhaps this canyon's namesake. This short passage ends at another one of the large quartz monzonite chockstones typical of Marble Canyon. The side canyon on the north side just above the third narrows has narrow passages and falls, some easy and fun to

Lower Marble Canyon		
	(miles)	(feet)
Cottonwood/Marble Canyon roads		
Stovepipe Wells	0.0	5
Cottonwood Canyon wash	8.6	720
Marble Canyon Road (junction)	10.8	1,180
First narrows (start)	13.2	1,760
Road's end (tightest spot)	13.4	1,815
Roadless canyon		
Road's end (tightest spot)	0.0	1,815
Side canyon	0.4	1,920
First narrows (end/chockstone)	1.1	2,110
Second narrows (start)	1.2	~2,150
Second narrows (end)	1.6	2,260
Third narrows (start)	4.0	2,860
Third narrows (end)	4.2	2,900
Dead Horse Canyon	5.1	3,115
Goldbelt Camp/Road	10.7	4,940

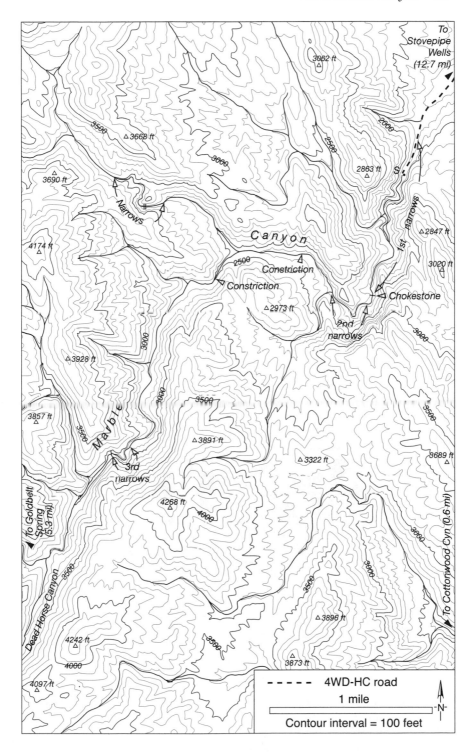

To
Stovepipe
Wells
(12.7 mi)

3062 ft

△3668 ft

3500

3000

2000

2500

2863 ft

S.

3690 ft

Narrows

1st narrows

△2847 ft

4174 ft

C a n y o n

2500

Constriction

3020 ft

Constriction

Chokestone

△2973 ft

2nd
narrows

3000

3000

△3928 ft

3000

3500

3500

3857 ft

Marble

3500

△3891 ft

△3322 ft

3689 ft

3500

3rd
narrows

4268 ft

4000

3000

To Goldbelt
Spring
(5.3 mi)

Dead-Horse Canyon

3500

To Cottonwood Cyn (0.6 mi)

3000

3500

3000

△3896 ft

4242 ft

3500

4000

3873 ft

4097 ft

- - - - - **4WD-HC road**

1 mile

N

Contour interval = 100 feet

climb. From here it's a short walk to Dead Horse Canyon. The area up canyon from this junction, which includes the fourth narrows, is described in the next section.

Hiking Suggestions

If you can drive to the end of the road, it is an easy walk to and through the first or second narrows, an easy day hike to the third narrows and back, and a long day hike to the fourth narrows and back. If you have a passenger vehicle, you will probably have to walk from the mouth of Cottonwood Canyon. It means a long day to the second and third narrows. The saving grace is that hiking in Marble Canyon is relatively easy due to its uncommonly gentle grades.

Marble Canyon has plenty of room for backpacking. An obvious route is from the canyon mouth to Goldbelt Spring, an easy two days one way. You can also do a nice loop via Dead Horse Canyon (see *Cottonwood Canyon*).

■

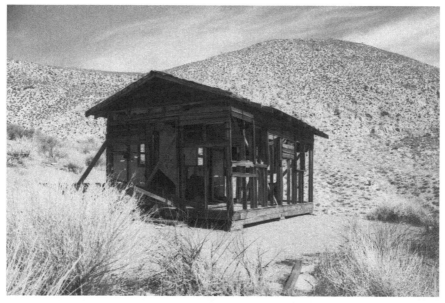

Cabin at Goldbelt Spring

UPPER MARBLE CANYON

> *What I like about this hike is the springs—of course Goldbelt Spring and its small mining camp, near the head of the canyon, but also the half a dozen nameless springs down canyon. One spring has a few tall cottonwoods; another one has thick tangles of willows and creeping grapevine. The unusual narrows at the bottom of this gentle canyon make a good goal for a moderate day hike.*

General Information

Road status: Essentially roadless; access by long primitive road
Shortest hike: Short strolls/easy
Longest hike: 8.2 mi, 1,140 ft one way (or more)/moderate
Main attractions: Mining camp, springs, narrows, mines, Sand Flat
USGS 15' topo map: Marble Canyon
USGS 7.5' topo maps: Harris Hill*, Sand Flat, Cottonwood Canyon
Maps: pp. 367*, 333

Location and Access

For the shortest route to this isolated canyon, deep in the south-western Cottonwoods, from Highway 190 drive the Saline Valley Road 15.7 miles to the Hunter Mountain Road (the right fork at the high saddle overlooking Panamint Valley). Drive this road 10.5 miles to the turnoff to the Quackenbush Mine (on the right), then 1.1 miles to the end of this spur at Goldbelt Spring. Park at the overlook above the old camp. Although there are a couple of steep grades around Hunter Mountain, in dry weather this route is easily manageable with a standard-clearance vehicle. Goldbelt Spring can also be reached from the north via the Racetrack Valley Road.

Mining History: The Mineral Wealth of Goldbelt

Despite its name, the Goldbelt area, near the head of Marble Canyon, never produced much gold. However, it holds a record of sorts for the number of precious metals and minerals it produced. Here, several generations of miners discovered gold and silver, then copper, later tungsten and talc, and finally wollastonite, each discovery triggering a small strike. It was Shorty Harris—perhaps the most popular single-blanket jackass prospector of the Death Valley mining era—who was said to have first discovered free-milling gold here at the end of 1904. During his long mining career, he was credited with no less than five major gold strikes, including Bullfrog and Harrisburg, although it has been suggested that he just happened to be at the right place at the right time, and later took undue credit. After his discovery at Goldbelt, the Goldbelt Mining District was organized, which stretched east to Death Valley and down to Cottonwood Canyon. The deposits did assay a fair value in gold, with a little silver to boot. Until at least 1910, efforts were made to develop a few gold claims, then copper claims. But as usual, their remoteness and the lack of capital stifled development. For a short time there was enough activity, however, that a camp was established, probably around the spring.

The area was then relatively quiet for a few years, until the war-induced increase in metal prices spurred renewed mining interest. In 1916 tungsten was discovered, again by Shorty Harris. By the next spring he had managed to ship out a few hundred pounds of tungsten ore worth about $1,500. He and others subsequently developed other small tungsten mines a few miles south of Goldbelt Spring, but they probably produced only an occasional sack of ore.

From the 1940s to the 1960s several small talc and other mineral claims were located in the area, and exploited off and on. The Quackenbush Mine is a good example. A small steatite-grade talc deposit first claimed by Beveridge Hunter and Shorty Borden in June 1944, it had produced only about 750 tons by 1955, and probably not much more in the 1960s when it was reactivated for a short time. After talc it was wollastonite, discovered in 1959 close to the spring. Known as the Calmet claims, these deposits were worked as late as 1976, which was the final mining activity in the area.

Historical records of the small mining camp that still stands near Goldbelt Spring today are scarce. The year it was built, its builders, and who occupied it over what period of time, are no longer known. The cabins' style suggests that it was built in the 1930s or 1940s and occupied by talc miners, and perhaps later on by workers at the Calmet claims. It was still active in 1959 (one of its residents was a cow, fenced in a small lot by the spring), and probably as late as the 1960s.

Route Description

Goldbelt Spring. The small mining camp at Goldbelt Spring is a picturesque site, nestled in a deep hollow overlooking the canyon. Its wooden cabin and dugout, bullet-ridden water tank, old truck, over-turned car, and decaying fences, are now a riddle to decipher. Goldbelt Spring has a thicket of wild rose. The hollow at the base of it sometimes has a small pool of algae-covered water. Except for a couple of seeps in higher forks, it is the only water in a long canyon. In June it supports a colorful display of roses. In the evening, after a long walk or drive, it is a peaceful place to rest, to watch birds drinking at the pool while the hills slowly turn to gold.

Goldbelt district mines. There are a few mines within a mile of the camp. The open pit with the red metallic sorter along the road 0.8 mile west of the spring, is one of the Calmet Mines (wollastonite). The Quackenbush Mine is 0.9 mile north of the camp, up a rougher road (an easy walk). It has a couple of small wooden headframes, a main shaft and a few timbered adits, and small talc tailings.

The Mule Tail Mine is harder to reach but more interesting. This small talc mine (with a little tungsten and gold) is believed to be the site of Shorty Harris' original strike that started this district. From the Quackenbush Mine, continue north down to the bottom of the road (0.7 mile), where the Mule Tail Mine Road forks to the right. This road first descends towards Sand Flat, then turns around, climbs into a side canyon of Marble Canyon, and ends shortly below the mine (4.1 miles, 1,140 feet up and down). With a standard vehicle one can drive the first 2 miles, but this road is so rarely visited it makes a great hiking trail. Joshua trees dot this entire route; look also for Mojave fishhook cactus, a relatively rare treat. About 500 yards before the mine, hike to the talc bin visible 150 yards to the right of the road. Behind the bin a foot trail ascends to the mine (0.5 mile). The site has four tunnels, some of them still timbered, a few prospects, a mine car and a decrepit ore chute. On

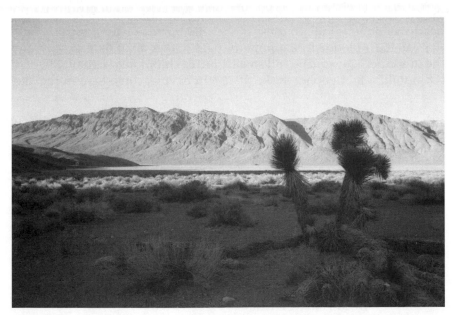

Sand Flat, a short walk from the Mule Tail Mine Road

the way back, extend this hike a mile or so down to Sand Flat, a beautifully desolate high-desert basin surrounded by stark mountains. An alternative is to return from the mine to Goldbelt Spring via a trail at the end of the road (see map) and some cross-country hiking.

Marble Canyon springs. From Goldbelt, hike down the wash that winds below the camp. For the next 4.8 miles Marble Canyon is a relatively narrow wash framed in high, steep hills. The highlights here are the springs—six of them, unnamed, unknown, all but one unmapped. The first one, a green thicket of willows plugging the wash, is a short distance down, at the confluence with Shorty Harris Canyon. Look for a steep, overgrown trail starting in a steep ravine on the left just inside Shorty Harris Canyon. In 0.8 mile, it climbs 800 feet to an old prospect near the top of Harris Hill.

The next springs are scattered along the wash down canyon. Although they don't usually have surface water, their small groves of willow and mountain mahogany are green a good part of the year, and they are restful areas for a break. One of the most pleasant springs has a lone stand of three old, tall and shady cottonwoods, whispering in a more open stretch of canyon. The largest spring, a little further, has a beautiful thick oasis of tall willow overgrown with grapevine. The narrows start about 0.7 mile further.

The wash is thickly vegetated with rabbitbrush, blackbrush, Mormon tea, sage, and many other high desert plants. Walking along the wash and on higher ground to avoid the springs is simplified by a nearly continuous trail, courtesy of the wild burros—trust these lazy animals to have plodded the optimum path. Other animals also seek out the moisture. I saw quails and smaller birds, chipmunks, cottontails, and a beautiful 4-foot gopher snake. If at all possible, come here in the late

Upper Marble Canyon		
	Dist.(mi)	Elev.(ft)
Goldbelt Camp (end of road)	0.0	4,940
Goldbelt Spring	(0.2)	5,070
Shorty Harris Canyon	0.6	4,705
Harris Hill	(0.9)	5,765
Spring (cottonwoods)	3.75	3,635
Largest spring (grapevine)	4.1	3,540
Fourth narrows (start)	4.8	3,315
Fourth narrows (end)	5.1	3,240
Dead Horse Canyon	5.6	3,115

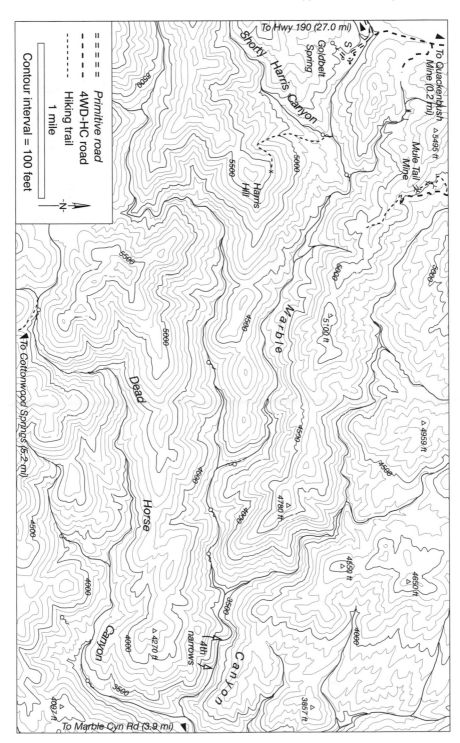

Legend:

= = = = = Primitive road
‒ ‒ ‒ ‒ 4WD-HC road
‒ · ‒ · ‒ Hiking trail

Contour interval = 100 feet

1 mile

-N-

To Hwy 190 (27.0 mi)

To Quackenbush Mine (0.2 mi)

△ 5495 ft

Mule Tail Mine

Shorty Harris Canyon

Goldbelt Spring

Harris Hill

5500

5000

5500

5500

5000

4500

4500

4000

Marble

△ 5100 ft

5000

5500

Dead

Horse

Canyon

△ 4270 ft

4000

3500

409 ft

To Cottonwood Springs (5.2 mi)

To Marble Cyn Rd (3.9 mi)

4500

4000

3500

4000

4500

4500

Canyon

4th narrows

△ 4550 ft

4650 ft

4000

3857 ft

△ 4780 ft

△ 4959 ft

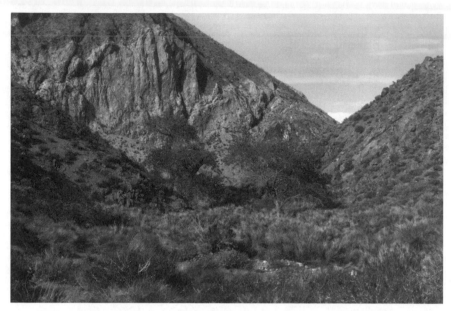

Cottonwoods at one of several unnamed springs in upper Marble Canyon

spring when wild flowers put on their show. I counted over 35 species and subspecies, some of them profusely covering the wash.

The fourth narrows. If the springs didn't do it for you, the narrows of upper Marble Canyon certainly should. They are quite different from the other narrows down canyon. Their sinuous path is lined with sheer walls, crystallized at places, strikingly banded further down, then polished and streaked with wavering calcite veins. The canyon gets quite narrow at places, but you may find yourself searching for patterns rather than constrictions. This beautiful passage has a few monzonite chockstones to surmount, large brecciated boulders, clumps of Panamint phacelia growing out of cracks in the walls, water pockets, and much more. Below the narrows, a windy defile, unusual for its varied geology, leads in 0.5 mile to Dead Horse Canyon, the end of the upper canyon.

Hiking Suggestions

For an easy half-day hike, make a loop along Shorty Harris Canyon to check out its springs (returning via Hunter Mountain Road), or hike to Sand Flat or Marble Canyon's largest spring. For a moderate day hike, go as far as Dead Horse Canyon, or hike the mines loop via the Mule Tail Mine Road. If you have a full day, loop back along rarely visited Dead Horse Canyon, which has narrows and springs.

■

COTTONWOOD CANYON

The popular primitive road through Cottonwood Canyon provides convenient access to a scenic canyon, a meandering gorge, and a few side canyons with tight narrows to explore on foot. The crowning jewel is the luxuriant springs beyond the end of the road, which give rise to intermittent creeks, swamps, and three thick oases of cottonwoods, willows, and grapevine. The hike to the largest oasis, irrigated by Cottonwood Springs, is a rare treat offering a glimpse at one of the hidden wonders of Death Valley.

General Information

Road status: Primitive road to and in lower canyon (HC)
Shortest hike: 1.1 mi, 200 ft / easy
Longest hike: 19.7 mi, 4,460 ft one way (or more)/ difficult
Main attractions: Springs, creek and lush oases, narrows, fossils
USGS 15' topo map: Marble Canyon
USGS 7.5' topo maps: E. of Sand Flat, Cottonwood Canyon*, Harris Hill
Maps: pp. 373*, 333

Location and Access

Cottonwood Canyon is one of the longest canyons in the Cottonwood Mountains. A primitive road, the Cottonwood Canyon Road, runs a good part of it to the first spring in the upper canyon. To get to it, drive this road from its start at Stovepipe Wells for 8.6 miles to the wash of Cottonwood Canyon (see *Lower Marble Canyon* for details). It is then 10.4 miles to the end of the road. Up to the Cottonwood Canyon wash the road is manageable with a passenger vehicle. The rest of it is in washes and generally requires high clearance.

Route Description

The lower canyon. Just above the canyon mouth the road goes through the first narrows, which start at an impressive gateway. For 0.4 mile it winds beneath some of the highest near-vertical surfaces in Death Valley. This deep passage ends abruptly, widening onto a broad valley framed in gold and rust-colored hills. Just past this point it is tempting to drive up the wide side canyon straight ahead (which is usually blocked off by a sign and a log), but the canyon road actually veers left and follows the south wall. The marked junction with Cottonwood Canyon is 0.8 mile past the head of the first narrows.

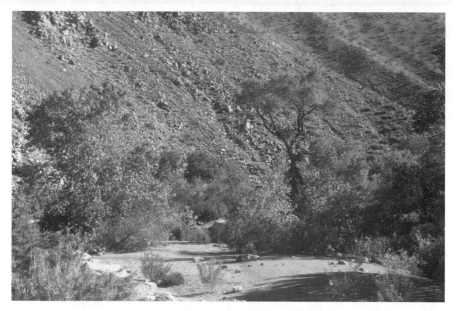

Cottonwood trees at middle spring in upper Cottonwood Canyon

From the junction it is 4.9 miles to the narrows, along a fairly wide, straight, and uneventful stretch. But the grades are uncommonly gentle, averaging only 200 feet per mile, and if you are walking you can travel at a pretty good clip. Don't miss the large cave in the east wall about 1 mile before the narrows. It is an unusual 70-foot deep overhang, probably formed by stream erosion, with large boulders protruding from the high ceiling. Fossils are common along this canyon.

The second narrows. These narrows are one of Cottonwood Canyon's best features. Although not very narrow, they have rugged walls and meander tightly for quite a distance. The scenery changes gradually along the way as the gorge first cuts through dark gray dolomite, then tilted strata of interbedded dolomite and limestone, and finally limestone. In the west wall about 0.6 mile into the narrows, there is a nice breccia made of angular blocks of black dolomite or limestone cemented by a white material, probably calcite. Because the breccia is located in an outer bend, it has been polished by the stream into a fine panel of black and white mosaic.

The side canyons. Cottonwood Canyon has about a dozen side canyons. They are often narrower and windier than the main canyon, and all very different. If you can't make the springs, a hike into one of them may well turn out to be the high point of your visit here.

My favorite side canyon is the one that enters on the west side just before the upper end of the narrows. This enchanting place has two beautiful narrows. The first one, just 0.1 mile from the road, is very narrow, trapped between high, tightly winding water-worn walls that will often limit your line of sight to less than 20 feet. Giant granite boulders occasionally block the way. The striking contrast between the gray boulders, the immaculate walls, and the panels of reddish brecciated dolomite, puts this place in a class of its own. Progress is soon interrupted by an imposing 30-foot fall for expert rock climbers only. To reach beyond, walk back to the entrance to the narrows and scramble up the steep and very loose talus on the south side. At the top of this 350-foot rise a faint game track climbs down the other side to the wash. The length of this bypass is about 0.25 mile. From here you can walk down canyon towards the narrows you just bypassed for more boulder climbing and pretty breccias. Going up canyon instead, in 0.8 mile you'll run into the second narrows, which begin with two 12-foot polished falls. At places no wider than 4 to 5 feet, they meander for the next half a mile, graced with white, gray, and brecciated dolomite and many artfully designed falls.

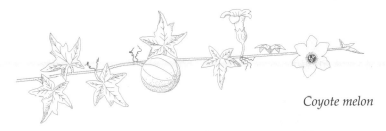

Coyote melon

Cottonwood Creek. The highlight of this canyon is doubtlessly Cottonwood Creek, an amazing little desert stream that supports several luxuriant oases. The first one starts right at the end of the road. In the shade of tall trees, grasses, cattails, cane, and willow shoots jostle for sipping rights along the creek. Few canyons in Death Valley offer this degree of lushness. After miles of barren desert, the sudden confrontation with this profusion of greenery may well seem like an illusion.

Along the next 4 miles there are three major springs. The lower one has several good stretches of flowing water, on the average a couple of inches deep and one or two feet wide. In late October I estimated its flow at 30 gallons per minute. The second spring, which is drier, forms dark, muddy swamps invaded by watercress. The third one, Cottonwood Springs, has a flow several times that of the lower spring. Each spring supports a thick oasis for some distance downstream from its resurgence, so that the upper canyon is a string of green oases separated by stretches of dry wash. At the upper end of each oasis, the transition from vegetation to desert is surprisingly abrupt. One second you are walking through a dark and humid grove, the next you emerge into bright waterless expanses.

Most of the large trees here are cottonwoods, easily identified by their round, pointed, silver-green leaves and deeply furrowed gray bark. The largest specimens exceed 3 feet in diameter. They are mixed with tall willows, while mesquite trees thrive on the edges of the groves. The trees are covered with thick canopies of hanging grapevine, which create a shady forest environment.

Generally, the walking is fairly easy, though at places you might get wet crossing the brush-choked stream. To circumvent the thick undergrowth (and prevent damaging this unique riparian system), follow the animal tracks on either side of the oases. The upper grove is very thick and best bypassed on a faint trail 30-50 feet above the wash on the west side. Towards its upper end, it squeezes between the walls of the narrowing canyon and requires some bushwhacking, but it is well worth it to reach gushing Cottonwood Springs.

Oases are magical places. In Cottonwood Canyon, they invite the visitor to take a pleasant stroll along a wooded stream, a rare

Cottonwood Canyon		
	Dist.(mi)	Elev.(ft)
Cottonwood Canyon Road		
Stovepipe Wells	0.0	0
Cottonwood Canyon wash	8.6	720
First narrows (start)	9.6	950
First narrows (end)	10.0	1,030
Marble Canyon junction	10.8	1,180
Second narrows (start)	15.7	2,120
Second narrows (end)	17.7	2,470
End of road	19.2	2,830
Roadless canyon		
End of road	0.0	2,830
Lower spring	1.1	3,030
Middle spring	1.7	3,160
Cottonwood Springs	4.0	3,630
Head	9.1	~5,180
Dead Horse Canyon	9.5	5,040
Hunter Mountain Road	14.6	6,500

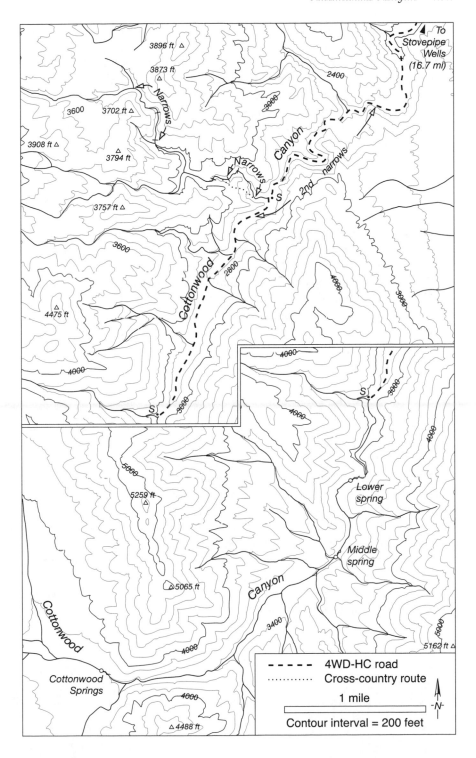

experience in this overwhelmingly dry land. In the summer you will find welcome shade, the tracks of coyote and bighorn sheep along sandy bottoms, and a surprising variety of birds. In the fall, look for the golden gourds of coyote melons, for large mushrooms called desert puffball near the swamps, for bright and fragrant flowering rabbitbrush, or a lone tarantula tiptoeing across the sand. Later in the season, the yellowing trees and carpets of dead leaves give a rare autumn flavor to this refreshing scenery.

Hiking Suggestions

If you have a high-clearance vehicle, drive to the end of the road and hike the upper canyon to explore the springs. Some of the side canyons in the mid-canyon offer exciting short hikes from the road. If you are looking for a good, long day hike, park below the narrows and hike to Cottonwood Springs (or a lower spring).

If you have a passenger car, chances are you will be able to drive only to the mouth of Cottonwood Canyon. It is then a long day hike to the second narrows and back. Unless you get a ride (which is quite possible on a long weekend), it will probably take an overnight hike to reach the springs. Camping is allowed anywhere in Cottonwood Canyon except within 200 yards of the springs. Water at the springs is abundant year-round, so for a change, water is not a problem. So that it does not become a problem, treat it before drinking.

For a longer trek, you may want to consider the popular, comparatively easy Cottonwood-Marble Canyon loop. From the junction between these two canyons, hike up Cottonwood Canyon to its head 5 miles beyond Cottonwood Springs, then down Dead Horse Canyon and back along scenic Marble Canyon (see *Lower Marble Canyon*). Marble Canyon can also be reached via one of the west-bearing side canyons of Cottonwood Canyon. This loop can be done in as little as three days. To avoid walking on roads, follow the same route to Dead Horse Canyon but then hike up canyon instead of down, to eventually join the old trail shown on the 15' map (which is definitely discontinuous) to Hunter Mountain Road. For a longer and wilder trek, you can also make a loop south from Cottonwood Springs to return along the north fork of Lemoigne Canyon (see *Lemoigne Canyon*).

■

LEMOIGNE CANYON

Lemoigne Canyon, named after a French miner who discovered a
small lead-silver deposit in it, is accessed by one of the worst roads in
the park. Driving there is an adventure in itself! Short narrows,
stands of Joshua trees, Lemoigne's cabin, and the numerous tunnels
and tailings left from nearly one century of mining are the main
objectives of a day hike into this isolated and forlorn canyon.

General Information

Road status: Roadless; accessed by very rough road (HC-4WD)
Shortest hike: 1.8 mi, 1,000 ft one way / moderate
Longest hike: 7 mi, 4,000 ft (or more) / difficult
Main attractions: Historical silver-lead mines, narrows, Joshua trees
USGS 15' topo maps: Emigrant Cyn, Marble Cyn, Panamint Butte*
USGS 7.5' topo maps: Emigrant Cyn, Cottonwood Cyn, Panamint Butte*
Maps: pp. 381*, 333

Location and Access

Lemoigne Canyon is one of the southernmost major canyons in
the Cottonwood Mountains. The Lemoigne Canyon Road starts on
Highway 190 6.2 miles west of Stovepipe Wells (or 2.9 miles east of the
Emigrant Ranger Station). Both the road and the road sign, posted a distance away from the highway, are easy to miss. If you are coming from
the valley and pass the pronounced dip in the highway (Emigrant
Wash), you've gone too far. Look for it again 0.4 mile east of the dip.

This road is so rough that it makes most of the park's backcountry roads look like freeways. A short distance in, it drops into Emigrant
Wash, and it takes some effort to find where the road resumes on the far
side. For the next few miles it dips steeply in and out of many small
washes, and a high-clearance 4-wheel-drive vehicle is imperative. After
4.3 miles there is an old turnout on the left, about 0.2 mile below the
canyon mouth. The road ends 1.2 miles further, at the first side canyon.

For those who don't have the right vehicle to tackle this road but
are determined to get there, hike the old Indian trail from the Emigrant
Campground (see *Kerdell Prospect*), which is shorter and more level than
the road. The mouth of Lemoigne Canyon is almost due west, near the
north end of the prominent dark basaltic flow capping the base of the
range. Follow this trail about 3 miles to its end, where it meets the
Lemoigne Canyon Road at the turnout mentioned above.

History

This canyon is named after Jean Lemoigne, a French prospector from the early mining days of Death Valley who discovered a small lead-silver deposit in the canyon's south fork. It was not a fabulous lode by any means, but somehow it ended up being worked intermittently for about 90 years, longer than just about any other mine in the park. It didn't make Lemoigne rich, but it did make him famous. Well-educated and well-mannered, Lemoigne belonged to a different breed of prospectors, more attuned to the land than to the publicity and material wealth that motivated most prospectors. He pursued a different kind of wealth—a peaceful and unhurried life in the desert he loved. Unfortunately, little of his life story is accurately known. The chroniclers who wrote about him somehow managed to disagree about almost every important event in his life, to the point where today everything you read about Lemoigne must be taken with a grain of salt. This includes the following account, which is most likely partly incorrect.

Lemoigne was born in France around 1857 under the name of Jean François de Lamoignon. Some references state he first came to Death Valley in the early 1870s after serving as a sailor. A more common and colorful version is that he arrived here around 1884 at the request of fellow countryman Isidore Daunet. Lemoigne was to supervise mining operations at Daunet's Eagle Borax Works, on Death Valley's salt pan. The story goes that he arrived around the time Daunet committed suicide, and turned to working in local mines to support himself.

What does appear to be well documented is that through the 1880s, after shedding his aristocratic name somewhere along the way, Lemoigne became involved in serious prospecting. In Europe he had been trained as a mining engineer, and although many prospectors fared well without a formal degree, Lemoigne did exceptionally well. For over a decade he prospected and mined all over eastern California and western Nevada. His name became associated with an impressive number of claims. However, the one discovery that literally put his name on the map is a silver-lead deposit in what is now Lemoigne Canyon. Accounts differ as to the date of his discovery, which ranges from 1882 to 1887. A possible source of confusion is that some years later, in 1896, he filed claims on a similar deposit in nearby Cottonwood Canyon. Nevertheless, the earlier claims were the ones to which he attached the most importance. Although they contained considerably more lead than silver, and mostly low-grade lead, Lemoigne liked to think they were the richest around, and he held on to them the rest of his life.

During his long stay in the area, Lemoigne worked his mine just enough to satisfy his minimal needs. His claims were so remote that large scale development was unthinkable, yet he still thought about it.

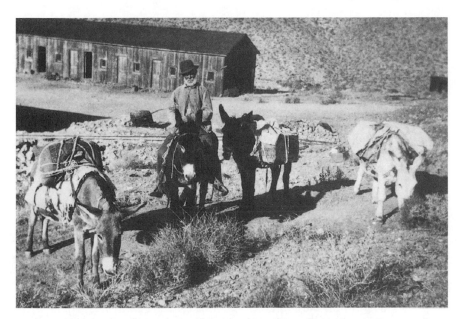

Jean Lemoigne leaving camp with supplies, February 1915
(Courtesy of the National Park Service, Death Valley National Park)

For a time, there was talk of a railroad extension to this isolated region to serve the copper mines of the Ubehebe Mining District and the gold mines in the Argus Range, but it never happened. During the feverish boom of Skidoo and Rhyolite, Lemoigne received respectable offers for his property, but none of them worked out. Some say he was offered payments by check, which he distrusted. Others argued that his asking price—up to $250,000—was much too high. In all likelihood, he was more interested in mining than selling out. He waited for the best part of a quarter of a century for a good offer or a railroad, both of which he probably knew would have required nothing short of a miracle.

According to Dane Coolidge, a traveler who chronicled turn-of-the-century life in the West, Lemoigne was "quite a different type of man from the ordinary burro-cursing prospector . . . calm, polite, philosophical; with polished manners, a ready smile and all the ways of a gentleman." Lemoigne entertained good relationships with other prospectors. A kind, generous, and hospitable man, he lived long enough to earn the respectable nickname of "Old John." When he died around 1919, alone with his burros near Salt Creek, he was probably still holding on to his dream—that he owned one of the largest silver-lead mines in the West.

But Old John's mine was not nearly as rich as he had loved to believe. For nearly 60 years after his death his claims were relocated, leased, bonded and sold, and probed by over 1,000 feet of tunnels, but they never produced a fortune. Development of his claims began almost right after his death, when they were relocated by Beveridge Hunter and Bill Corcoran. After sinking a 25-foot tunnel, the two men realized how much work was needed and began looking for financial backing. By the summer of 1920 a rich ledge assaying as much as 61% in lead had been exposed, which an optimistic engineer estimated at no less than two and a half million dollars. In spite of this flattering figure, it took two fruitless attempts before they managed to interest the right party—two local men, W. R. McCrea and John Reilly, who took a lease on the property with an option to buy. For several months they worked the claims diligently, driving a crosscut tunnel to intersect what was then the richest known ledge. Their efforts paid off. In May 1924, they hit a rich vein larger than any previously exposed on the property.

As usual this new strike triggered grand visions. In a short time the two men had made plans to turn the property into the largest lead mine in the West. A year later Reilly had acquired the property from Hunter and Corcoran for a large amount of cash and stock, and organized the Buckhorn Humboldt Mining Company. McCrea, the main stockholder, became the company manager, then the president after Reilly's death in the spring of 1925. The access road to the canyon was built around that time to connect the mine to the main Trona-Beatty road. The following few years saw the heyday of the Lemoigne Mine. For a change, Old John's quiet hideout was hopping. The property attracted the attention of as many as 10 leasers, who worked on adjacent claims. One of them, the Lemoigne South Extension Mining Company, uncovered ore worth up to 80% in lead. The Buckhorn Humboldt Mining Company worked its rich ledge, and later on opened a second mining area, deeper in the south fork. During this period two trucks left the mine every day, hauling ore some 50 miles to Beatty. Around 150 tons were shipped in 1925, and another 80 tons in 1927. Most of it was high grade and fairly rich, reportedly averaging 10% to 50% in lead, as well as 5 ounces of silver and 0.5 ounce of gold per ton.

Unfortunately, the high-grade lode was just too small to sustain even this modest production for very long. With trucking costs alone running as high as $18 per ton, mining the extensive lower grade deposits was unprofitable. When operations were discontinued around 1928, the total return was only $20,000. The Buckhorn Humboldt held on through 1948, but its mines were idle much of this time. Further work was carried out in 1953 and in the early 1960s. The last mining took place in the mid-1970s when previously unexplored ground yielded ore with up to 14 ounces of silver per ton. But all these attempts did not even double the 1920s production figure. Had Old John not been so attached to his mine, he would have made a fortune selling a few high-grade pockets that at one point in time he had several prospective buyers convinced was the legendary Lost Gunsight Lode.

Geology

In the Jurassic, the intrusion of the granitic pluton that became Hunter Mountain dramatically altered the stratigraphy of this region. A huge slab of Bonanza King Formation dolomite, 1,500 feet thick and at least 15 square miles in area, was displaced along a thrust fault by more than a mile, covering all younger formations. Erosion carved Lemoigne Canyon in this strata, but it barely made a dent in it. With the exception of the Owens Valley Formation along the meanders, the only rocks exposed for miles consist of this displaced Cambrian formation.

Route Description

The first side canyon. To start with, you may want to check out the side canyon on the left at the end of the road. You'll walk through an eerie defile of smooth white walls punctured with egg-shaped cavities and small arches in very soft basaltic pyroclastic rock. At the end of this passage there is a hollowed-out high cliff of the same rock straight ahead. An easy shortcut leads up to the low saddle to the right of this cliff and down the other side into the south fork above the narrows.

The narrows and the meanders. The lower canyon is the most scenic part of the south fork. It starts with short narrows typical of the southern Cottonwoods—shallow and tortuous, with bulging walls of dark dolomite. There are a few short falls, all of them easy because in the past they were filled with rocks to accommodate trucks. The narrows lead into a trench-like passage that extends a short distance past the confluence with the north fork. About 0.5 mile further, the south fork enters a narrower area that twists around six tight meanders. These meanders are not true narrows, as they are mostly walled in on one side only, but they are rugged and windy, lined by thick, broken limestone walls.

The mid-canyon and Lemoigne's cabin. The following stretch to the mines is stark and desolate. Joshua trees grow in number up canyon, at first confined to the north-facing slopes, gradually spreading to the hotter south-facing slopes at higher elevations—a good example of the trade-off between elevation and exposure. Eventually a scant forest covers the canyon slopes up to the highest ridges, reinforcing the eerie atmosphere of this area.

The mining area begins at the fourth side canyon, which is on the south side. This side canyon contains Lemoigne's cabin, an odd structure of stone masonry, boards, and corrugated metal. It is a tiny one-room house, barely high enough for standing room. It is difficult to imagine anyone living in it for any length of time. Yet Lemoigne apparently managed to make it liveable, if not cozy, reportedly stocking it with literature classics. Unfortunately, time is inexorably taking its toll. The back wall has collapsed and the cabin is now filled with rubble. This historical site is also spoiled by a large corrugated metal house of more recent vintage. A few rusted artifacts are scattered around—spring mattresses and bed frames, boards and cans. A couple of crude rock shelters can be found nearby in the canyon walls.

The mines. Most of the 1920s production of the Buckhorn Humboldt company came from the mines above this side canyon. Their tailings are clearly visible from the cabins, at the top of the western ridge. A trail used to climb along this ridge to the mines, but it is now just a trace and you will need to climb to find it. The portal of the main mine level is on the west side of the ridge, above the ore chute at the top of the mine tailing. It goes clear across the ridge to the east side, where it emerges next to an open cut. Do not attempt to walk through it: between the east and west portals the tunnel is interrupted by a 20-foot vertical shaft (not to mention several inclined drifts along the way).

Lemoigne Canyon		
	Dist.(mi)	Elev.(ft)
Lemoigne Canyon Road		
Highway 190	0.0	1,285
Turnout/trail to Emigrant R. S.	4.3	2,350
Emigrant Ranger Station	(~3.0)	2,130
Road's end (1st side canyon)	5.5	2,800
Roadless canyon		
Road's end (1st side canyon)	0.0	2,800
Narrows (start)	0.4	2,980
Narrows (end)	0.6	3,040
Confluence (north fork)	0.7	3,080
Meanders (start)	1.2	3,350
Meanders (end)	1.8	3,780
Second side canyon	2.1	3,940
Fourth side canyon	3.3	4,700
Lemoigne's cabin	(0.1)	4,800
Lemoigne Mine	(0.5)	~5,200
Fifth side canyon	3.6	4,860
Head	5.8	6,780

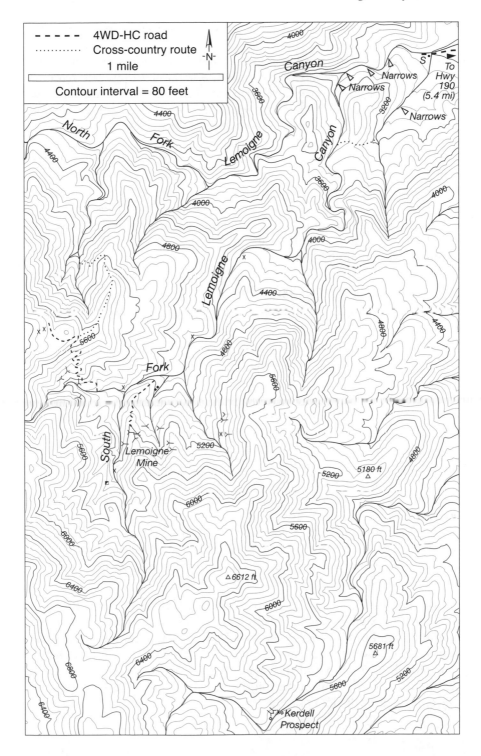

4WD-HC road
Cross-country route
-N-
1 mile
Contour interval = 80 feet

Canyon
Narrows
Narrows
To Hwy 190 (5.4 mi)
S
Narrows
Canyon
North
Fork
Lemoigne
Lemoigne
4400
4000
4800
4400
4000
4000
Fork
4800
Lemoigne
Mine
South
5200
5180 ft
6000
5600
6400
6000
△6612 ft
5681 ft
6800
6400
5600
Kerdell
Prospect

All other mines and prospects are located in this and the follow-ing side canyons. Several old trails still climb up to them. Records dis-agree as to the location of Lemoigne's Mine. USGS maps place it on the north side of the fifth side canyon, while some geology publications claim it is the mines above the fourth side canyon. This confusion may reflect the probable fact that Lemoigne discovered and worked several deposits. The location of the cabin suggests that the fourth side canyon may be the site of the original discovery.

If you are intrigued by old mines, you will want to spend a little time around here. Most of the remnants date from the 1947-1953 period. In general, the lead and silver ore occurred in fissures in the form of small, high-grade bodies of mostly massive galena. Very little ore is now exposed in any of the tunnels, except for small amounts of galena, cerus-site (lead carbonate), and bright yellow tabular crystals of wulfenite (an oxide of lead and molybdenum).

Hiking and Backpacking Suggestions

The south fork. The mining area is an easy goal for a day hike if you start from the end of the road, a full day hike if you start from the Emigrant Ranger Station. You can also do a shorter loop heading out via the first side canyon and returning down the narrows.

The north fork. With its long, wildly meandering course, this fork is well worth a visit. A nice way to see its lower portion is to make the following full-day loop. From the confluence, go up the south fork to the fifth side canyon. Climb the old trail north to the ridge above the mines. From where the trail crests the ridge, it is a steep descent on the far side into the north fork. From the ridge to the confluence is about 4 miles.

A more extensive trip is to retrace the old route to Cottonwood Canyon, across one of the park's largest roadless areas. From the conflu-ence, it follows the north fork to the crest of the mountains, a rolling plateau with thick stands of Joshua trees. It then drops into the upper drainage of Cottonwood Canyon, cutting through Jurassic quartz mon-zonite down to a broad alluvial basin and Cottonwood Springs. There is flowing water along the next 4 miles to the road.

Lemoigne's grave. If you were touched by Lemoigne's life, you may want to pay homage to his grave. It is located near where his body was found, about 1.5 miles west of Beatty Junction. The cross that marked his grave is gone (probably another brilliant act of vandalism), but with the 7.5' map and the nearby USGS marker you can locate it within a few yards. Out in the middle of Death Valley, it is a lonesome place, perfect for the loner he was.

■

THE KERDELL PROSPECT

> *This offbeat destination is included here mostly for the benefit of desert rats. To find it takes a lot of walking in next to no shade, and lonesomeness is perhaps its most remarkable feature. But hardy hikers will find here a plethora of delightful features, from winding gorges to narrows, falls, a wide variety of plants and wild flowers — and the mine itself, abandoned in a scenic forest of Joshua trees.*

General Information

Road status: Roadless; hiking from paved or 4WD/HC road
Shortest hike: 1.7 mi, ~250 ft one way (or less)/moderate
Longest hike: 7.9 mi, ~3,700 ft one way/difficult
Main attractions: Indian trail, remote canyon and lead mine
USGS 15' and 7.5' topo maps: Emigrant Canyon, Panamint Butte
Maps: pp. 385*, 381, 333

Location and Access

The Kerdell Prospect is located in the nameless canyon south of Lemoigne Canyon. The beginning of this hike is along the Emigrant-Lemoigne trail, which starts at the Emigrant Campground, 9.1 miles west of Stovepipe Wells on Highway 190. From the campground, the mouth of the canyon is just behind the prominent ridge to the west-southwest, 2 miles away. Park at the nearby Emigrant Ranger Station and follow the directions to the trail given below.

History

Not much is known about the history of the Kerdell Prospect. It was a latecomer, first worked in March 1949, when two adits and some drifts were developed to exploit a lead deposit. The area was relocated in December 1954 by Roy Hunter as the Lone Ear Prospect. Even then supplies and water had to be packed in to this remote and hopelessly dry location. Most of the ore was galena found in the limestone of the Owens Valley Formation, with traces of gold and copper minerals. Although the workings eventually amounted to a few hundred feet of tunnels, they did not lead to any known commercial production. The mine was reached by a 6-mile cross-country hike from a trail connecting Lemoigne Canyon and what is now the Emigrant Ranger Station. This trail is said to have been originally an Indian trail, later used by miners and prospectors.

383

Route Description

The Emigrant-Lemoigne trail. This trail starts in the middle of the campground boundary furthest from the road. It heads straight across the fan, roughly west the whole way, but at first it is narrow and vague, and it's easy to lose it. Small cairns mark its location (they are potentially historical; do not destroy them or add stones to them). At the first large wash crossing (0.9 mile), the trail resumes a little further up the wash as a wider road lined with rocks, easier to track. If you lose it, aim for the foot of the ridge, which is a more tedious but slightly shorter route. The vast field of heavily varnished boulders covering the fan is olivine basalt. They originate from the Pliocene flow capping the foothills of the Cottonwood Mountains to the southwest. After about 1.7 miles, you will reach a wide wash. Head up this wash to go to the Kerdell Prospect. To go to Lemoigne Canyon instead, continue on the trail on the far side of the wash 1.3 miles to its end at the Lemoigne Canyon Road.

The canyon. The route proceeds up the broad and uneventful lower canyon, then into its second main side canyon, on the north side 1.5 miles above its mouth. With its changing character, this fork is far more interesting, and a great place to explore the many facets of the desert. It soon enters a small gorge—neither very deep nor narrow, although framed by vertical walls—which winds through the Pliocene basaltic flow. After 1.5 miles the wash goes through a short plug of reddish fanglomerate, then enters the thick limestone beds of the Owens Valley Formation and the second gorge. This one is longer, quite different from the first gorge, with short narrows at one point. The grade is moderate and the walking generally easy, except in the gorges where progress is slowed down by thicker vegetation and many falls. There is a total of 13 falls 6 feet or higher, the highest one about 18 feet, and several shorter ones. Only two of the falls, in the second gorge, require technical

	Dist.(mi)	Elev.(ft)
The Kerdell Prospect		
Emigrant Campground (trail)	0.0	2,140
Main wash	1.7	~2,260
Lemoigne Canyon Road	(1.3)	2,350
Canyon mouth	2.6	~2,640
Fork	4.1	3,240
First gorge (start)	4.5	3,540
Second gorge (start)	6.9	5,230
Kerdell Prospect (camp)	7.8	~5,680

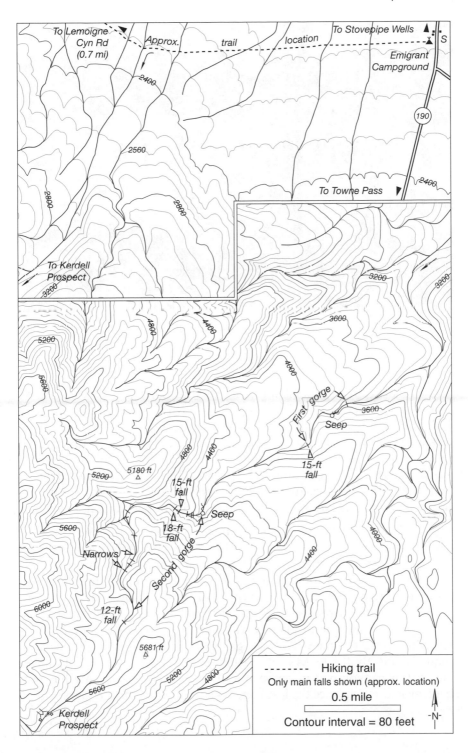

To Lemoigne Cyn Rd (0.7 mi)

Approx. trail location

To Stovepipe Wells

S

Emigrant Campground

190

To Towne Pass

2400

2560

2800

2800

3200

To Kerdell Prospect

3200

5200

4800

4400

5600

3200

3600

First gorge

3600

Seep

15-ft fall

5180 ft

4800

4400

15-ft fall

5200

18-ft fall

Seep

4000

Narrows

Second gorge

4400

6000

12-ft fall

5600

5681 ft

Hiking trail

Only main falls shown (approx. location)

0.5 mile

5200

4800

Kerdell Prospect

Contour interval = 80 feet

-N-

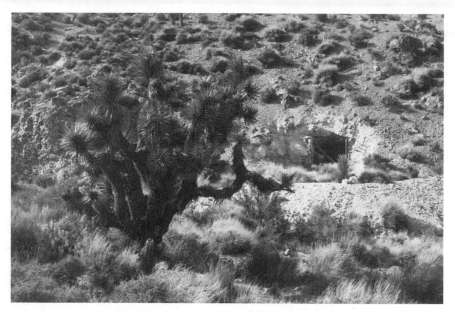

Adit used as a shed at the Kerdell Prospect

climbing or a short bypass. Past the second gorge, the canyon remains open the rest of the way (0.9 mile) to the mine.

This canyon is outstanding for its unusually diverse vegetation. In the spring many wild flowers grace its wash, including mohavea, Indian paintbrush, indigo bush, Mojave aster, locoweed, globemallow, larkspur, rosemary eriogonum, and purple sage. I also came upon a number of uncommon plants, such as miner's lettuce at shaded dry seeps, Panamint phacelia and rock spiraea on the walls of the narrows, and Mojave fishhook cactus above the second gorge. Swallows, ravens, hummingbirds and hawks can be sighted in the upper canyon.

The Kerdell Prospect. This all but forgotten lead mine is located deep in the upper canyon, among Joshua trees and within sight of timberline—another botanical treat. Its two main tunnels are at the top of the large tailings looming above the wash. Just below them are the remains of two small camps, one of them sheltered by a large pinyon pine, and a shallow prospect once used as a shed. It's a long walk to this mine, but it is unique in many ways. I truly enjoyed its isolation, not knowing ahead of time what I was going to find there, and what I eventually found. By the looks of it, except for the mine itself, I could have sworn this canyon had never seen a human being. It certainly has not been visited much since the last miners abandoned it decades ago.

∎

PART VIII

PANAMINT MOUNTAINS

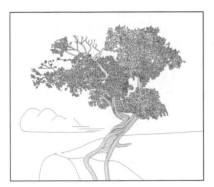

WEST OF DEATH VALLEY the land gathers itself into a long and high mountain range known as the Panamint Mountains. Covering an area of about 820 square miles, they are the largest in the park. They are also by far the highest: near the center of the range, Telescope Peak culminates at 11,049 feet, almost a mile above the Black Mountains to the east. At their northern end is Tucki Mountain, a large turtleback reaching 6,726 feet above sea level. South from here the crest has several high peaks reaching above 10,000 feet. Between Wildrose Peak and Porter Peak, a distance of 15.5 miles, the elevation hardly drops below 8,000 feet. From Porter Peak south the crest drops rapidly towards the Owlshead Mountains. The lowest elevation, at the foot of the fans, is around -250 feet along Death Valley and about 1,200 feet along Panamint Valley, on the west side of the Panamints.

Unlike most mountain ranges of comparable elevation, the Panamint Mountains are devoid of extensive foothills. From base to summit the central range is one long unobstructed slope. The distance between Telescope Peak and the edge of Death Valley's salt pan is just under 12 miles. This is one of the longest slopes this steep in North America. The difference in elevation between these high and low points exceeds 2 miles. It makes Death Valley the deepest depression in the coterminous United States, nearly twice as deep as the Grand Canyon.

Access and Backcountry Driving

The Panamint Mountains are circumvented and accessed by numerous roads, yet because of their size accessibility varies greatly. Tucki Mountain is within easy reach of Highway 190 and Emigrant

Canyon Road. The east side of the Panamints is accessible from Highway 190, the Badwater Road, and the West Side Road. Access can also be gained from the Emigrant Canyon Road and the primitive roads to Skidoo and Aguereberry Point. By ascending to the crest of the range at 8,133-foot Mahogany Flat, the Wildrose Canyon Road provides the easiest access to the high Panamints.

Several primitive roads climb part way into western canyons from the Panamint Valley and into eastern canyons from the West Side Road. As a general rule, these roads are relatively good up the alluvial fan to the canyon mouth, and a 2-wheel-drive vehicle is often adequate. Inside the canyons they deteriorate and usually require high clearance and/or 4-wheel drive. Only Warm Spring Canyon has a through road. This road climbs up to Warm Spring and Butte Valley, then goes over Mengel Pass and down Goler Wash to Panamint Valley. Past Warm Spring this road requires high clearance, and the Goler Wash Road requires 4-wheel drive as well on both sides of Mengel Pass.

In the past, the West Side Road was closed from about late May through October, although car travel was still permitted on a limited basis in that season (see *Seasonal Road Closure* in *Desert Hiking Tips*). Since this policy is not widely known, if it is still in effect and you decide to come here in the summer, you may well have the eastern Panamints all to yourself!

Geology

The Panamint Mountains were formed by upthrust along a north-south trending fault line that extends along their western side. Numerous shorter faults run along the eastern front. The steepest escarpment occurs on the thrust side, which has been rising at the fault line along Panamint Valley. The side facing Death Valley has been tilted eastward around a general axis located at the alluvial fan level, so that the lower part of the mountains has been sinking while the upper part has been uplifted. As a consequence, the most abrupt canyons in the Panamints are generally located on the western scarp, places such as Hall and Big Horn canyons, which climb from the Panamint Valley floor 1,000 feet per mile for several miles. Along Death Valley the canyons start from a lower elevation, are generally longer and not quite as steep.

Alluvial fans almost completely surround the Panamint Mountains. Their physiography reflects the general eastward tilting of the range. They are comparatively short on the west side, especially along Panamint Dry Lake, but miles long and massive on the east side. From south to north the foot of the range becomes more and more deeply buried in its own alluvia, perhaps from a slight northward tilt of the mountains. Blackwater and Tucki washes, near the north end, are broad rivers of gravel, whereas further south Six Spring and Galena canyons start immediately as relatively narrow canyons.

Most of the Panamints are composed of marine deposits dating as far back as the Precambrian. They have been eroding for such a long time that much of the younger strata have been stripped off, exposing much older rocks over most of the mountainous area. With few exceptions, from Tucki Mountain to Warm Spring Canyon the youngest rocks are Devonian, at least 360 million years old. Most of the central portion of the range was deposited in the Cambrian. Older, Precambrian formations occur along the upper west side and around Galena and Warm Spring canyons. Other than the Quaternary alluvial deposits, younger rocks are exposed in four major areas. The relatively lower elevations south of Warm Spring Canyon down to the Owlshead Mountains comprise primarily Tertiary volcanic rocks, and Pliocene and Pleistocene nonmarine deposits. From the northwestern tip of Tucki Mountain down to Wildrose Canyon and west to Panamint Valley, a large deposit of Plio-Pleistocene rocks is exposed. Volcanic rocks of probable Oligocene age occur in isolated areas along the eastern foot of the mountains, especially north from Trail Canyon. Finally, a large, early Tertiary granitic intrusion covers several square miles near the head of Hanaupah Canyon—a relatively uncommon occurrence in Death Valley.

Hydrology and Vegetation

The Panamints are high enough that they capture a little of the moisture from the Pacific Ocean that has made it over the Sierra Nevada, and they receive a fair amount of precipitation. The average yearly rainfall is at least 9 inches at 7,000 feet, and up to 15 inches in the high Panamints. Every year snow usually blankets the highest summits until March and sometimes as late as May. In the winter, ice can make the highest crests inaccessible without proper equipment—ice has probably claimed more human lives than the heat.

Thanks to this relative abundance of moisture, many canyons have a little surface water year-round, usually in the form of springs or even running creeks. These springs are fed by rain and snow melt that has percolated downward and is routed to the surface by nearly horizontal thrust faults. Compared to typical springs in this desert, their flow is usually fairly substantial. Reflecting this higher precipitation and the broad range of elevations, the vegetation of the Panamints is one of the most varied in the park, and it encompasses most of the local plant zones. Even Joshua trees can be found here, though mostly in the White Sage Wash area. The high Panamints also support the most extensive woodland belt in the park, and the only limber pine and bristlecone pine forest.

Hiking

Because of their wide range of elevation and geological diversity, the Panamint Mountains offer an unusual variety of sceneries, from barren slopes to dense forests, dry washes to spring-fed oases, and wide-open valleys to narrow canyons. Combined with a colorful history, this diversity makes this range one of the most interesting hiking areas around Death Valley.

Some of the most scenic hiking destinations in the Panamints are the canyons of Tucki Mountain. Except for Telephone Canyon, all of these are roadless. The most popular ones, Mosaic and Grotto canyons, are easily accessible and provide the visitor with a good exposure to the basic elements of desert canyon hiking. All other canyons can only be reached by hiking several miles from a paved road. Canyons on the east side of Tucki Mountain, south from Little Bridge Canyon, are among the most remote in the park. The only one that is named, Trellis Canyon, is well worth exploring.

The canyons draining the eastern Panamints tend to be broader, at least near their mouths. However, they are among the best places in the park to see a desert stream, which makes up for the general lack of narrow gorges. South from Trail Canyon, most major canyons have at least one sizeable spring, if not several springs and/or a perennial creek supporting a few acres of lush riparian vegetation. Much of the southern Panamints witnessed a lot of mining activity, and old mines and camps can still be found at many locations, in particular in Trail, Galena, Warm Spring, and Anvil Spring canyons. The Goler Wash Road, a beautiful, rugged route prized by 4-wheel drive enthusiasts, gives access to several isolated springs, mines, tramways, as well as a lovely desert stream, before reaching Mengel Pass and Butte Valley. The forested belt of the high Panamints gives an unusual character to the upper reaches of several of the major canyons. These more shaded areas provide cooler hiking grounds in the summer, as well as fragrances and wildlife found nowhere else in the area, and expansive views of Death Valley.

Yet the most striking features of the canyons of the eastern Panamints are perhaps their length and remoteness, and the countless possibilities for exploration that they offer. Places like Death Valley, Chuckwalla, and Starvation canyons, and scores of unnamed drainages, are far from any road. Six Spring Canyon is another one, and some of its side canyons have very good narrows. There is plenty of space out there for hikers seeking solitude.

■

Suggested Hikes in the Panamint Mountains					
Route/Destination	Dist. (mi)	Elev. change	Mean elev.	Access road	Pages
Short hikes (under 5 miles round trip)					
Arrastre Spring	0.5	510'	5,440'	H/6.6 mi	446-448
Grantham Mine*	~0.6	<100'	~2,100'	Graded	443-444
Greene-Denner-Drake Mill	1.0	510'	4,770'	Paved	472
Grotto Canyon (first grotto)	1.2	390'	610'	P/1.0 mi	405-407
Grubstake Spring	0.3	200'	3,440'	H/3.5 mi	446
Hanaupah Cyn (1st narrows)	2.2	1,160'	3,740'	H/9.3 mi	430-432
Hanaupah Spring	1.7	840'	3,590'	H/9.3 mi	430-431
Hummingbird Spring	1.0	910'	6,860'	H/1.8 mi	516
Hungry Bill's Ranch	1.8	830'	4,290'	F/10.1 mi	437-440
Jayhawker Spring	2.4	1,100'	3,550'	Paved	463-464
Journigan's Mill	0.2	60'	4,400'	Paved	468-469
Malapi Spring	1.5	700'	4,690'	Paved	469-470
Montgomery Mine	2.2	1,240'	3,650'	H/1.8 mi	445-446
Mosaic Canyon (25-ft fall)	1.7	970'	1,440'	Graded	400-402
Mosaic Cyn (fourth narrows)	2.5	1,490'	1,700'	Graded	400-405
Mud Spring	2.2	960'	3,590'	Paved	516
Panamint Mine loop*	3.5	1,450'	1,700'	Graded	443
Pink Elephant Mine	0.5	300'	2,570'	Graded	444-445
Saddle Rock Mine	2.5	1,540'	4,310'	Paved	458
Skidoo mines loop*	2.2	~200'	5,700'	P/7.4 mi	460
Stretched-Pebble C. (15' fall)	2.3	1,470'	1,185'	Paved	396-398
Striped Butte	1.4	980	4,160'	P/9.0 mi	448
Telephone Arch and Spring	0.4	190'	2,730'	H/2.6 mi	451-452
Trail Canyon, confluence to					
Broken Pick Millsite	0.3	140'	3,530'	H/9.3 mi	420
Morning Glory Camp	1.5	860'	3,850'	H/9.3 mi	423-426
Old Dependable Mine	2.4	1,420'	4,130'	H/9.3 mi	423-425
Smith and Polson Camp	1.9	1,020'	3,970'	H/9.3 mi	420-421
Warm Spring	0.1	130'	2,430'	Graded	444
Intermediate hikes (5-12 miles round trip)					
Dripping Spring	3.0	1,880'	4,400'	H/9.3 mi	420-422
Grotto Cyn (to amphitheater)	3.4	2,110'	1,470'	P/1.1 mi	405-408
Grotto Canyon 3rd side cyn	3.7	2,400'	1,340'	P/1.0 mi	405-408
Hanaupah Cyn (3rd narrows)	4.5	3,400'	4,740'	H/9.3 mi	430-434
Jayhawker Canyon narrows	3.3	1,490'	3,750'	Paved	463-466
Johnson Cyn (fourth spring)	2.7	1,560'	4,650'	H/10.1 mi	437-440

Route/Destination	Dist. (mi)	Elev. change	Mean elev.	Access road	Pages
Intermediate hikes (5-12 miles round trip) (cont'd)					
Johnson Cyn (Panamint Pass)	5.1	4,200'	5,970'	H/10.1 mi	437-440
Little Bridge	3.3	1,900'	900'	Paved	412-414
Little Bridge Cyn (to head)	4.5	3,080'	1,490'	Paved	412-414
Montgomery Mine	4.0	1,700'	3,270'	Graded	445-446
Morning Glory Mine loop*	8.2	2,880'	4,860'	H/9.3 mi	423-426
Skidoo via Saddle Rock Mine	5.2	2,450'	4,850'	Paved	458-460
Stretched-Pebble Cyn (head)	3.5	3,190'	2,040'	Paved	396-398
Telephone Arch and Spring	2.9	1,020'	2,500'	Paved	451-452
Trail Canyon, north fork	3.5	2,550'	4,700'	Graded	418-419
Tucki Mine	2.8	1,060'	4,530'	P/7.1 mi	452-454
Twin Springs	3.8	3,210'	2,560'	Graded	400-405
Wildrose Peak	4.5	2,100'	8,010'	Graded	517-520
Long hikes (over 12 miles round trip)					
Aguereberry Point Road to					
Dripping Spring	6.6	4,470'	4,550'	Graded	418-422
Morning Glory Mine	7.3	5,430'	4,780'	Graded	418, 423
Jayhawker Cyn to Pinto Peak	9.3	4,510'	5,250'	Paved	463-466
Pinto Peak trail to Pinto Peak	7.9	2,190'	6,410'	Paved	466
Porter Peak	6.6	5,230'	6,190'	H/10.1 mi	440
Saddle Rock Mine (via cyn)	7.7	3,280'	3,380'	Paved	451-452
Skidoo (via Telephone Cyn)	10.4	4,180'	3,940'	Paved	451-452
Squaw Spring	7.8	1,860'	3,060'	Paved	448
Summit Camp (via canyon)	8.1	3,900'	4,950'	Paved	463-466
Telescope Peak					
from Mahogany Flat	6.7	3,150'	9,600'	P/1.6 mi	520-522
from Hanaupah Cyn Rd	8.5	7,920'	6,900'	H/9.3 mi	430-434
Tucki Mine	10.3	3,300'	3,470'	Paved	451-454
Overnight hikes (over 2 days)					
West Side Rd to Ballarat via					
Johnson & Surprise cyns	28.6	15,330'	3,410'	Graded	437-440
Johnson & Pleasant cyns	28.7	17,390'	4,060'	Graded	437-440
Shorty's Well to Telescope Pk	16.8	11,294'	4,320'	Graded	430-434
Trail Canyon (road to road)	12.8	6,220'	2,860'	Graded	417-419
Wildrose Cyn-Trail Cyn-					
Aguereberry Point Road	12.6	4,400'	6,000'	Graded	417, 517

Key: P=Primitive (2WD)   H=Primitive (HC)   F=Primitive (4WD)
*=Total distance and elevation change (ups + downs) for loops

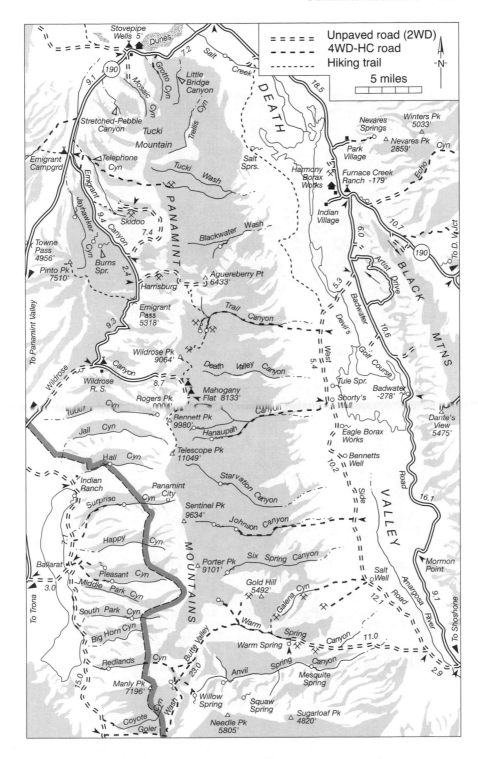

Unpaved road (2WD)
4WD-HC road
Hiking trail

5 miles

-N-

Stovepipe Wells 5'
Dunes
7.2
Salt Creek
DEATH
18.5
190
9.1
Mosaic Cyn
Grotto Cyn
Little Bridge Canyon
Trellis Cyn
Stretched-Pebble Canyon
Tucki Mountain
Nevares Springs
Winters Pk 5033'
Nevares Pk 2859'
Echo Cyn
Emigrant Campgrd
Telephone Cyn
Tucki Wash
Salt Sprs.
Park Village
Harmony Borax Works
Furnace Creek Ranch -179'
Emigrant
Jayhawker Cyn
9.4
Skidoo
7.4
Blackwater Wash
Indian Village
6.0
10.7
To D. VJct
190
Towne Pass 4956'
Burns Spr.
2.4
Harrisburg
Agutreberry Pt 6433'
PANAMINT
Artist Drive
BLACK
Pinto Pk 7510'
Emigrant Pass 5318'
Trail Canyon
West 5.4
Devil's
5.3
Golf Course
10.6
MTNS
9.3
Wildrose Pk 9064'
Death Valley Canyon
To Panamint Valley
Wildrose Canyon
Wildrose R. S.
8.7
Rogers Pk 9994'
Mahogany Flat 8133'
Tule Spr.
Shorty's
Badwater -278'
Dante's View 5475'
Tubur Cyn
Rennett Pk 9980'
Hanaupah
Canyon
Eagle Borax Works
Jail Cyn
Hall Cyn
Telescope Pk 11049'
Bennetts Well
10.2
Indian Ranch
Surprise
Cyn
Panamint City
Starvation Canyon
VALLEY
Happy Cyn
Sentinel Pk 9634'
Johnson Canyon
Side
16.1
Mormon Point
Ballarat
3.0
Pleasant Cyn
Middle Park Cyn
Porter Pk 9101'
Six Spring Canyon
Salt Well
Amargosa
9.1
To Trona
South Park Cyn
Gold Hill 5492'
Galena Cyn
12.1
Road
To Shoshone
MOUNTAINS
Big Horn Cyn
Warm
Spring
Canyon
11.0
Redlands Cyn
15.0
Butte Valley
23.0
Warm Spring
Anvil Spring
Canyon
Mesquite Spring
2.9
Manly Pk 7196'
Willow Spring
Squaw Spring
Sugarloaf Pk 4820'
Coyote
Goler
Cyn
Wash
Needle Pk 5805'

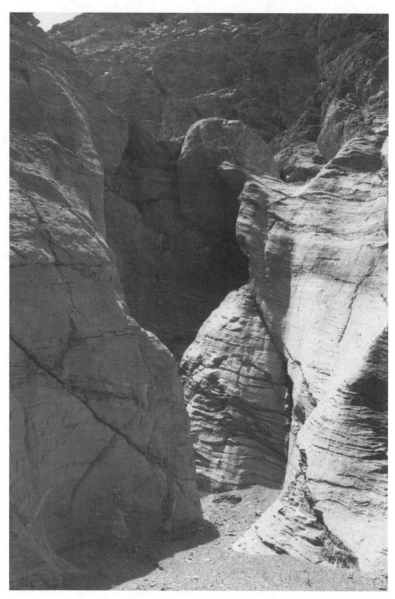

*Impressive chockstones challenge climbers
along Stretched-Pebble Canyon*

STRETCHED-PEBBLE CANYON

This fun little canyon is perhaps best described as different from most. Narrow the whole way, studded with falls, it is bounded by strangely metamorphosed rocks probably deposited during an ice age over half a billion years ago. Some of the falls are high and dangerous: without rock climbing experience you may not go very far.

General Information

Road status: Roadless; hike from paved road
Shortest hike: 1.2 mi, 490 ft one way / moderate
Longest hike: 4.0 mi, 4,100 ft one way (or more) / moderate
Main attractions: Long, tight narrows, falls, rock climbing, geology
USGS 15' and 7.5' topo maps: Stovepipe Wells
Maps: pp. 397*, 393

Location and Access

Stretched-Pebble Canyon is the third canyon west of Mosaic Canyon, on Tucki Mountain. Start from Highway 190 3.3 miles west of Stovepipe Wells (or 5.8 miles east of the Emigrant Ranger Station).

Geology: Precambrian Ice Age

The rocks exposed on the northwest slope of Tucki Mountain, which includes this canyon, were tentatively assigned to the Kingston Peak Formation. Of all the local formations, this is one of the most unusual, not so much for its composition as for the mystery surrounding its origin. About half of it is made of a conglomerate called diamictite, a wild mixture of rocks of all sizes ranging from sand to large boulders. What is puzzling about this formation is that it is sandwiched between two formations made primarily of dolomite, a rock typically formed in warm seas. What could have caused such a radical change?

This dolomite-conglomerate sequence is found in other late-Proterozoic formations around the world, which all record a profound transformation in the Earth's environment. The most appealing theory is that the Kingston Peak Formation was formed during an ice age. Only glaciers, it has been argued, can move around such chaotic combinations of unsorted rocks. According to this scenario, around the beginning of the formation the weather changed dramatically, and what was perhaps a tropical seascape turned to a frozen landscape. On at least two occasions, glaciers advanced and withdrew, each time dumping into shallow rift valley basins the hodgepodge of odd-sized sediments that became the Kingston Peak diamictite. Evidence of glaciation includes isolated boulders reminiscent of those shed by today's icebergs, and stones faceted and striated by advancing ice sheets. In the Jurassic and Cretaceous, large portions of the formation were metamorphosed by granitic intrusions. At places the metamorphism was so intense—as much as 3,000 atmospheres and 650°C—that individual rocks were flattened like pancakes, producing what is known as stretched-pebble conglomerate. In Nemo Canyon, for example, diamictite boulders were compressed by three times their original size.

The tentative identification of the Kingston Peak Formation in Tucki Mountain has never been confirmed, so possibly none of this is relevant to this canyon. But then is it just a coincidence that the canyon walls are lined with wildly deformed boulders?

Route Description

The fan. The canyon mouth is about 1.2 miles southeast up the fan, just to the right of the grayish hill at the foot of Tucki Mountain. In about 0.5 mile you should run into the wide wash that leads up to the canyon. The grade is moderate and the walk fairly easy.

On the high points of the fan, the exposed surfaces of many of the rocks have suffered from several forms of erosion, fairly common on alluvial fans. In more water-soluble rocks, wind-driven rain has etched fine wormy rills. Samples containing alternating layers of different compositions exhibit parallel grooves where the more soluble material has been preferentially dissolved. Other rocks show pitting caused by wind-blown particles. In comparison, the rocks' protected undersides are fairly smooth. Rocks lying in the washes do not show any of these features. Because they are periodically rearranged by floods, they are never exposed long enough to be affected by these slow weathering processes.

Another interesting feature along the way is the old Rhyolite-Skidoo telephone line (see *Telephone Canyon*). If you hike on the fan west

Stretched-Pebble Canyon		
	Dist.(mi)	Elev.(ft)
Highway 190	0.0	450
Mouth	1.2	940
15-ft fall	2.3	1,920
Fork	2.8	2,360
Head	3.5	~3,640

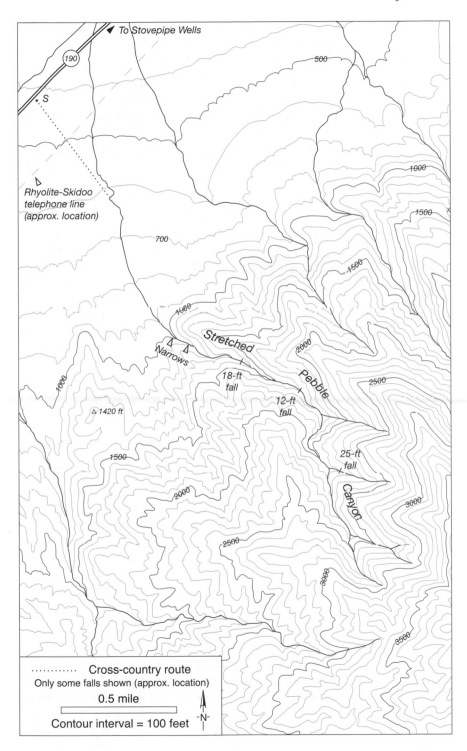

To Stovepipe Wells

190

● S

△

Rhyolite-Skidoo
telephone line
(approx. location)

500

1000

1500

700

1500

Stretched

Narrows

18-ft
fall

2000

Pebble

2500

12-ft
fall

△ 1420 ft

25-ft
fall

1500

Canyon

3000

2000

2500

3000

3500

············ Cross-country route
Only some falls shown (approx. location)

0.5 mile

↑
-N-
↓

Contour interval = 100 feet

of the wash you will cross it about 0.35 mile from the highway. Decaying pole stumps and two metal wires lying on the ground still point to their original destination: Stovepipe Well.

The lower canyon. The exciting thing about this canyon is that it is one serious constriction. From just above its mouth to the fork 1.6 miles in, and beyond, you will be wandering through passages not so deep but consistently narrow, occasionally widening just enough, it seems, to close down even more a little further. At the tightest spots, the walls are only a few feet apart. The course is often so windy that it will keep you guessing as to what is in store ahead.

The strongly foliated rocks this canyon cuts through give it quite a distinctive character. The near-vertical walls are occasionally adorned by mosaics and wavy patterns where polished. These deformed strata create an odd landscape, a contin-

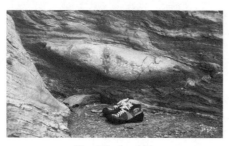

Stretched pebble

uously changing visual treat. The most unusual exposures are the stretched-pebble conglomerate exposed at several places in the canyon. Large, sturdy boulders of dolomite and quartzite trapped in the walls, originally a foot or more across, were squashed into ellipsoids several times longer than they are thick.

Everything would be simple but for one delightful detail: this place is an obstacle course. Up to the fork, about 18 falls and chockstones between 5 and 25 feet high challenge the way. If you enjoy climbing, you will probably find them the highlight of this hike. The falls are generally less than vertical and offer good-size holds. However, there are often chockstones wedged at their top, which makes the last move risky. All high falls can be circumvented except for the 15-foot fall about 1.1 miles in. Topped by a large chockstone, it must be climbed, and it will stop quite a few hikers. The climbs are never worse than about 5.7, generally easier than in Grotto Canyon, but some of them are fairly exposed, and the rock is often flaky. Be careful, especially coming back.

The upper forks. The two branches past the fork are short and shallower, but they are quite narrow and well worth exploring. The grade gradually increases and falls become more frequent. The left fork has the highest fall in this canyon. The right fork, longer and more interesting, goes through several tight passages and about half a dozen high falls before ending at the foot of a small bowl overlooking Death Valley.

■

MOSAIC CANYON

For its diversity of scenery, easy walking, and convenient access, Mosaic Canyon is one of the most popular hiking destinations in the park. If Death Valley is new to you, the lower canyon is a good introduction to the unexpected delights of desert canyons. It has tortuous narrows with colorful mosaics, finely polished marble, and interesting geology. The upper canyon, far less visited, will appeal even to seasoned desert rats for its sculpted narrows, rugged canyons, and hard-to-reach Twin Springs.

General Information

Road status: Roadless; good graded road to canyon mouth
Shortest hike: 0.5 mi, 230 ft one way/easy
Longest hike: 3.8 mi, 3,210 ft one way (or more)/strenuous
Main attractions: Narrows, mosaics, polished marble, falls, springs
USGS 15' topo map: Stovepipe Wells
USGS 7.5' topo maps: Stovepipe Wells*, Grotto Canyon
Maps: pp. 403*, 393

Location and Access

Mosaic Canyon is at the north end of Tucki Mountain, at the apex of the alluvial fan behind Stovepipe Wells. Just west of the motel a signed road leads in 2.4 miles to a small parking area at the mouth of the canyon. The road is well graded and good enough for just about anything on wheels.

Geology

The main formation exposed in lower Mosaic Canyon is called the Noonday Dolomite. Its characteristic tan-colored dolomite forms the canyon's flat, strongly tilted west wall, clearly visible from the road and the parking area. This formation was deposited in the late Proterozoic, well over half a billion years ago, when this area was flooded under the Pacific Ocean. It was later buried to great depths under the Precambrian and Cambrian formations now forming the east wall. In the process, some of the dolomite was subjected to elevated pressures and temperatures and was metamorphosed into marble. During the far more recent uplift of Tucki Mountain, the entire sequence of formations on the east side broke loose along a large fault. Erosion carved Mosaic Canyon along this fault, exposing the marble all along the narrows.

Route Description

The first narrows. A good thing about Mosaic Canyon is that it closes down into narrows almost right away. Along the first half a mile it winds tightly between walls of white marble or the mosaics that inspired its name. The marble bedrock has been chiseled by stream erosion into a succession of whirlpools and grooved chutes polished to a slick finish. The mosaics are breccia, small rock fragments bound in a natural cement. Two main types can be found here. The first, dominantly pale yellow, is made mostly of angular chunks of Noonday dolomite and marble. Look for samples on the east side just before the narrows. The second type, more common, is composed of a greater variety of rocks in a grayish cement. Entire walls are made of this colorful mosaic.

The narrows are quite tight, often no more than a few feet wide, but not very deep. Every other decade a major flood comes along and buries the narrow inner channel under several feet of gravel and mud, and it then takes several years for minor storms to scoop it all out again. Major floods happened here in the summer of 1950 and in the mid-1970s. Prior to this last event, the narrows were much deeper. They had one sizeable fall, high enough that a railing and metal steps had to be anchored in the wall to help hikers. Look for their rusted remains in the east wall 150 yards into the narrows. But the narrows will deepen again; it's only a matter of time.

You may want to visit the pretty side canyon on the right at the upper end of the first narrows. It goes through a narrow defile of fanglomerate, then runs into a few falls and interesting polished marble bedrock with deep potholes. Beyond all this there is a 20-foot fall, and a boulder-filled wash above it, ending at a small amphitheater.

The open wash. Past the first narrows the main canyon widens between cut banks of alluvia. The soaring flanks of Tucki Mountain provide a scenic backdrop along this more open stretch. It is a short walk to the next narrows (although in the summer it seems forever). A little before the second narrows, the wash splits around a prominent island of slanted marble. Here you have two choices, either to go along the wash or to take the rim trail, which bypasses the second and third narrows.

The rim trail. This trail starts at the marble island, up the ravine bank on the east side. It climbs to a low ridge, then drops (and vanishes) into the wash of a side canyon (325 yards). (The other option is to take this side canyon where it starts just past the island; either climb the 10-foot fall—low 5s—or bypass it on the slanted ledge on the left). Pick up the trail again 175 yards up the wash, just before it makes a sharp left, in the first ravine on the right (look for cairns on two large boulders). The trail, very faint at first, is eventually well defined as it climbs to the high rim of Mosaic Canyon, then follows it before dropping into the main wash just above the third narrows. Although this bypass route (about 1.25 miles) is not shorter than the canyon route, it provides quicker access to the upper canyon and offers impressive vistas.

The second narrows. You will have walked just over a mile by the time you reach the second narrows, which start at a 9-foot boulder jam, easy to negotiate. This scenic passage is made of a series of constrictions, stretches of polished bedrock, tight curves, hollowed walls, and colorful mosaics. Rock climbers may want to bring climbing shoes, as there are some good traverses, boulders, and slabs here and in the first narrows, often with good landings in soft gravel.

Eventually the wash enters a long, straight corridor which dead-ends at an 18-foot slanted fall—the end of the second narrows. Although the fall can be climbed (low 5s), it is safer to bypass it. Walk back about

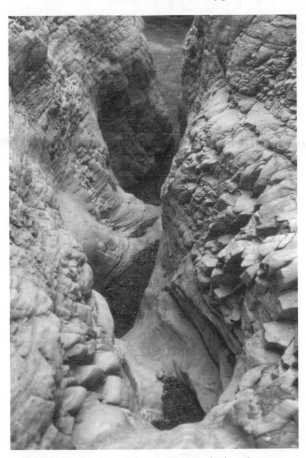

Polished chutes along Mosaic Canyon's fourth narrows

120 yards to the beginning of the straight corridor and hike up the small ravine on the west side (look for cairns). It climbs gently to a trail along the edge of the corridor that leads to the wash just above the fall.

From here on up the canyon is broader for another 500 yards, although it goes through two short narrow stretches. Between them, at a sharp left turn in the wash, there is another pretty side canyon on the right side. Narrow, choked with boulders and brushes, it has several colorful falls. After 300 yards the route is impeded by a high chockstone, more tricky to climb. In the right wall of the alcove above it, look for rare boulders of cemented ventifacts, probably fan material worn by erosion and later cemented by hot springs. In another 250 yards this side canyon becomes essentially impassable at a high-rising wall.

Back at the main canyon, the wash soon runs into a 25-foot fall, in a small amphitheater with walls coated with thick, candle-like mud drippings.

The third narrows. The 25-foot fall is the gateway to the third narrows, a deep, twisted gorge bounded at its upper end by another high fall. The fall climb is probably only a 5.8, but it is quite high and the rock is usually dusty. If the "heavy" traffic in the lower canyon bothered you, don't give up just yet. Most hikers don't go any further, and from here on it's pretty quiet.

To continue, walk back 120 yards to just before the last narrow stretch, and look for a faint trail on the steep slickrock on the east side.

	Mosaic Canyon	
	Dist.(mi)	Elev.(ft)
Parking area/mouth	0.0	950
1st narrows (start)	0.1	~1,000
1st narrows (end)	0.5	1,180
Side canyon #2/rim trail	0.9	1,340
2nd narrows (start)	1.1	1,480
2nd narrows (end at 18-ft fall)	1.4	1,680
Side canyon #3	1.6	1,790
3rd narrows (25-ft fall)	1.7	1,920
3rd narrows (end)/rim trail	2.1	2,080
Fork (side canyon #4)	2.2	2,150
Grotto	2.5	2,440
Side canyon #5	2.9	3,020
Twin Springs	(0.9)	4,160
Head	4.7	5,370

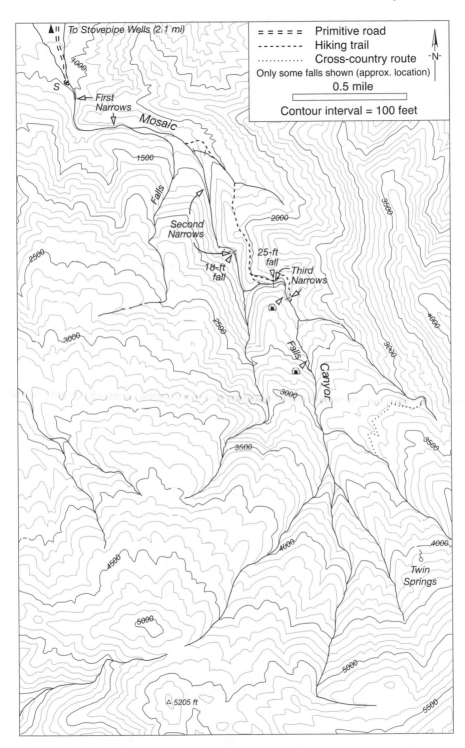

To Stovepipe Wells (2.1 mi)

= = = = = Primitive road
- - - - - - - Hiking trail
. . . . Cross-country route

-N-

Only some falls shown (approx. location)

0.5 mile

Contour interval = 100 feet

S

First
Narrows

Mosaic

4000

1500

Falls

Second
Narrows

2500

18-ft
fall

25+ft
fall

Third
Narrows

2000

3500

3000

2500

Falls

4000

3500

Canyon

3000

3500

3500

4500

4000

4000

Twin
Springs

5000

5000

5000

5500

△ 5205 ft

This trail climbs a very steep, loose talus to the rim trail (~0.15 mi). Turning left on this trail will take you back to the marble island (1 mile). Turning right will take you to the head of the third narrows (0.25 mile). Along the way, you will walk along the rim of the narrows, glimpsing 80 feet down at a virgin wash framed by sheer walls. Hikers with climbing experience can try to get down to the bottom. An easy route is near the low point in the trail, where a promontory on the right overlooks the narrows. The ravine on the north side of this overlook can be down-climbed without too much effort. The narrow slit a short distance up the narrows has a slick chimney that can be friction-climbed to an impressively deep grotto. Climbing down canyon instead will take you past a few easy falls to the brim of the 25-foot fall.

The upper canyon and Twin Springs. Shortly past the third narrows, the canyon forks. The right fork is the main canyon, the left fork the fourth major side canyon. One of the greatest challenges here is little-known Twin Springs, high on the ridge separating these two forks.

The main canyon route is the most difficult. From the fork it leads shortly through some good narrows, terminated by a beautiful grotto with a 40-foot high ceiling. Beyond it, the wash steepens markedly. Progress becomes increasingly difficult, slowed down by other falls requiring bypasses. Where the wash opens up again, about 0.4 mile past the grotto, look for a shallow side canyon on the east side (side canyon #5). In 0.5 mile it peters out in front of a very steep slope. The springs are almost directly to the south, and almost overhead. The final 600-foot ascent is extremely steep. Bring the 7.5' map for guidance.

The other route starts at the left fork. This fork, fairly narrow, winds between colorful bluffs. It is consistently steep but has only one high (11 feet) but passable fall. The sharp ridge on the west side in the middle of the last major bend (elev. 3,090') is the easiest place to strike a cross-country route to the springs. After about 0.4 mile of talus scrambling and ravine crossing, you will reach the fifth side canyon. The rest is the same as the first route.

Both routes involve a strenuous 1.5 to 2-mile, 2,000-foot climb from the fork, most of it scrambling on steep, unstable slopes, and potentially dangerous. If you are in shape, this is a good target for a day hike. If you decide to backpack instead, remember that camping is prohibited along the first 2 miles of Mosaic Canyon, which is past the third narrows. The reward is a green oasis graced with desert columbines, and grand views of the deep swath of Mosaic Canyon and northern Death Valley. Rarely visited, this is a precious haven for the bighorn sheep. If you are lucky, you may encounter one.

■

GROTTO CANYON

> *When the Rock Climbing Goddess created Grotto Canyon, she was obviously working overtime. Together with its three main forks, it forms a wild system of labyrinthine canyons graced with beautifully carved grottoes and many tight narrows. All forks have many closely spaced polished falls, from 5-foot chutes to high drop-offs. Scaling them requires anything from a scramble to hard technical climbs. If you have an inclination for rock climbing, you will want to return over and over to this seemingly endless maze.*

General Information

Road status: Essentially roadless; access by primitive road
Shortest hike: A short stroll/very easy
Longest hike: 3.4 mi, 2,100 ft one way (or more)/difficult, with rock
    climbing
Main attractions: Several narrows, grottos, falls, great rock climbing
USGS topo maps: Stovepipe Wells (15'), Grotto Canyon (7.5')
Maps: pp. 409*, 413, 393

Location and Access

Grotto Canyon is the next main canyon east of Mosaic Canyon, on the north slope of Tucki Mountain. From Stovepipe Wells drive Highway 190 east for 2.4 miles to the marked road to Grotto Canyon on your right (drive slowly; it's easy to miss). This road goes about 0.9 mile to the wash of Grotto Canyon, drops steeply into it, and continues up the wash for 1.1 miles to end just before the first grotto. The first mile is easily passable with a standard-clearance vehicle. In the wash the road has deep gravel, and if you don't have a high-clearance vehicle you'll need to walk. It's a pleasant hike anyway, along abrupt conglomerate walls fluted by erosion.

Route Description

Much of the pleasure of discovering this special place is that few people know exactly what is there. As you enter the first grotto there is tremendous excitement in knowing that you are crossing the threshold into largely unknown territory. I have tried to preserve this invaluable characteristic by purposely omitting many natural features. Distances are difficult to assess; consequently, the chart is approximate. However, distances don't mean as much in this canyon as elsewhere, as climbing slows down progress to a mere mile per hour. But there is no need to rush through this wonderland of rocks.

The first grotto. Grotto Canyon was first named in the 1890s by officials of the Pacific Coast Borax Company, who were probably the first immigrants to see this place. It's a well-suited name, as it does have several grottoes, scattered along the main and side canyons. One of the many delights of this hike is to look for these awesome caves carved in the rock. On a hot summer day they offer cool shade in which to rest. The first grotto, located just beyond the end of the road, is accessible to all. Hollowed walls converge overhead to form a cave so deep that it is rarely penetrated by sun rays. Here and all along the canyon, look for slickensides (see *Red Wall Canyon*). There are some good exposures on the east side along the last 100 yards before the first grotto.

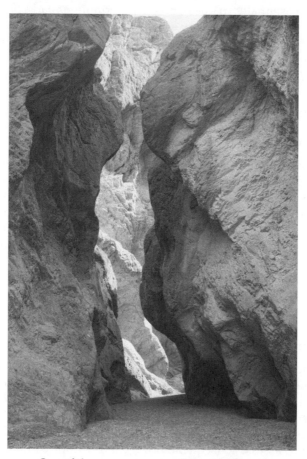

One of the many narrows of Grotto Canyon

Just inside the grotto, dwarfed by the soaring walls, there is a steep, 12-foot fall blocking the way. Just beyond it is another fall, about 8 feet high and overhanging. The lower fall is a slab climb (at most a 5.6), and the upper one a 5.6-5.7 climb. Hikers with little climbing experience encounter various difficulties here. These two falls are certainly the most difficult of the first few falls, so if you can overcome them, it's likely to be a home run—for a while. Even if you decide to turn around here, the first grotto, the erosional features along the wash, and the great views of the sand dunes still make this short hike well worth it.

The main canyon. The main canyon is the westernmost branch, the fork you will naturally take if you follow the widest and lowest wash. For 2.4 miles past the first grotto, it is a wonderful succession of winding narrows filled with smoothly polished falls and giant chockstones. I counted eight narrows, although the exact figure is a matter of definition, as they often run into each other. Some of them are so tight and abrupt that they appear to be mere cracks, and it often comes as a surprise that they actually go through. These narrows are thrilling places, mysterious and intimate like the slit canyons of the Colorado Plateau. Their contorted paths give little advance warning about the falls they contain. Yet there are many along the way—about 27 higher than 5 feet. Three of them are too high to be climbed and must be bypassed. The ultimate fall, at the end of the canyon, is a towering drop-off at the head of a vast, wall-framed amphitheater, much too high for free climbing for almost anyone.

The succession of falls and narrows produces an ever-changing scenery, and yet it is repetitious enough to challenge your memory and sense of orientation. After wandering for a few hours, you may not remember exactly what you saw earlier, and discover on your way back territory you could swear you never crossed before. Progress is slow, and you may find your sense of time strangely altered. These odd distortions of time and space are one of the attributes of mazes, and a most striking feature in Grotto Canyon.

The grottoes, narrows, and falls were created by stream erosion in the very hard and thick Bonanza King dolomite. The rock varies in color from light to dark gray, and under the right light it brightens to a silvery sheen. Along the floor and walls of the narrows, bowls, scoops, and chimneys have been hollowed out in this resistant rock.

If you come here in late winter or early spring, you will find bright pockets of wild flowers blooming along the more exposed walls. Mexican bladdersage (*Salazaria mexicana*), an interesting shrub with pale spherical calyces like Japanese lanterns, thrives in the wash. Stay alert for tarantulas, chuckwallas, and scorpions, which I spotted in this canyon, and sidewinders, which I was told like to hang around here.

The side canyons. Grotto Canyon has three major side canyons, all on the east side. Scenic and challenging in different ways, they are as worthy of a visit as the main canyon.

My favorite is the third one, which starts as an inconspicuous slit in the eastern wall. It is not much more than a mile long, but it has one of the most amazing narrows in the park. It starts immediately as a very narrow polished corridor snaking around a couple of extremely tight 180° bends. The walls are so close that you can touch them simultaneously without fully stretching your arms. There is a pretty grotto at the end of this corridor, backed by a high fall (about 5.10a) and three similar falls above it you'll need to bypass. The rest of the way is essentially one long narrows punctuated with beautiful carved falls. At mid-canyon, erosion has cut through a bed of dolomite tilted at 60°, forming an unusual slanted corridor with small polished basins. Then there is a 90-foot fall, twisting high into a cliff of finely banded dolomite, the gateway to perhaps more wonders.

About rock climbing in Grotto Canyon. This system of canyons has more climbable falls than any other I have visited in the park. If you have little rock climbing experience, refer to *Rock Climbing* in *Desert Hiking Tips* before coming here. Bring a friend, and a short rope or webbing to help each other up or down tricky falls. If you are an adept climber, this small climbing heaven may well become your favorite. Bring your climbing shoes, and for a change you will use this activity as a means to an end as well as a pleasure in itself. Most of the falls are short, between about 5 and 12 feet, with difficulty ranging up to 5.8. There are also several higher falls, in the range of 30 to 100 feet, upward from 5.9 in difficulty, which need to be bypassed.

If you come here to climb, you may have to get rid of rock piles some hikers insist on leaving at the base of some falls as a climbing aid, especially in the lower canyon. It's fine to set up such aids, but it is

Grotto Canyon		
	Dist.(mi)	Elev.(ft)
Mouth (edge of wash)	0.0	415
Road's end	1.1	780
First grotto	1.15	800
1st side canyon	1.35	900
2nd side canyon	2.3	1,440
3rd side canyon	2.6	1,695
Amphitheater	3.4	2,520

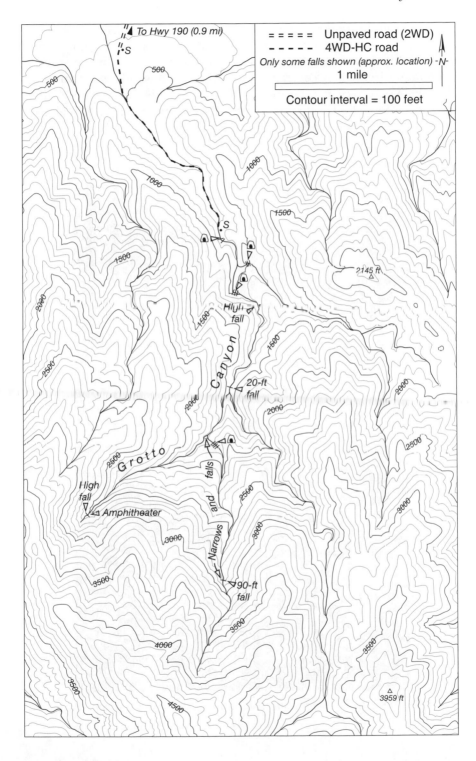

To Hwy 190 (0.9 mi)

= = = = = Unpaved road (2WD)
- - - - - 4WD-HC road

Only some falls shown (approx. location) -N-

1 mile

Contour interval = 100 feet

inconsiderate to others to leave them behind. Please destroy them on your way back. This is one of the few good canyons for climbing in the park, and it should be left so for climbers to enjoy. Also make sure to obliterate cairns when you return. It will give other hikers a chance to find their own passage. Besides, if they came this far, they probably don't need to be told which way to go. These simple measures will also preserve the wildness of this exceptional canyon.

■

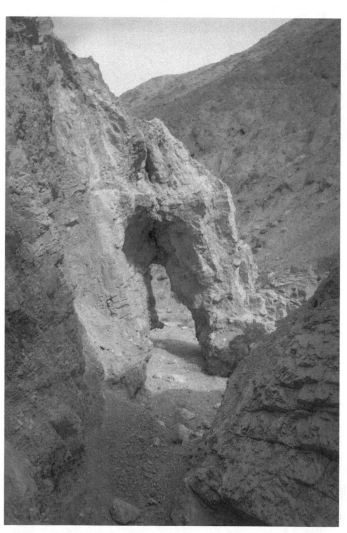

This narrow bridge spans the wash of Little Bridge Canyon.

LITTLE BRIDGE CANYON

> *This out-of-the-way canyon packs in many features over a short distance and is perfect for a short day hike. Its namesake is a graceful rainbow of stone arching down over the canyon wash. The geology is good, the fossils are hard to find but beautiful, and the narrow slots in its half dozen side canyons are challenging places to explore.*

General Information

Road status: Roadless; hiking from paved road
Shortest hike: 3.3 mi, 1,860 ft one way / moderate
Longest hike: 4.5 mi, 3,000 ft one way / moderate
Main attractions: Natural bridge, slot canyons with falls, geology, fossils
USGS topo maps: Stovepipe Wells (15'), Grotto Canyon (7.5')
Maps: pp. 413*, 393

Location and Access

Little Bridge Canyon is on the eastern slope of Tucki Mountain, just east of Grotto Canyon. Start on Highway 190 near the east end of the sharp bend about 3.1 miles east of Stovepipe Wells (or about 4.1 miles from the Scotty's Castle Road).

Geology: Ordovician Marine Fossils

Both the Pogonip Group and Ely Springs Dolomite exposed in the lower part of Little Bridge Canyon contain fossils of Ordovician sea animals, including corals, gastropods, and brachiopods. The latter were marine animals that lived in a shell, some of which resemble today's bivalves. Their shell has a vertical plane of symmetry, like a scallop's. They are one of creation's most enduring phyla. Brachiopods first became important in Paleozoic seas, thrived through the Permian, and although several orders were wiped out during the Permian extinction, they are still represented today by over 200 species.

The Ely Springs Dolomite contains strophomenids, an order of hinged brachiopods. Their shell has a wide hinge line, and because of their shape and flattened appearance they are sometimes called petrified butterflies. The upper member of the Pogonip Group is also known to contain large fossil gastropods. You may want to try your luck at finding some of these pretty fossils, although they are a little difficult to locate (start looking on the fan). Remember that this is a national park: you are welcome to look all you want, but not to disturb or collect anything.

Route Description

To get there. From the highway it's a little over 2 miles to the canyon mouth. The most interesting route is up a little ravine right along the eastern base of Tucki Mountain. This ravine starts just past the transmission line south of the highway. It sinks progressively deeper below the surface of the fan to eventually form a miniature canyon with steep fanglomerate walls. In 0.6 mile the ravine climbs back up to the top of the fan and you will need to drop into a second, larger wash. Follow it up for 400 feet, then bear left at the fork. The upper half of this fork is a shallow cleft littered with boulders and occluded at one point by a nice fall in fanglomerate. It eventually leads back up to the fan on a 25-foot high bank overlooking the mouth of Little Bridge Canyon. Look back at the views of the Funeral Mountains and the stark Death Valley Buttes.

Pay close attention on this hike. Some hikers wander off into the mountain too soon. If you do, retrace your steps, climb east out of the wash as soon as you can, and follow the fan route described below.

The fan route is less exciting but more straightforward. Follow a course parallel to the ravine and a few hundred yards east of it. This route crosses a few ravines, especially near the top of the fan. The inch-size, reddish, prickly plant growing profusely on the fan gravel is spiny chorinzanthe. It is quite common in the Mojave Desert but is often over-looked—until you inadvertently touch one! In the spring you might find shredding evening primrose and Death Valley mohavea in bloom. For a change of scenery, walk the ravine on the way up, and walk the fan on the way back for panoramic views of the dunes.

The lower canyon. Little Bridge Canyon begins as a moderately narrow passage. The rust-streaked walls are made of Ely Springs Dolomite, formed between approximately 460 and 438 million years ago. In 0.3 mile, just after the canyon veers left and straightens out, this formation stops abruptly on the west side at a conspicuous vertical strata of

Little Bridge Canyon		
	Dist.(mi)	Elev.(ft)
Highway 190	0.0	-30
Mouth	2.1	1,160
Quartzite strata	2.45	1,370
Window	2.7	1,500
Little Bridge	3.3	1,830
Fork	4.0	2,180
Head (amphitheater)	4.5	~3,000

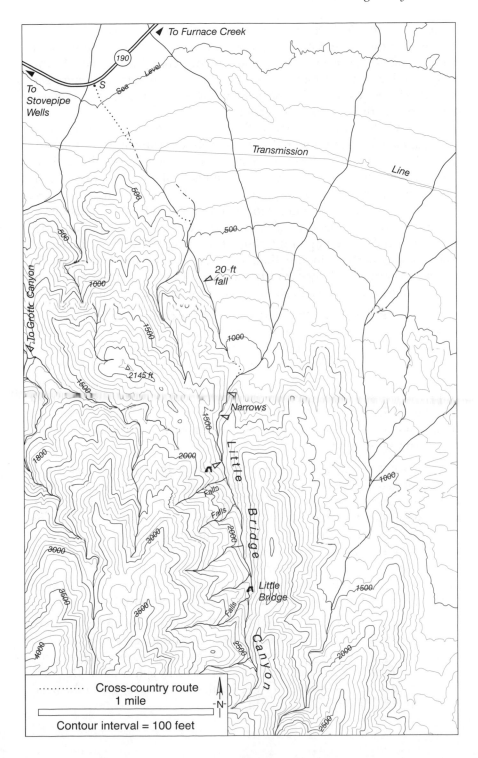

To Furnace Creek

190

To Stovepipe Wells

S

Sea Level

Transmission

Line

500

20-ft fall

500

1000

To Grotto Canyon

1000

1500

1000

2145 ft

Narrows

1500

1800

2000

Little

2000

Falls

Falls

Bridge

1000

3000

3000

2000

Little Bridge

1500

3500

3500

Falls

4000

2500

Canyon

2000

2500

Cross-country route

1 mile

N

Contour interval = 100 feet

white quartzite. This formation is called Eureka Quartzite. It occurs throughout the Panamint Range, and because it is so much lighter than most formations it constitutes a convenient geological marker. In this canyon, it has been strongly tilted by folding, to the point of being nearly vertical, and deformed by shearing, which crushed the rock and made the formation thinner than elsewhere.

Past the Eureka Quartzite, the wash runs parallel to the geologic formations, which are oriented approximately north-south on this side of Tucki Mountain. Different formations are exposed on either side of the wash. For about 1.2 miles the east wall is straight, sheer, quite colorful and wonderfully carved at places. It is made of Ely Springs Dolomite. It is then replaced by a younger formation, the Hidden Valley Dolomite (Silurian and Lower Devonian). The west wall is composed of an older formation called the Pogonip Group (Lower and Middle Ordovician). The Eureka Quartzite, intermediate in age, is sandwiched between these formations and should occur right along the canyon, but the wash was eroded along this weakened strata and only scattered exposures remain.

Little Bridge. In the west wall not far past the quartzite strata there is a narrow vertical window tucked in a purplish, tightly folded anticline. It is a little arch, but one of this canyon's secrets is that it does not have one, but two such formations. The canyon's namesake is about 0.6 mile further, in the middle of a short jog in the canyon. It is an impressive and graceful bridge eroded through a small fin of Eureka Quartzite. The upper end of this 20-foot thick span of rock is spawned by the canyon wall, while its lower end rests on the canyon floor, so that the wash passes underneath it.

Slot canyons. Another attraction here is the side canyons. There are about half a dozen of them, all draining the steep western wall, most of them mere slots blocked by high falls. None of them extends very far, but collectively they make up in number what they lack in length. The falls are smoothly polished, looming walls of naked stone trapped in claustrophobic spaces. When the light is right they glow with warm shades of orange and red. The falls are all difficult to ascend, but they are made of relatively strong dolomite. Climbers will be able to scale a few of them, and in some places a few other falls beyond them.

The upper canyon. Beyond Little Bridge the canyon has more to offer, including a dazzling white gateway in Eureka Quartzite, shallow narrows and more slot canyons. About 0.7 mile past the bridge is the first major fork. The east fork quickly steepens and peters out in 0.5 mile. The west fork climbs through a steep boulder-strewn ravine to the head of the canyon at a walled-in amphitheater.

■

TRAIL CANYON

The steep road through rugged Trail Canyon offers a scenic ride deep into the Panamint Mountains. One of the attractions here is the 250-million-year geological record displayed along its walls, which gives a chance to browse for interesting fossils of ancient sea animals. The roadless upper canyon and its south fork contain several mines and colorful camps, springs, narrows and eventually panoramic views from the thickly-forested slopes of Wildrose Peak. If you are walking, the spectacular 2,500-foot descent along the old trail in the north fork offers a peaceful alternative route to the heart of the canyon.

General Information

Road status: Primitive road in main canyon (HC); upper canyon roadless
Shortest hike: Short strolls/easy to moderate
Longest hike: 12.8 mi, 6,220 ft one way (or more)/difficult
Main attractions: Mining camp, scenic canyon, geology, wild flowers
USGS 15' topo maps: Furnace Creek, Emigrant Canyon*
USGS 7.5' topo maps: Devil's Speedway, Wildrose Peak*
Maps: pp. 421*, 427, 393

Location and Access

Trail Canyon is located on the east side of the northern Panamint Mountains. The Trail Canyon Road starts off of the West Side Road, 5.3 miles south of the Badwater Road (it is marked). The first 4.4 miles, up to just inside the canyon mouth where the road drops into the wash, are passable with a passenger car. In the canyon the road requires high clearance. About 5.3 miles above the canyon mouth the road branches out at the confluence, where the north and south forks meet the main canyon. The main canyon and the two forks have a short spur road in their lower end.

If you can't drive into Trail Canyon, the shortest way to hike into it is down the north fork. This fork used to have a road, which connected the Trail Canyon Road to the Aguereberry Point Road and Emigrant Canyon. This road was seriously washed out in the mid-1970s (doubtlessly an act of God) and now it is practicable for less than a mile up from the confluence. To get to the head of this fork, drive the Emigrant Canyon Road 11.8 miles south of the Emigrant Ranger Station (or 9.3 miles north of the Wildrose Canyon Road) to the Aguereberry Point Road. Follow this good graded road across Harrisburg Flat. (After

415

1.4 miles, stop at the Aguereberry Camp where Pete Aguereberry lived while mining the Eureka Mine, on the south side of the hill, until his death in 1945.) About 3.6 miles further, you will get to a spur on the right marked by a post. This is the upper end of the old Trail Canyon Road. Drive it a very short distance to a locked gate and hike from here.

History: Mining in Trail Canyon

In its day, this canyon witnessed a fair amount of mining, betrayed today by numerous sites. First it was gold, which involved three companies—the Death Valley Wonder Mining and Milling Company, the Wild Rose Mining Company, and the Trail Canyon Mining Company—all as small as they were short-lived. Created between March and November 1906, they all quickly developed a few tunnels on their property. Although good gold assays were reported, as well as silver in some cases, these efforts were probably stimulated more by the nearby gold rush at Skidoo than by the actual value of the claims. Little is known about production, but chances are it did not amount to much. By the spring of 1907 all three companies had folded. The owners of the Wild Rose Mining Company may have been the luckiest: they reportedly sold to a Boston syndicate for about $300,000, probably just before the market crash of March 1907.

Trail Canyon came alive again thirty-some years later, this time for antimony. From 1939 to 1941, around $50,000 were invested in mining developments and in the construction of a road and camp in the south fork for the Old Dependable Antimony Mine. It produced about 70 tons of high-grade ore before the operations were suspended during the war. In 1948 the claims were relocated as the Old Dependable Group, and the following year a new party repaired the road to mine a small open cut. But the remoteness and small size of the deposit made exploitation unprofitable. The open cut only produced an 11-ton high-grade pod before the Old Dependable closed down for good.

Gold mining did not work so well, and antimony was not such a winner either, but it didn't stop miners from looking one last time—for tungsten. Tungsten deposits are rare in Death Valley, and since Trail Canyon inherited several of them, it attracted a lot of attention. Tungsten was mined in the main canyon at the Sheepshead and Victory group of mines, near the mouth of the north fork at the Tarantula Mine, and in the south fork at the Morning Glory Mine. There were others: Jack Smith and John Polson's Ronald "A" claims; the AA Placer, which covered almost 22,000 acres; the Blackwater Mine and its several hundred claims; promotional claims such as the All Mine and the Lucky Find claims in the south fork, which saw little actual mining; and a few downright fake claims. At the peak of the excitement, miners even tried to have the National Monument abolished to make their life easier! But other than peace and quiet, there was nothing much here to harvest. Most of the active claims were worked for short time, and none of them turned up appreciable quantities of ore. The Sheepshead and Victory Mine had shipped only one ton of high-grade ore by 1943. It was reported idle in 1951, and in all likelihood was abandoned much earlier. The Morning Glory Mine, far up the slope of Wildrose Peak, was so hard to reach that steep switchbacks had to be constructed to get to it. A long tramway was strung across the canyon rims to transport the ore down to the road in the south fork. The Morning Glory camp was relocated at a later time as the Lucky Find Millsites #1 and #2. In spite of all this concerted effort, most of what this mine produced was ornamental rock. The Tarantula Mine, operated in 1958, was probably the only profitable tungsten mine in Death Valley in the 1950s. The Aguereberry Point Road was built at that time to access it. In later years the Tarantula was relocated as the Broken Pick Mine. Tungsten mining was still ongoing in the south fork as late as 1971, but it is doubtful that the financial return was ever substantial.

Geology: A 250-million-Year Record

One of the main attractions of Trail Canyon is the long geological record exposed on its walls. For over 5 miles above its mouth the stratigraphic sequence contains all nine formations from the Ely Springs Dolomite (late Ordovician) to the Stirling Quartzite (late Proterozoic), a time span of around 250 million years. The formations run roughly parallel to each other and perpendicular to the canyon, so that the road conveniently crosses all of them. As a result of the Panamint Mountains' uplift, the formations dip towards Death Valley and get older up canyon. They represent a sizeable fraction of the park's geological history and occur in most of its ranges. If you intend to do some serious exploring in this region, this is a good place to learn to identify them.

The first formation, exposed on both sides starting shortly after the road drops in the wash, is the Ely Springs Dolomite. The interbedded limestone and dolomite exposed for a couple of miles roughly in the middle of the canyon—and where the road comes closest to the north wall—belong to the Bonanza King Formation. The last one, the Stirling Quartzite, ends at the confluence. Refer to the stratigraphic column in *A Few Basic Facts* as a guide to identify the other formations.

Route Description

The lower canyon. From its mouth up to the confluence Trail Canyon is wide and fairly straight. Native Americans took advantage of this unobstructed passage much before we did: in the spring they used it to migrate from the hot valley to the cooler mountains. If you are driving you'll find the place relatively scenic. If you are hiking, although the road makes the walking easier than when it was an Indian trail, it is a long and uneventful hike to the confluence. Even the wash material is average. One saving grace is the dense cover of brittlebush in the lower canyon, which turns to a bright yellow sea in the spring. If your goal is a day hike into the upper canyon, definitely try to come down the more scenic north fork.

If you are interested in geology, you will probably look at all this differently. One of the things to do here is to look for fossils. If you have never indulged in this activity before, you may find that it is, if nothing else, an incentive to inspect places you would not even have noticed otherwise. Several of the steep ravines and side canyons draining into Trail Canyon provide access to fossiliferous beds. Animal fossils are found only up to the two main side canyons facing each other (where the Wood Canyon Formation, the oldest formation bearing animal fossils, is exposed). The Pogonip Group contains abundant large gastropods. This formation is well exposed in the side canyon on the north side, about 0.6 mile up from where the road drops into the wash. Look near its mouth on the east side. The Nopah Formation contains trilobites and echinoderms in breccia, and linguloid brachiopods in shale. Try the next side canyon on the north side, before the constriction in the main canyon. The Bonanza King Formation contains two light brown sandy shale layers less than 50 feet thick and about 200 feet apart. The upper layer contains linguloid brachiopods and well-preserved trilobites. Although some of these fossiliferous beds are relatively easy to find, most of them require a lot of walking and scrambling, which may not be all that much fun past the month of April.

Hiking access via the north fork.   From the Aguereberry Point Road, the old Trail Canyon Road drops steeply into the canyon. Although washed out at several places, its switchbacks are convenient to negotiate the precipitous slope. The views are spectacular, encompassing forest-clad Wildrose Peak, the deep V of Trail Canyon, a wedge of salt pan and the distant Black Mountains. The road is so steep that the wash of Trail Canyon, several thousand feet below and less than 2 air miles away, is visible most of the way down. After 1.1 miles the road ends abruptly at the wash of a side canyon of the north fork, which leads down to the confluence.

Because of the large elevation change in this fork, plants are unusually varied. In late May I counted over 35 perennials and annuals in bloom (and probably missed many more). The slopes were dotted with masses of lupine, Indian paintbrush, purple sage, and lavender

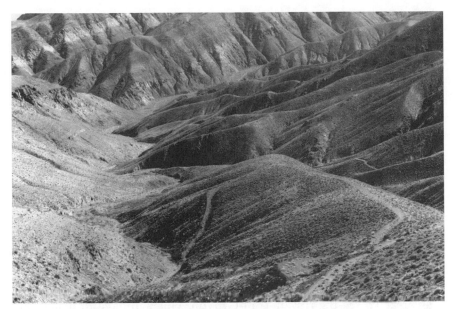

Looking down at Trail Canyon from the switchbacks in the north fork

Death Valley penstemon. Bright yellow desertgold and carpets of purplish red bigelow mimulus thrived in the rocky wash. The stingbush,
recognizable by its uncanny habit of sticking tenaciously to whatever
brushes it (socks, shoes, pants, and human skin alike) exhibited its
showy greenish yellow flowers everywhere (if you get snagged, try
using a comb to remove stingbush leaves). There were also spotted langloisia, desert prickle poppy, and the magnificent magenta flowers of
beavertail cactus. If you are into desert flowers, this will definitely be a
highlight.

The rocks along this fork are dominated by shales, with some
quartzite, sandstone, and dolomite, all from the Proterozoic Johnnie
Formation. Look for the impressive landslide of large quartzite cobbles
at the mouth of the first side canyon on the right. A little further there is
a colorful outcrop of shale in a bend in the west wall—greenish grading
into purple, folded and shattered. There is a short constriction in the
wash 1.5 miles below the road, where polished bedrock of orange shale
is exposed between low vertical walls. Below it the old road resumes as
a trace and continues for the last 0.9 mile to the confluence. Before getting there, check out the Broken Pick Mine, in the last side canyon on the
west side, about 300 yards before the confluence. The remains are minimal, but there is a nice little spring nearby. There is also a small spring
with a trickle of water in the main canyon just below the confluence, a
short distance up the first ravine downhill from the small adit.

The Broken Pick Millsite.   About 0.3 mile above the confluence, a short access road on the left leads to the Broken Pick Millsite, a picturesque camp cradled in a small bowl ringed by low hills. The history of this camp spans many years, having been active first in connection with the Nichols Mine and Millsite, later relocated as the Broken Pick Mine and the Small Hill Millsite. Being one of the most recent camps in the park, it is also one of the most extensive. It has quite a few standing structures, obviously from very different eras. The old wooden shack and outhouse may date back from as early as the 1930s, while the bunkhouse and 40-foot trailer—still partly furnished, with bathrooms and even showers—are from the 1950s or 1960s. Water for these lavish facilities was trucked in from the valley. Add a few collapsed adits and tailings, a couple of beat-up trucks, a water tank, and a colorful junkyard, and you'll get a fair picture of the place.

Smith and Polson Camp and the Ronald "A" Mines.   The canyon road ends at the Broken Pick Millsite. It was washed out several times since Trail Canyon's last mining hurrahs, and it is now part of a wilderness area. To see the rest of Trail Canyon, you will have to walk. The wash is wide and fairly steep, but it's only 1.5 miles to the next mining area.

Trail Canyon		
	Dist.(mi)	Elev.(ft)
Trail Canyon Road		
West Side Road	0.0	-253
Grade down to wash	4.4	1,260
1st set of side canyons	7.8	2,660
2nd set of side canyons	8.5	2,960
Confluence with north fork	9.3	3,420
Lower end of old road (hike)	(2.4)	5,090
Gate off Aguereberry Point Rd	(3.5)	5,970
Broken Pick Millsite/End of rd	9.7	~3,600
Roadless canyon		
Broken Pick Millsite/End of rd	0.0	~3,600
Ronald "A" No. 1 Mine	1.5	4,380
Ronald "A" No. 4 Mine	(0.25)	~4,520
Smith and Polson Camp	1.6	4,480
Side Canyon	2.6	5,240
Spring	(0.25)	~5,560
Dripping Spring	2.7	5,340

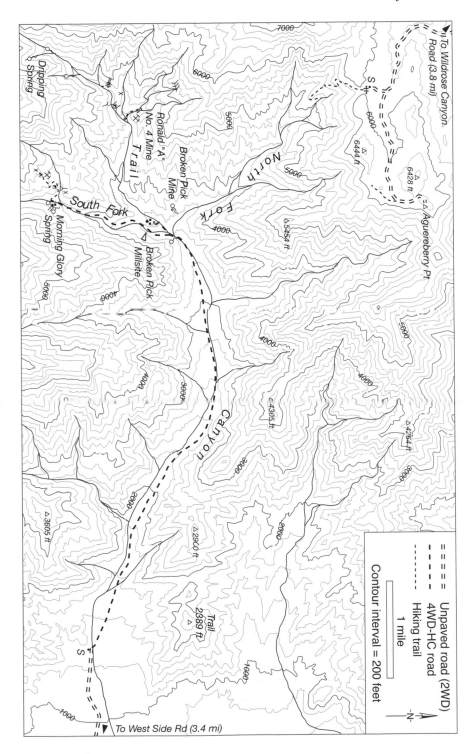

To Wildrose Canyon Road (3.8 mi)

7000

Dripping Spring

6000

5000

Ronald "A" No. 4 Mine

Broken Pick Mine

Trail

6444 ft

6428 ft

North

Fork

5454 ft

South Fork

4000

Broken Pick Millsite

Aguereberry Pt

Morning Glory Spring

5000

4000

5000

4000

4000

4305 ft

4264 ft

3605 ft

3000

Canyon

2000

2000

3000

2900 ft

2589 ft

Trail

4000

1000

S

To West Side Rd (3.4 mi)

Unpaved road (2WD)

4WD-HC road

Hiking trail

1 mile

Contour interval = 200 feet

-N-

There are many mines here, both along the main canyon and in the two side canyons on the west side. Somewhere in there are the Sheepshead and Victory Mine, the Blackwater Mine, and others, although unfortunately after three generations of mining it is hard to tell which is which. The main site at the junction with the two side canyons is the Ronald "A" No. 1 Mine, which was worked by Jack Smith and John Polson. The large tailing high above the mouth of the first side canyon is the Ronald "A" No. 4 Mine. An old road in this side canyon leads up to its open cut, which worked a large, nearly vertical vein of tungsten-bearing milky quartz. Smith and Polson camp was on the leveled area by the lone cottonwood just up canyon.

There is much to see here. The camp has one of the best stocked junkyards around, the blue-green ore discarded on some of the tailings is almost as pretty as at the Morning Glory Mine, and there are many tailings to check out. But be careful. A few of the tunnels have deep hidden pits near their entrance, and most of them are very crumbly.

Dripping Spring. This rarely visited spring is a little over a mile further up this fork. Towards the end of this stretch the canyon finally tightens a little. There are actually three small springs in this area. The first two springs are about 0.2 mile into the next two side canyons on the east side. The third one—the largest—is a little further in the main canyon. From this point on the canyon steepens and narrows considerably, and this is as far as most people explore.

Hiking and Driving Suggestions

If you have the right vehicle, Trail Canyon is easy to access and a fun place to go canyon exploring on wheels. In a day, you can drive to the confluence and hike to Dripping Spring (about two hours round trip), or explore one of the other forks. You can also camp at the confluence and use it as a hub to launch day hikes into the forks (see *South Fork of Trail Canyon*).

If you can't drive further than the mouth, try hiking up to the Broken Pick Millsite, just past the confluence. The round trip takes a short day. Because it is a long walk to the confluence, it pays to make it a whole-day trip and to include one of the forks. If you hike in via the more scenic north fork, it is a long day to go through the main canyon, or to Dripping Spring, and return. Except for long weekends and holidays, motorized traffic is minimal in the main canyon and hikers should have it all to themselves. If the West Side Road continues to be closed in the summer, it is the quietest time of all.

■

SOUTH FORK OF TRAIL CANYON

The south fork is the most scenic part of Trail Canyon. In the lower canyon the colorful Morning Glory camp, its small spring, and the Old Dependable Antimony Mine are all a short distance from the main canyon road. The best part is the old Morning Glory Mine, on a high, forested ridge at the far end of the south fork's rugged narrows. With its unlikely tramway, spectacular mining road and beautiful ore, it is one of Death Valley's hidden gems.

General Information

Road status: Rough road in lower fork (4WD-HC); roadless beyond
Shortest hike: 1.5 mi, 860 ft one way / moderate
Longest hike: 4.4 mi, 2,880 ft (or more) / strenuous
USGS 15' topo maps: Furnace Creek, Emigrant Canyon*
USGS 7.5' topo maps: Devil's Speedway, Wildrose Peak*
Maps: pp. 427*, 421, 393

Location and Access

From the confluence in Trail Canyon, the south fork climbs southward towards Wildrose Peak. Refer to *Trail Canyon* for driving and hiking directions to the confluence. There is a road along the first 1.5 miles of the south fork. It is in poor shape, gets worse farther up canyon, and requires high clearance.

Route Description

Morning Glory Camp and Spring. There is nothing exceptional in the lower part of this fork—high-rising slopes, and a wide, coarse, and steep wash. The going is slow, although the road helps a little. The Morning Glory mining camp, about 1.5 miles in, makes it all worth it. Built on a long bench above the wash, it is one of the few relatively well-preserved camps in Death Valley. Used in the days of the Morning Glory Mine and the Lucky Find claims (see *History* in *Trail Canyon*), it still has several standing structures. One of them is a small cabin, still furnished with a bed, cupboards, and shelves. It even has a separate bathroom with a sink and toilet. There is also a long, wooden, garish green house with a stone fireplace and an eclectic mess of furniture, a headframe, and an open shed with work benches. The carcass of a 1950s-vintage Dodge is resting on a heap of rusted cans, its chrome grid still grinning in the sunlight. At least one good-sized flash flood ripped

423

through this fork since the 1950s. It severed the frame of a small truck, now largely buried under gravel in the middle of the wash.

Morning Glory Spring, marked by a few honey mesquites, is at the upper end of the camp. Water pools up under a small cluster of cane, then flows down a short manmade trough before dropping and vanishing into the wash. The system of tanks and pipes below was used to collect and distribute the spring water to the camp.

Across the wash from the camp a steep road, badly washed out at the start, bypasses the side canyon and leads to a small mine. The mine adit is buried in rubble and little else is left, but it has good views of the abrupt forested slopes of Wildrose Peak and the stratified northern wall of Trail Canyon. It makes a pleasant base camp, within walking distance of water.

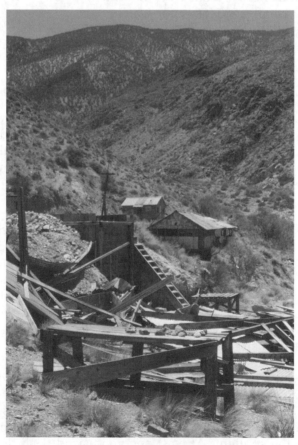

Morning Glory Camp

The Old Dependable Antimony Mine. For another mile past the camp the wash remains wide (and roadless). Things start to pick up at the next side canyon, which marks timberline, with scattered junipers and pinyon pines thickening up ahead. Just beyond there is a small cave at the foot of the west wall, with a ceiling blackened by campfires—an Indian site, a miner's shelter? The next (third) side canyon, on the west side, starts with a series of falls in a fairly deep and narrow stretch, and may warrant further exploration. The Old Dependable Antimony Mine (see *History* in *Trail Canyon*) is a little further on the east side, about 60 feet above the wash. A short road circles up around the tailing to the open cut and the two adits mined in the past. The wooden chute and ore bin are still in place above the tailing, along with more modern mining equipment. The ore occurred in thin lenses and pods of stibnite (antimony sulfide) in gray limestone. Look for the weathered outcrop of limestone at wash level just south of the tailing, in which erosion has etched rows of upside-down spires and a small window.

The narrows and the tramway. About 0.3 mile past the Old Dependable, look for an old gate on the right. It guards the rough grade to the Morning Glory Mine, about 1,400 feet above. The loop hike to this remote mine is definitely the most scenic area of the south fork. The best approach is to hike up to it along the canyon to see the narrows, and to return down this spectacular road.

Past the gate, the canyon soon becomes choked with boulders, then forks. The right fork is the main canyon. The aerial tramway of the Morning Glory Mine is first visible here, hanging about 100 feet overhead, an old bucket still attached to it. The stretch of canyon from here to the mine is mostly steep and narrow. Bedrock has been scooped into a series of unusual orange polished chutes, falls, basins and whirlpools. Passages barely 5 feet wide alternate with slightly wider areas invaded by trees and brush, and the feeling of confinement is constant. Most of the falls are easy to negotiate. Climbing out of the shallow canyon to bypass the most difficult ones will bring you close to the tramway, its rudimentary towers and old ore buckets. Few of the original towers are still standing. The cable lies on the ground most of the way, spanning the canyon at a few places. The forest thickens up canyon; a rare opportunity to rest under fragrant and shady pines.

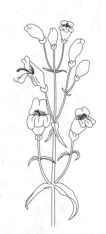

Death Valley penstemon

The Morning Glory Mine. The ultimate reward of this strenuous hike is the old tunnels of the Morning Glory, perched high on an open ridge below Wildrose Peak. The ore is milky quartz brightly stained with gray, green, and deep blue. Samples can also be found in the narrows, especially below the cable crossings. The rough terrain you have just crossed emphasizes the hard work involved in the development of this remote mine, more than a mile above Death Valley. The views are exhilarating, and the name of the mine quite appropriate. The miners did not strike it rich, but they most likely found finer treasures.

A place for bird lovers. The higher elevation and proximity of springs make this fork and upper Trail Canyon a haven for birds. In late May, I spotted wrens, falcons, hawks, hummingbirds, and the usual forlorn ravens perched high on rocky spurs. Cliff swallows fluttered up and down the canyon walls, while above timberline Steller's jays fought their endless territorial wars. The most endearing encounter I made was with a quail that had nested under a bush by the road below the camp. I walked right by her nest, and in the stillness of the canyon her noisy takeoff startled me as much as I had startled her. She flew 30 feet away and proceeded to be as vocal as she could to drive me away. She was obviously guarding something far more precious than an empty nest, and sure enough, moments later a couple of tiny chicks came scampering out from under the bush. I had already created enough of a trauma, and quickly walked away to let her regroup her family.

Hiking and Driving Suggestions

If you drive to the end of the road in the south fork, it is a short day to visit this fork up to the Morning Glory Mine. If you drive only as

South Fork of Trail Canyon		
	Dist.(mi)	Elev.(ft)
Confluence with north fork	0.0	3,420
Morning Glory Camp	1.5	4,280
2nd side canyon	2.2	4,670
3rd side canyon	2.3	4,730
Old Dependable Mine	2.45	4,840
Road to Morning Glory Mine	2.6	4,940
Morning Glory Mine (via road)	(1.8)	6,300
4th side canyon	2.8	5,060
Morning Glory Mine	3.8	6,300

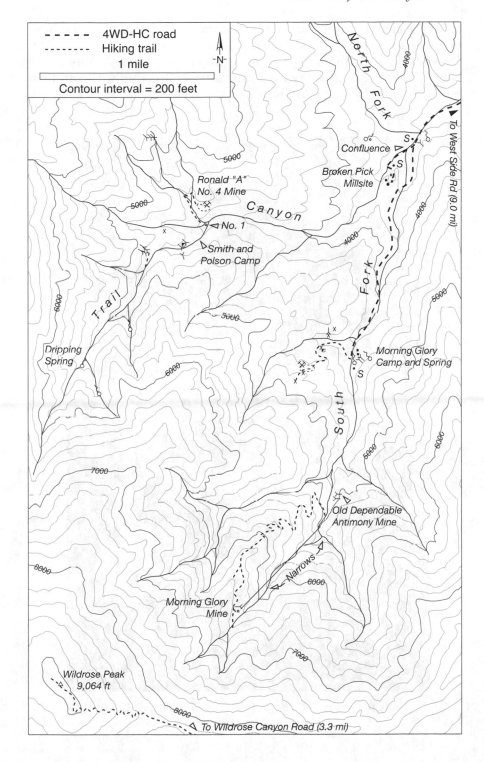

far as the confluence, it takes a full day; start early, or camp at the confluence. If you hike in via the north fork, it is a long day to the Old
Dependable Mine and back. For most people the Morning Glory Mine
would be too far for a day hike. Consider an overnight trip to this
remote site, or beyond to Wildrose Canyon.

■

*Pools and slickrock in the first narrows of Hanaupah Canyon
(Photo by Marc Fermigier)*

HANAUPAH CANYON

The south fork of Hanaupah Canyon is rugged but one of the best. The oasis beyond the end of the long, rocky canyon road is a desert wonder, lush with grapevine, willows, and mesquite trees irrigated by a perennial stream. Further on, the wash enters enchanting narrows where waterfalls plunge into clear pools beneath luxuriant rock-wall gardens. Still further, the canyon squeezes through an imposing chasm carved in massive plutonic rock, to eventually wind into the high-mountain woodland. The sky is the limit: from the salt pan Hanaupah Canyon leads all the way up to Telescope Peak, the highest vertical climb under 20 miles in the lower 48 states.

General Information

Road status: Rough road to first spring (HC); roadless beyond
Shortest hike: 1.7 mi, 840 ft one way / moderate
Longest hike: 8.5 mi, 7,920 ft one way (or more) / grueling
Main attractions: lush springs, creek and waterfalls, wet narrows,
        woodland, spectacular peak climb
USGS 15' topo maps: Bennetts Well, Telescope Peak*
USGS 7.5' topo maps: Hanaupah Canyon, Telescope Peak*
Maps: pp. 433*, 521, 393

Location and Access

The three forks of Hanaupah Canyon drain the eastern slope of the Panamints, below Telescope Peak. A road runs up into the lower part of the south fork, branching off the West Side Road 10.7 miles from its northern end (or 25.2 miles from its south end). Up to the mouth (4.9 miles) it is in relatively good shape, although at times it may require high clearance. Along the way you will cross the Hanaupah Fault scarp, a long and abrupt 10 to 30 foot step in the fan parallel to the mountains, formed by block faulting during the sinking of Death Valley. At the mouth of the canyon the road drops sharply into the wash along a steep grade cut in the bank. High clearance is definitely needed for the 3.4 miles of rough canyon road beyond.

History: Shorty Borden

As with most places in North America, the Indians discovered this canyon first. The name Hanaupah almost certainly has a Shoshone origin. It has been suggested that *Pah*, which means water in

Shoshonean, had something to do with this name. A more likely origin was supplied by Frederick Coville, who headed the 1891 Death Valley biological survey. He reported that the Indian name for this canyon was *Wishi Honopi*. *Wishi* is the word for Indian hemp (*Apocynum Cannabinum*), a plant with tough stalk fibers the Indians made into twine. *Hoon no pee* means canyon or gorge.

Limited mining activity took place in Hanaupah Canyon. A few small silver strikes occurred near the lower spring in the south fork around 1889, in 1905, and finally in the 1920s. Each time the availability of water and wood was viewed as a major advantage of this site, as it would have facilitated developments and made camp life somewhat comfortable. But little is known about the extent of these mining efforts.

Most of what is known about this canyon's history is associated with Alexander "Shorty" Borden, a prospector who came to Death Valley in 1887, reportedly to search for the Lost Breyfogle Lode. Failing to find it, he prospected far and wide in the Panamints, achieving some degree of notoriety not for his strikes, which were minor, but for being a friendly, hospitable old-timer, and later on for having a spring named after him—Shorty's Well. When he discovered (or perhaps rediscovered) a small silver lode in Hanaupah's south fork, he decided to develop his find. In September 1932 he began constructing the present canyon road to his mine. Shorty was a great walker, familiar with the hardships of the desert. Using hand tools, burros, and a little dynamite, he completed this amazing 10-mile road in only six months, reportedly at the age of 66! He also dug what is now Shorty's Well in mesquite thickets at the lower end of his road. His heroic efforts were probably never redeemed. In spite of the road, the cost of shipping still exceeded the value of the ore, and Shortly eventually abandoned mining. After the creation of the monument in 1933, he lived off the slowly increasing tourist population, sharing his meager prospector's diet of coffee and beans in return for more substantial food from the wealthy visitors who stumbled upon him in the middle of nowhere.

Route Description

Shorty Borden's camp and mine. From the end of the road, it is 1 mile up a deep and scenic portion of the canyon to Shorty Borden's camp. Sometimes there is a little water flowing in the wash along the way, but vegetation is sparse until you reach the lush stream-flooded area where the canyon opens up. Shorty Borden's base camp was on the south side of the wash. A three-room house and a shower house stood here until at least the end of the 1970s, but they are now gone, and most years the site is overgrown. What is left is a little junk, and the carcass of a bug-eyed car up canyon. The short, steep grade just east of the camp leads to a timbered mine entrance, which may have been a small work-shop. There are two groups of mines in the vicinity. The first one, on the north canyon slope, is reached by the overgrown upper end of Borden's road (0.8 mi, 600 ft). The other group, above Hanaupah Spring, can be reached via the road on the south side of the camp (1 mile, 440 feet). Except for great vistas, little remains at either mining area.

The creek. One of the most striking features of Hanaupah Canyon is the unlikely stream and oasis just past the old camp, a sight to behold as one of the desert's most precious gifts. For 0.7 mile a vigorous stream plunges over boulders, bubbles into watercress and algae-covered pools alive with water-skimmers, swarms of larvae, and toads. Fed by rain and snow from the high Panamints, it has the largest flow I have seen in any Death Valley canyon. At various times I have estimated it at 50 to 200 gallons per minute. It supports acres of dense willows, mesquites, and grapevine. In the late summer and early fall, look for the small blue grapes on the wild vines, an edible fruit that was part of the Panamint Indian diet. Many other plants thrive along the creek—cane, grasses, Mormon tea, blackbrush, sacred datura, coyote melon, sage, cliffrose, and carpets of pricklypear cactus on the higher banks.

The thick vegetation makes walking in the wash tedious. To avoid damaging this sensitive oasis, hike the old mining road on the north side to Hanaupah Spring, where the vegetation ends. It is a little tricky to find: look for small trails connecting to it northwest of the camp area. Although badly damaged and overgrown with creosotes and mesquites, it makes walking easier, and you will still be treated to the alluring sound of rushing water. After a few hundred yards look for a narrow trail dropping back down to the wash.

Hanaupah Spring. The stream is fed by Hanaupah Spring, one of the most lush canyon springs in Death Valley. It is a cliff spring, rising from an horizontal fault in the steep south wall tens of feet above the wash. The geological formations were visibly displaced along the fault by shearing (the top portion shifted westward), probably during the uplift of the Panamints. The slick wall below the fault is covered with luxuriant hanging gardens draped with wide sheets of water. Signs of burros, bighorn, and coyote are plentiful all around.

The first narrows. Past the spring the canyon is dry for a short distance, but at the next bend it abruptly becomes lush again as it enters one of the most exceptional narrows in the park. This 0.3-mile passage starts with a double waterfall, an idyllic spot where water tumbles over dark blue dolomite into clear basins shaded by cliffs and willows. A little further there is a long polished slide interspersed with white-rimmed pools, then a 10-foot cascade in a small grotto, livened up by dragonflies, birds and frogs. High on the south wall, water trickling from a crack supports a green rock-wall garden of maidenhair fern, grasses, and Indian paintbrush. Still further the narrows are choked with high brush and willows. To make it through takes some heavy-duty bushwhacking—a rare chance to get your feet wet while hiking in Death Valley!

This corridor ends at an impressive 25-foot fall recessed in a deep grotto. The falls up to here are fairly easy, but this one will stop a lot of people. It can be climbed, preferably with climbing shoes, either in the deep vertical crack on the left or up the wall just to the right of it (5.5-5.6/exposed). If you can't make it, the shortest bypass is probably the road south of the camp—a long way back. Just above the fall is the little spring that feeds the narrows, a colorful spot marked by small willows and orange pools lined with showy Panamint prince's plume.

The second narrows. For the next 0.8 mile the canyon remains wide and offers excellent views of Telescope Peak, just a few air miles away. The steep wash, sprinkled with the first conifers, is a chaotic field of giant boulders and large water-worn logs. The boulders come from a large intrusion of monzonite and quartz monzonite called Granite at Hanaupah Canyon, widely exposed south and west from here.

Beyond this open area the canyon goes through the second narrows. They start as a deep channel carved out of monolithic monzonite, occluded within sight by a majestic 45-foot fall. This slick fall, essentially

Hanaupah Canyon		
	Dist.(mi)	Elev.(ft)
Hanaupah Canyon Road		
West Side Road	0.0	-245
Steep grade to wash/mouth	4.9	~1,700
North/South Fork confluence	6.2	2,200
End of road	8.3	3,160
Roadless canyon		
End of road	0.0	3,160
Hanaupah Spring	1.7	4,000
First narrows	1.9	4,160
25-ft fall	2.2	4,320
Upper spring	2.3	4,410
Second narrows (start)	3.1	5,000
Timberline (end 2nd narrows)	3.4	5,240
Third narrows (start)	4.5	6,560
Telescope Peak	~8.5	11,049

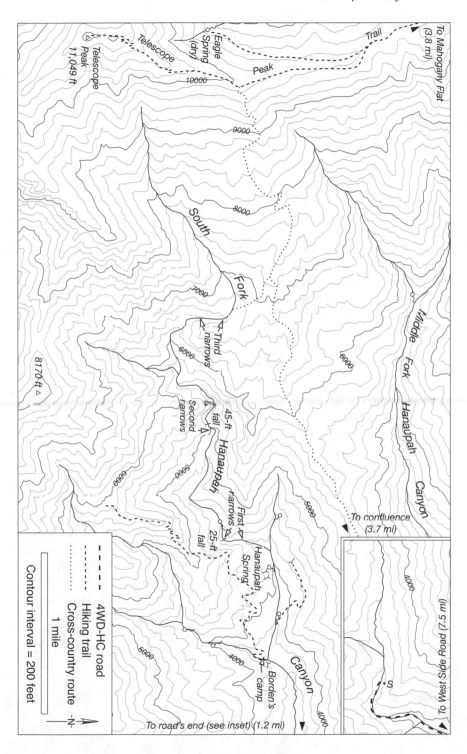

To Mahogany Flat
(3.8 mi)

Trail

Telescope
Peak

Eagle
Spring
(dry)

10000

Telescope
Peak
11,049 ft

9000

8000

South

Fork

7000

Third
narrows

6000

6000

Second
narrows

8170 ft

45-ft
fall

Hanaupah

First
narrows

25-ft
fall

5000

6000

5000

To confluence
(3.7 mi)

Middle Fork Hanaupah Canyon

5000

Hanaupah
Spring

Borden's
camp

Canyon

4000

4000

5000

4000

4000

To road's end (see inset) (1.2 mi)

4000

S

To West Side Road (7.5 mi)

4WD-HC road
Hiking trail
Cross-country route
1 mile
Contour interval = 200 feet
-N-

unscalable, can be avoided by scrambling about 150 feet up the boulder talus on the north side. Further on the narrows continue, encased in towering walls, choked with giant boulders. Timberline is a short distance away, just above a steep slickrock gouged with deep potholes—signs of ancient running water. For the next 1.1 miles you will go through an increasingly thick forest of pinyon pines and junipers. Progress is not always easy, but if you trudge far enough you may find forgotten little figures of red men and deer still dancing on a wall.

The upper canyon. At the upper end of the second narrows the canyon turns to a steep ravine. From here the goal is Telescope Peak, about 4 miles distant and 4,500 feet higher. The terrain is very rough, often unstable, clogged with trees, and very steep—from 1,500 feet per mile to over twice as much near the crest. The easiest way is to climb to the ridge between the south and middle forks as early as possible (perhaps as far back as the confluence for backpackers), and to follow it to the Telescope Peak Trail about 1.3 miles north of the peak (elev. ~9,920'). It is grueling, but the ultimate reward is unequalled. Few sensations are as exhilarating as reaching the highest mountain around Death Valley after trudging across this rough canyon. From two miles up, the blinding salt flats and the succession of desert ranges marching to the horizon form an awe-inspiring scenery likely to remain with you for a long time.

Hiking Suggestions

Hanaupah Canyon can be discovered in many ways. If you can only drive as far as the canyon mouth, you can walk to the first spring, a moderately difficult day hike. Otherwise, from the end of the road it is a short day hike to and through the first narrows. Count on a long day to reach the end of the second narrows and back. The southern ridge road from Borden's camp is a good hiking trail offering spectacular vistas.

The trek up what I call "The Wall," from Shorty's Well up to Telescope Peak, is one of the most challenging hikes in Death Valley. The elevation gain is 11,300 feet over only 17 miles. Crossing the Grand Canyon in one day is much easier—it's half as much climbing up, and there is a trail. Only a chosen few can do this hike in a day (I am not one of them, yet), and even fewer can cram the round trip between sunrise and sundown. Since from the summit it is still 6.5 trail miles to the closest road (see *Wildrose Peak and Telescope Peak*), most people will want to take at least two days, and cache food and water along the trail. The same hike downhill is less taxing, but it's hard on the knees and still best done in two days. The spring helps the water problem (do purify it, though), as does the snow on Telescope Peak, if you time it right.

■

JOHNSON CANYON

> With its mile-long stream and luxuriant oasis of grapevine and willow, Johnson Canyon is one of a kind. A popular hiking goal is the historical remains of Hungry Bill's Ranch, originally established to provide vegetables to booming Panamint City. In the thickly wooded upper canyon beyond the ranch, you can pick up the "fresh vegetable route" to spectacular Panamint Pass, then down the other side to legendary Panamint City and well-watered Surprise Canyon.

General Information

Road status: Primitive road into lower canyon (HC); roadless beyond
Shortest hike: 1.2 mi, 570 ft one way / difficult
Longest hike: 5.1 mi, 4,200 ft (or more)/strenuous
Main attractions: Desert stream, oases, Hungry Bill's Ranch, history
USGS 15' topo maps: Bennetts Well, Telescope Peak*
USGS 7.5' topo maps: Mormon Point, Galena Canyon, Panamint*
Maps: pp. 439*, 393

Location and Access

Johnson Canyon is in the south-central Panamint Mountains. It is accessed by a primitive road that starts on the West Side Road 20.9 miles from its north end (15 miles from its south end). It climbs the fan for 6.4 miles, then drops steeply into the broad and rocky canyon wash and continues up canyon for 3.7 miles. It ends at Wilson Spring, a scenic cluster of willows and tall cottonwoods irrigated by a little creek.

On the fan the road has a few rough spots, some at the very start, which require high clearance. As usual things get much worse in the wash, where lighter vehicles may need 4-wheel drive as well.

History: Hungry Bill's Ranch

Hungry Bill's Ranch, once a green pocket of terraced gardens and orchards, is tied to the discovery of silver in Surprise Canyon, just on the other side of the Panamints from Johnson Canyon. The strike occurred in 1873, a time when spirits were inflamed by major silver bonanzas in western Nevada. The rush was so frantic that by the time news of the strike reached civilization, 20 square miles had already been staked. The boom gave birth to Panamint City, a roaring camp that quickly swelled to a population of over 1,000, and gained the reputation of being one of the toughest towns in the West. It was to satisfy the

435

town's growing need for fresh produce that an enterprising man named William Johnson started a ranch a few miles to the east, in the well-watered canyon that now bears his name. In the mid-1870s, Johnson moved in on the Shoshone Indians who then lived in the canyon, built terraces and irrigation channels, and planted gardens of beans, squash, melons, and corn, and a fruit and nut orchard. His harvest was hauled over the rugged pass to Panamint City. He made a profit on the vegetables, but the trees hardly had a chance to mature before the boom was over. By the spring of 1876 the most promising mines had started to run out. That summer, a devastating flood wiped out most of Panamint City. Less than a year later the last mines had closed down, and Johnson took his business elsewhere.

Some years later, a Shoshone named Hungry Bill took over the abandoned ranch. Hungry Bill was a quiet, 6' 4" giant with an insatiable appetite. It has been said that either he, his father, or both, witnessed the struggle of the first white men across Death Valley in 1849 (see *Jayhawker Canyon*). In their younger years, he and his brother Panamint Tom made headlines by making periodic raids as far as Los Angeles to steal horses and provide meat for their tribe. As waves of miners later swamped Death Valley, they established a peaceful relationship with the immigrants. During the glory days of borax mining, they were hired to gather mesquite wood near Furnace Creek to fuel the boiler at Harmony Borax Works. Hungry Bill and Panamint Tom also helped build the road across the salt pan for the 20-mule-team wagons.

The Panamint Mountains were part of the Shoshones' ancestral territory. Johnson had built his ranch on the site of *Puaitungani*, one of at least five main Shoshone villages in the southern half of Death Valley, then still in use. Panamint Tom had a ranch at a village called *Pabuna*, in Warm Spring Canyon. Another probable pre-settler site was in Panamint Valley near Warm Sulphur Spring. In the late 1800s a famous Indian known as Indian George kept a ranch there, and supplied miners at the nearby camp of Ballarat with fruit. So when Hungry Bill took over the ranch after Johnson's departure, he was probably just returning to his tribe's former land. He and his family cleared a few additional acres, planted more trees, and tended vegetable gardens. In 1897, a thunderstorm wiped out Tom's ranch, and he moved in with Hungry Bill's family. Although the government did not officially approve their application for a homestead until well into the next century, they lived here for many years. The ranch was abandoned soon after Hungry Bill passed away, probably in 1919. Until at least the 1950s his grandson made seasonal trips to the ranch to harvest fruits for his family, who then lived in the valley. Now, after decades of neglect, the few trees that still bear fruit only feed the coyotes.

Route Description

The lower springs. The most unusual and exciting part of this canyon is undoubtedly its intermittent creek and luxuriant oasis. This area is easily reached from the end of the road by a well-defined trail on the south side of the wash. About 0.1 mile in, look for a well-preserved stone arrastre on the left side of the trail. There are two others, about 0.5 and 1 mile further, on the same side; the second one has an interesting stone flume, used for water collection. The first willows and pools appear 0.3 mile from the road, where the canyon squeezes between vertical, rocky walls. Isolated trees soon thicken to a wall-to-wall oasis; pools swell to a singing stream with a generous flow of several gallons per minute. For the next 2 miles, you will be crossing one of the lushest and wettest springs in Death Valley.

There is only one problem, difficult to reconcile with sparsely-vegetated Death Valley: the oasis is so dense it is almost impenetrable. Unless you like trekking through jungles, you will want to avoid the wash and follow the higher trails along the gorge's rims. These trails are not the most well behaved. Steep and rocky, they tend to split or to sneak back to the creek while you are not paying attention and disappear in a hopeless tangle of brush. It can be a pain; you may even forget you are supposed to be having a good time. To minimize frustration, stay on the south side, which has the most continuous trail system. The

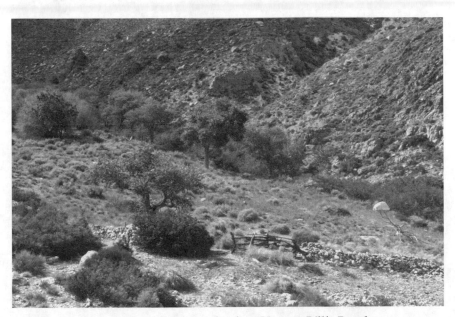

Abandoned field and orchards at Hungry Bill's Ranch

exception is the sharp jog in the canyon, where the creek must be crossed twice in close succession. Also, don't take the cairns too seriously: they indiscriminately point to good and bad trails. Even with these pointers in mind it will be slow going. It's still a great hike, overlooking the green ribbon of shrubs, grapevine, and trees winding down the bottom of the rocky gorge, within earshot of the hidden creek. In the late spring, blooming grizzly bear pricklypear and other cacti brighten the dusty trails. Occasionally, you will be able to drop down to the cooler creek side and enjoy a small waterfall or pockets of watercress and mint.

Hungry Bill's Ranch. The old ranch sprawls on both sides of the wash, just past the head of the second spring. Its most visible signs are several large cleared fields enclosed by monumental stone walls, which give this area an unexpected rural flavor. Several feet high, as much as 6 feet thick and hundreds of feet long, these walls are works of art. Although not mortared, they are extremely sturdy and still intact. No one knows who constructed them, Indians or settlers, though they were probably erected to keep livestock out of farmed areas. The first set of large walls, on the north side, is thought to have been the historic camp of Hungry Bill. The largest field, a little further up canyon on the south side, was Swiss Ranch, the site of Johnson's ranch, and probably the place later cultivated by Hungry Bill and his family. Covering about 10 acres, surrounded by an almost continuous wall, it is still lined up with

Johnson Canyon		
	Dist.(mi)	Elev.(ft)
Johnson Canyon Road		
West Side Road	0.0	-248
Mouth (top of rise)	6.4	2,320
South fork	9.1	3,380
Wilson Spring (road's end)	10.1	3,870
Roadless canyon		
Wilson Spring (road's end)	0.0	3,870
2nd spring	1.2	4,440
Hungry Bill's Ranch	~1.8	~4,700
Porter Peak (via trail)	(~4.8)	9,101
3rd spring	2.4	5,000
4th spring	2.7	5,425
Old road (fresh vegetable route)	4.1	6,800
Panamint Pass	5.1	8,070
Panamint City	(2.0)	~6,300

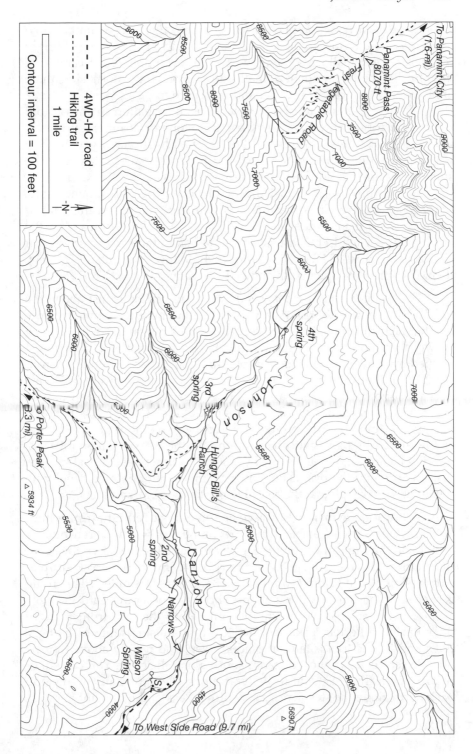

Legend:
- – · – · 4WD-HC road
- – – – – Hiking trail
- · · · · · · Hiking trail

1 mile

Contour interval = 100 feet

-N-

To Panamint City (1.6 mi)

Panamint Pass
△ 8070 ft

Fresh Vegetable Road

8000
8500
8000
7500
8500
7500
7000
9000
6500
6500
7000
7000
6500
6000
6500
7500
6500
6500
6000
6500
6500
6000
5000

4th spring

3rd spring

Johnson

Canyon

Porter Peak
(8.3 mi)
△ 5934 ft

5500
5000
5000

Hungry Bill's Ranch

2nd spring

Narrows

Wilson Spring

4500
5000
5000
5000

△ 5690 ft

4500
4500

To West Side Road (9.7 mi)

the old orchard trees—apple, apricots, peach, figs and walnuts—now overgrown and dying. In the late spring the field turns to a sea of bright red desert globemallow, a scene worthy of an impressionist canvas. A little further, at the mouth of a small side canyon on the north side, there are two large terraces, possibly abandoned gardens.

There is much to discover here, from irrigation ditches to old fences and forgotten trails. A few smaller stone enclosures with doorways suggest living quarters, although the Shoshones lived here in wickiups well into the 1900s. Watch out for rattlesnakes. They love the stone walls, and the one I bumped into was particularly obnoxious.

The third spring, past the ranch, is essentially impenetrable. Masses of hanging vines coat the sheer canyon walls, and the narrow wash between them is choked with willows. A trail bypasses it on the north side, starting in the last steep ravine before the narrow passage. It climbs to a rim 50-100 feet above the wash, follows it for about 500 feet, then drops into the open wash above the spring.

The upper canyon to Panamint Pass. Timberline is just above the third spring, and with it starts a very different, more temperate canyon. For the next mile walking is easier, along narrow game trails winding between granitic rocks, in the partial shade of a healthy conifer forest livened by birds and rodents. Sample this sharp change in the environment up to the next spring, a thick willow grove at a main fork. Hikers in search of offbeat routes may want to go deeper into Johnson Canyon. The hiking is strenuous, along a steep, boulder-strewn wash. You'll eventually run into a trail on the right side, a remnant of the "fresh vegetable route." Its tight switchbacks climb all the way to Panamint Pass, offering increasingly fine views of the surrounding forested peaks. From Wilson Spring to the pass is only about 5 miles, but don't let it fool you: the going is so rough that the round trip takes a long day.

Backpacking routes. For a scenic three-day overnight trip, continue along the "fresh vegetable route," beyond the pass down Frenchman's Canyon to the ruins of Panamint City. You can then hike down the beautiful narrow drainage of spring-fed Surprise Canyon to be picked up at either Chris Wicht Camp (~6 miles) or Ballarat (~11.4 miles). This route is special—it has more water than just about any other in Death Valley.

Another possible overnight route is up the trail from Hungry Bill's Ranch to Porter Peak. Look for it on the hillside south of Hungry Bill's Ranch. The trail is faint at places, steep, and mostly above timberline. Porter Peak is a short distance south along the crest. You can either return down the west side to Ballarat along Pleasant Canyon, or loop back north along the steep crest via Sentinel Peak and Panamint Pass.

■

WARM SPRING CANYON

Warm Spring Canyon is a fun place to explore by car, especially if you are interested in old mines. There is here a plethora of tunnels, ore bins, arrastres, tramways, and other paraphernalia associated with talc, gold, silver, and even fluorite mining. In the lower canyon the highlights are the talc mines, lush and well-watered Warm Spring, and its mining camp. In the upper canyon, hikers can visit the Montgomery Mine, Arrastre Spring, or hard-to-reach Gold Hill, one of the oldest mining areas around. Still beyond, Butte Valley and Anvil Spring Canyon offer secluded old camps and isolated springs.

General Information

Road status: Road graded to spring; primitive beyond (HC-4WD)
Shortest hike: Short strolls/very easy
Longest hike: ~20 mi, ~7,300 ft one way (or more)/strenuous
Main attractions: Talc and gold mines, camp, springs, backcountry road
USGS 15' topo maps: Wingate Wash*, Manly Peak, Telescope Peak, Bennetts Well
USGS 7.5' topo maps: Anvil Spring Canyon East, Anvil Spring Canyon West*, Manly Peak, Panamint
Maps: pp. 447*, 393

Location and Access

Warm Spring Canyon is in the southern Panamints. A road runs through its entire length, starting from the West Side Road 2.9 miles from its southern end (or 33 miles from its north end). Up to Warm Spring, it is graded and easily passable with a passenger car. Further on it is rough and requires high clearance, if not four-wheel drive at places.

History: Talc Mining

Although prospectors combed the Death Valley region for precious metals from as early as 1860, it was more prosaic minerals like talc and borax that produced the biggest bonanzas. However, Death Valley's talc deposits were not recognized and developed until the 1930s, when the demand for talc from several industries was on the rise.

The discovery of talc in lower Warm Spring Canyon is credited to Louise Grantham and Ernest Huhn, who located between 1931 and 1935 the 11 original claims that were to support decades of productive mining. The claims covered a continuous strip along the wash starting just inside the canyon. Although more than 50 claims were also located in the area in the 1950s, the original claims turned out to be the richest.

Much of the mining activity centered on the richer south-side deposits, and most of the production came from the lowest ones, the Big Talc and Warm Spring No. 5 deposits, later known as the Grantham Mine. As elsewhere in the region, these deposits occur only in the late Precambrian Crystal Spring Formation (see *Ibex Spring*). The gently dipping talc bodies occur in fault-bounded strata tens to thousands of feet long and a few to 20 feet thick. They were mined underground along drifts and inclined tunnels. To avoid costly timbering, a room-and-pillar method was employed. The talc was extracted along a grid of perpendicular tunnels dug into the talc-bearing layer. The large blocks of undisturbed vein (the "pillars") between the tunnels were left in place to support the roof. A map of the mine looks something like a city map.

In the early days, talc was extracted from a single drift, loaded into mine cars and trammed to the surface. After 1955 ventilation was improved to accommodate more efficient diesel loaders and trucks. Over the years more drifts were sunk, deeper into the main talc layer, producing a steady supply of high-grade talc. By 1972 the Grantham Mine had been in operation almost continuously for nearly 30 years, and had produced more talc than any other mine in California.

In 1973 the mines were acquired by the Johns-Manville Products Corporation. Because of tight ventilation requirements and long hauling distances, the Grantham Mine was deemed uneconomical and shut down in December. In 1974 deposits further up canyon were mined by open pit—first Warm Spring No. 3, then the Warm Spring deposit. The latter produced until 1975, at which point it had reached a depth of 80 feet and had become too steep and poor for further exploitation. In subsequent years the Grantham Mine was re-opened intermittently as ownership of the mines changed. It was never as good as in the old days, but it still turned out to be the biggest money maker. When it finally closed down in the late 1980s, its total dollar production was one of the highest in Death Valley, perhaps only exceeded by borax mining.

The other major talc deposit was Montgomery Mine, further up canyon. It started more slowly, but it was also a winner. The original claims, located by Owen Montgomery and Harry Gower around 1940, were leased by the Sierra Talc Company, which developed the mine underground. Most of the small, early production took place during the Second World War, when high-grade talc was reserved for strategic applications and the lower-grade talc from this mine was sold for commercial use. After 1946, further underground mining required expensive timbering and the area was mined only intermittently. In 1972 the Cyprus Industrial Minerals Company resorted to surface mining to open a rich, deeply buried deposit. Over the next few years, more than one million tons of rocks were removed to reach the talc veins hundreds of feet below the surface. By 1975, the Montgomery had produced over $5 million, and it kept on producing for years. When the deposit played out in the late 1980s, it was one of the last active mines in Death Valley.

Route Description

The Panamint Mine. The washed-out road to this small talc mine takes off on the south side of the canyon road just before it drops into the wash of Warm Spring Canyon. This area was first located by Ernest Huhn in 1935, and later acquired by the Southern California Minerals Company (see *Saratoga Spring*). It produced intermittently a modest 4,700 tons between 1952 and 1957. After 0.25 mile there is a faint fork in the road to the right. If you are driving a standard-clearance vehicle, or if you are looking for a short, moderate hike, park here and walk the 3.5-mile loop to the two mine sites.

The main road (straight) ends in 2.0 miles at a tunnel, a decaying ore chute, and an open pit that has since then been covered up. Exploited in the mid-1950s, it produced most of the talc from this group of mines. From the highest working you can walk over the short rise to the north, follow a faint, nearly level trail for a few hundred feet, then climb down to the second mine site (~0.6 mile). You can also reach it by returning to your starting point and hiking the 0.9 mile right fork in the road. This second mine, which has more extensive remains, was worked underground in the early 1950s. Though its centerpiece—an unusual three-chute ore bin—unfortunately partly collapsed, it is still an interesting site, with its split-level ore chute cascading down from the tunnel, and its rail loading bridge supported by trestles.

The lower talc mines. The first large mine on the south side of the road is the Grantham Mine. To visit this extensive site, drive or walk 0.25 mile north of the parking area, past the towering loading structure, and take a stroll up the road that winds into the mining area. It first goes by a large talus displaying the many varieties of talc and tremolite that came out of the mine. The adit just behind the loading structure, which has been obstructed by rubble, is Warm Spring No. 5. The deposits are made of three talc-rich layers separated by a 15-foot layer of silicate-carbonate rock. The 15-foot lower layer, which was the thickest, richest, and most regular, was worked the most extensively. The open portal 250 yards further, across from the middle access road, is Big Talc. Connected underground to Warm Spring No. 5, it was the largest producer. From this portal, many drifts fan out into the lower talc-bearing layer, reaching half a mile underground and covering more than 10 miles of slanted tunnels. The leveled south end of the site has a small junkyard and heaps of massive slabs of talcose rock.

For the next couple of miles the road passes by several mines. Most of the mines on the south side were operated until fairly recently, while the mines on the north side are historical and more interesting. For example, try Warm Spring No. 6. Its adit and ore bin are across the road from the Grantham Mine. The next stopover is the giant pit of the Warm Spring Mine, marked by large tailings 0.7 mile past Big Talc. It is worth a look, if only to see what even moderate open-pit mining can do to the land. The dark exposure along the far wall of the pit is diabase. The old machinery and dark gaping tunnel at White Point, 100 yards before the camp, give a good idea of the scale of these operations.

Warm Spring. With its abundance of water and luxuriant vegetation, this spring has a busy history of human occupancy. As early as the 1880s it was used sporadically by miners. In the early 1930s Louise Grantham established a camp here to serve her mines. Besides her own residence, it had a shop, a mess hall, generator, dormitory, and several houses with showers and flush toilets. The superintendent at the time acknowledged it as one of the finest camps in Death Valley. Later on, it only housed the mine office and facilities for vehicle maintenance.

Today, half a dozen more recent buildings remain, partially furnished, surrounded by decaying walkways, stairways, irrigation pipes, and fenced gardens. The last thing you might expect to find here is a large and inviting deep blue swimming pool, replenished by water from the spring. After a long dusty drive, this is a peaceful place to rest, shaded under tall cottonwoods, oleanders, saltcedars, and fig trees. Behind the camp short trails lead up either side of a steep ravine, choked with well-watered grapevine and cane, to the spring, where warm water gushes out of two seeps at the base of the cliff.

The Gold Hill Mill, between the camp and the road, is one of the most interesting historical structures in the area. It was built in the late 1930s, probably to process ore mined at Gold Hill, in the upper canyon. It is unusual for its anachronic combination of recent and old technologies—a power-driven stone arrastre, cone and jaw crushers, a ball mill, a diesel engine, and a complex system of flywheels, pulleys, and belts. Besides being a good example of an early processing plant, this complicated agglomerate of machinery is a lot of fun to try to decipher.

The Pink Elephant Mine. This small mine, high on the steep slope north of the camp, is one of the very few fluorite mines in the park. The original claims were located in 1937 and 1939. Assessment work was carried out for an unknown period of time, probably spanning several years. The exploratory tunnel at the lower level is said to change direction ten times in the course of its 700-foot length—as the mine's name suggests, some hallucinating may have been going on! Around 1946 some thought was given to installing a mill on the site, but the ore bodies were so scattered and the site so remote that mining was never profitable and was likely never seriously undertaken.

The old road to the mine starts across from the camp. Its junction with the canyon road is washed out, but the road is easy to see from the camp. It is now a foot trail, climbing in about 0.5 mile to the timbered lower adit. As an alternative, you can take a direct route up the fan, aiming for the tramway visible from the camp. Although marginal, this little mine has its own charm, inspired by the small aerial tramway connecting its three levels, the short railway spur at the third level, and its fine views. Besides its psychedelic name, what is special about it is that it is dug in the oldest known rocks in Death Valley. These ancient quartz-mica-schist and granitic gneiss belong to the metamorphic core of the Panamints and have been dated at about 1.7 billion years old. It's a good place to touch a rock a full one third as old as the Earth itself.

The mid-canyon (no map). The next point of interest is about 1.8 miles beyond the camp, at a faint junction marked by two posts. The windy road on the right, now a foot trail, ascends to the Montgomery Mine, the westernmost talc mine. The interesting older mine, with its four-chute ore bin and rail spur, dates from the 1940s. Look around for

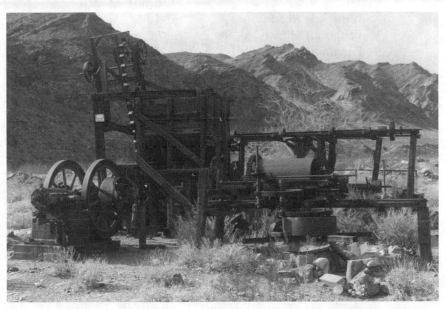

The Gold Hill Mill, near the mining camp at Warm Spring

white or green, greasy steatite, a soft rock also known as soapstone Native Americans carved into utensils and ornaments.

Back to the junction, the main road gradually climbs through a less-than-spectacular upper canyon. A point of interest along this stretch is Grubstake Spring, a small seep tucked away in a side canyon on the south side, 3.5 miles from the camp. As the road nears the pass into Butte Valley, it goes through a field of large granitic boulders, both visually interesting and a potential bouldering site.

Arrastre Spring. To reach this historic site, turn north on the road to Gold Hill, 4.4 miles west of the camp. In 0.2 mile there is a faint spur on the left, which dead-ends in 2.2 miles in sight of Arrastre Spring, pinned to the steep slope of the ravine ahead. According to some historians, it is here that on February 14, 1850, one of the immigrants from the Bennett-Arcane party spoke the famous words "Good-bye, Death Valley," which gave Death Valley its name. When this episode took place, the party had just gone through nearly four weeks of waiting and privation at a small spring along the west side of Death Valley—a site known today as Bennett's Long Camp—while two of its fittest members,

	Dist.(mi)	Elev.(ft)
Warm Spring Canyon		
West Side Road	0.0	-219
Panamint Mine turn-off	7.3	1,290
Panamint Mine loop (hike)	(4.0)	~1,760
Mouth	7.5	1,255
Grantham Mine*	8.9	1,760
Warm Spring pit*	9.7	1,955
Warm Spring camp	11.0	2,420
Pink Elephant Mine (hike)	(0.5)	~2,720
Junction to Montgomery Mine	12.8	2,880
Montgomery Mine (hike)	(2.2)	~4,120
Junction to Gold Hill	15.4	3,645
Arrastre Spring	(2.8)	5,560
Pass into Butte Valley	18.0	~4,300
Anvil Spring Junction	22.5	4,160
Willow Spring	(1.9)	3,580
Squaw Spring (hike)	(9.3)	2,370
Mengel Pass	24.7	4,330
Wingate Road	34.0	1,115

*Elevation at road level

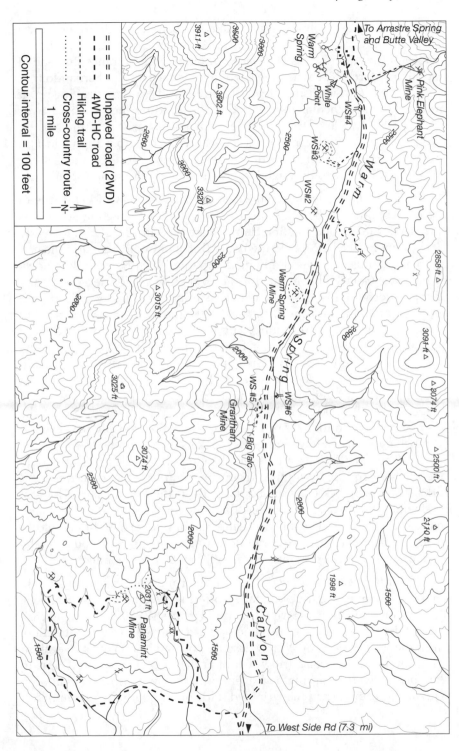

William Manly and John Rogers, walked to San Fernando to look for a feasible route and bring back supplies. This is a moving page in the history of the American West, a story of faith and endurance that ended happily in March 1850 when the party finally reached San Fernando.

It's well worth the steep, 0.5-mile walk to Arrastre Spring, if only for the spectacular views of the surrounding mountains. It was named after two arrastres, reportedly used as early as the 1890s by Indians employed to transport gold ore by burros from the Gold Hill mines to the spring for reduction. These primitive ore-grinding stone mills are still in place, although largely invaded by the spring's willows.

Gold Hill (no map). To the east of the spring is Gold Hill, one of the earliest areas to be mined in Death Valley. Prospecting started as early as the 1870s, and the first claims were filed in 1889. Until the early 1900s, minor strikes triggered the usual flurry of excitement and the creation and demise of several mining companies. In spite of these modest beginnings, Gold Hill continued to generate interest for decades. Many parties intermittently tried their luck at mining gold, silver, lead, and copper until fairly recently. In the 1930s and 1940s some of the old claims were leased, then acquired, by Louise Grantham and associates. They mined the Red Eagle claims for lead and silver, and shipped a few hundred tons of gold ore from the Panamint Treasure between 1931 and 1941. Some of these older claims, as well as new ones such as the Bullet claims, located for gold in 1942 and 1956, continued to be sporadically active in the 1950s and as late as the mid-1970s. Although one of the original mines sold for $207,000 in 1900, Gold Hill probably never yielded much more than a few high-grade pockets of gold and silver.

The Gold Hill area is reached by a very rough road, now only open to foot traffic. Two miles from the main canyon road, this road forks. The north fork ends in about 1 mile at the Bullet claim. The east fork winds up a wash to the Red Eagle claim. Most of these sites are marked by a few stone walls, tent sites, claim markers, and mine workings. Others, however, have very interesting mining rigs. If you have the stamina and an interest in mines, you will not be disappointed.

Butte Valley (no map). The main road continues into Butte Valley, a secluded high-desert valley offering several interesting hikes. Try a climb up colorful Striped Butte (1.4 miles, 980 feet), or a stroll around the three historic camps and springs near Anvil Spring Junction. From the nearby oasis of Willow Spring, you can also take an overnight hike down the old road (now a foot trail) into scenic Anvil Spring Canyon to Fivemile Spring and eventually Squaw Spring, a small seep with an old cabin lost in the wrinkled folds of the southern Panamints.

∎

TELEPHONE CANYON

The main attractions of this broad wash are its unusual arch and the intriguing arrastre at Telephone Spring. They make a fine destination for a half-day hike, or for a stroll if you can drive the canyon road. For a longer walk, hike the main canyon along what used to be the Rhyolite-Skidoo Road to the legendary town of Skidoo. For a different kind of experience, drive and/or partly hike the long road in the north fork to remote Tucki Mine.

General Information

Road status: Primitive road in lower canyon and north fork (HC)
Shortest hike: 0.3 mi, 150 ft one way / easy
Longest hike: 10.4 mi, ~3,150 ft one way (or more) / difficult
Main attractions: Tucki Mine, Arch, Telephone Spring arrastre,
       backcountry road, offbeat hike to Skidoo
USGS 15' topo maps: Stovepipe Wells, Emigrant Canyon*
USGS 7.5' topo maps: Stovepipe Wells, Emigrant Canyon*, Tucki Wash*
Maps: pp. 453*, 459, 393

Location and Access

Telephone Canyon drains the northwestern slope of Tucki Mountain, east of Emigrant Canyon. The Tucki Mine Road winds into the lower canyon and up the canyon's north fork to Tucki Mine, just beyond the crest of the Panamints. This road starts on the east side of the Emigrant Canyon Road, just downhill from the constriction at the canyon mouth, or about 1.5 miles from Highway 190 (or 7.9 miles from the Skidoo turnoff). This junction is easy to miss and the road is a little tricky at first. From the paved road it first goes up the wash, then turns around and climbs to the top of the fan. The rest is straightforward.

The Tucki Mine Road is generally not so bad, except that it has a thick crown of vegetation and a few short rough spots. The first rough area is the wash crossing, at the very start. The second one is a few short staircase steps in the road between 2.4 and 2.6 miles past the main fork. The two rocky spots about 1.6 and 2.0 miles further are the last and worst. Four-wheel drive is certainly not needed, but high clearance is preferable. If you are driving a standard-clearance vehicle, don't mind a rough road, and have experience with it, give it a try. It is possible to go all the way to the mine, although you'll have to drive very slowly and carefully to minimize scraping the bottom of your car.

History: The Rhyolite-Skidoo Telephone Line

The namesake of this canyon is the Rhyolite-Skidoo telephone line, which once connected the town of Skidoo, at the head of Telephone Canyon, to Rhyolite, about 50 miles away on the far side of the Grapevine Mountains. Skidoo and Rhyolite were the two largest, most famous and colorful mining towns the region ever had, and in their glory days communication between them became important enough to justify the painstaking installation of a telephone line. The line was completed in the spring of 1907. It went from Skidoo through this canyon on its way to a telephone station at Stovepipe Well, then ascended the Amargosa Range to Rhyolite. Later on, transportation problems at Skidoo were alleviated by grading a freight road in the canyon wash, which was a significant shortcut to Rhyolite compared to the previous route through Emigrant Canyon. In 1910 plans were made to surface the road in Telephone Canyon with mesquite to accommodate a mail and passenger car service, but it is not known whether they were ever implemented. The road and the telephone line have now been obliterated in this canyon, but remnants of the latter can still be traced part of the way today, in particular on the fan on the north side of Tucki Mountain (see *Stretched-Pebble Canyon*), and near Kit Fox Canyon (see *The Kit Fox Hills*).

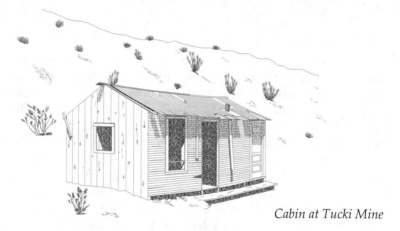

Cabin at Tucki Mine

History: Tucki Mine

This isolated gold mine, located at the head of Tucki Wash at the end of the steep Tucki Mine Road, has a long history of intermittent activity. Claimed first in 1909, then in September 1927, it was operated off and on until the 1970s. History and production records from these marginal gold deposits are scant. Over its lifetime the property, which encompassed the four main Tucki claims, was leased and worked by at least half a dozen parties. The ore, mined underground, was treated at Roy Journigan's Mill in Emigrant Canyon until around 1938, and afterwards at a small cyanide plant at the mine. In April 1939, after selling his mill, Roy Journigan became part owner of the mine, which eventually became the family's property (see *Burns Spring and Journigan's Mill*). Although nearly $18,000 was produced in 1941, the average production over other active years was likely more modest. After the early 1950s mining activity was sporadic, until in 1975 Russ Journigan and a few partners installed a crusher and a modern leaching plant at the site to extract gold from old tailings. The operation only recovered a few dozen ounces of gold before it shut down and the equipment was removed in March 1976.

Route Description

The arch and Telephone Spring. The lower canyon cuts through the fanglomerates of the Nova Formation. The reddish rock has eroded into a subdued topography of rolling hills dissected by gullies and ravines. Shortly after it enters the canyon, the road goes through shallow narrows, at one point passing under a small overhang. The narrows end in 0.3 mile, just below the main fork in the canyon. The road goes on straight ahead up the north fork. The right fork—the main canyon—is where the Rhyolite-Skidoo Road used to go, but it is now roadless.

The arch is a short distance up the main canyon. This is a scenic area, framed on the east side by a long cream-colored cliff. Coincidentally, the arch, punched through the cliff and overlooking the wash, is shaped like a telephone! Although only about 15 feet high by 20 feet wide at the base, this fragile formation, carved out of crumbly siltstone/fanglomerate, is an unlikely and rare occurrence.

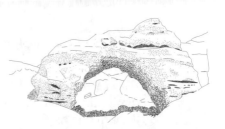

Telephone Arch

Telephone Spring is just past the arch, on a low outcrop plugging the middle of the wash. During Skidoo's gold rush, this was one of the stops on the Rhyolite-Skidoo Road. There is no longer water here, but the interesting remains of an old mill, dating probably from the 1930s gold mining revival. The centerpiece is a beautiful and fairly well-preserved power-driven arrastre, a circular trough lined with polished slabs of limestone, marble, and granite. Above the arrastre stand the concrete foundations that used to hold the mill's machinery. The masonry a few yards to the left is probably old pilings for a water tank. The narrow, rock-lined channel to the right diverted the slurry from the arrastre into three small settling ponds held by crude rock dams, still in place in the small wash below. I always find this site intriguing, for its odd location at a dry spring, its mysterious origin and unknown history. Where did the water come from? Why did it dry up?

The Rhyolite-Skidoo Road. This hike follows the route of the historical Rhyolite-Skidoo Road, which no longer exists in the canyon wash. (Purists may even want to pick up this segment of the old road at its start, on Highway 190, 0.9 mile east of Emigrant Junction; it's about 2 miles along this brush-invaded track to the mouth of Telephone Canyon.) From Telephone Spring, the route follows a broad canyon for 1.1 miles to the confluence of three forks, all of which ascend the steep edge of the plateau to Skidoo. The west fork is the main canyon and the easiest approach. After following it for 1.6 miles, just past a low saddle along the west side ridge, you'll pick up the faint trace of the Rhyolite-Skidoo Road as it climbs onto that ridge and soon joins the Saddle Rock Mine trail. It is then 1.9 miles up this steep road to its end, and 2.5 cross-country miles to Skidoo (see *Skidoo* for details).

The north fork and Tucki Mine. From the confluence the road winds up the mountain for 7.4 miles to Tucki Mine. The first 3.8 miles of the north fork of Telephone Canyon are open and uneventful. The road then traverses the only relatively narrow and deep part of the canyon,

Telephone Canyon		
	Dist.(mi)	Elev.(ft)
Tucki Mine Road		
Emigrant Canyon Road	0.0	2,660
Mouth (via road)	1.7	2,370
Main fork (start of hike)	2.5	2,630
Roughest spot in road	~7.1	~4,040
Junction/Pass	9.3	4,890
Tucki Mine	9.9	~4,680
Roadless canyon		
Main fork	0.0	2,630
Telephone Arch	0.3	~2,780
Telephone Spring	0.4	~2,820
Saddle Rock Mine trail	3.4	4,045
Saddle Rock Mine	5.1	~5,080
Skidoo (downtown)	7.8	~5,680

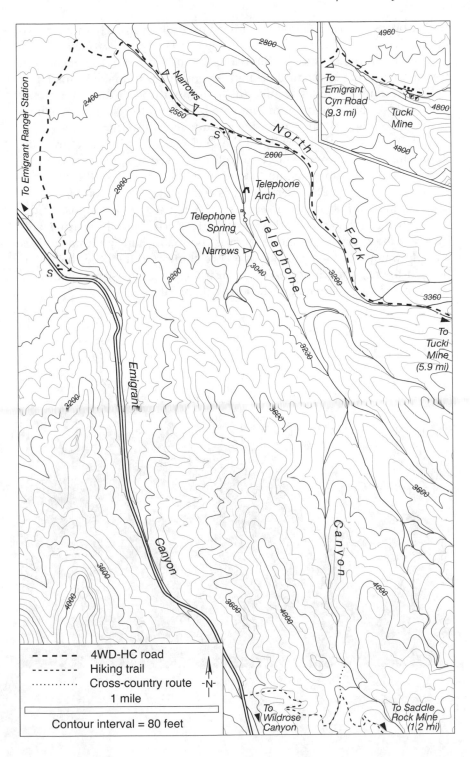

2800

4960

To
Emigrant
Cyn Road
(9.3 mi)

Tucki
Mine

4800

4800

Narrows

2400

2560

2800

North

Fork

Telephone
Arch

Telephone
Spring

Narrows

3040

3360

To
Tucki
Mine
(5.9 mi)

To Emigrant Ranger Station

2800

S

3200

Telephone

3200

3200

Emigrant

3200

Canyon

Canyon

3600

3600

3600

4000

3600

4000

4000

4000

4000

4000

- - - - - 4WD-HC road
- - - - - Hiking trail
· · · · · · · · Cross-country route   -N-
1 mile

Contour interval = 80 feet

To
Wildrose
Canyon

To Saddle
Rock Mine
(1.2 mi)

which opens up again about 1.7 miles before the pass. The mine is 0.6 mile down the east side of the pass, at the head of a fork of Tucki Wash.

The roughest spot in the road is 0.6 mile into the deeper canyon. If you are driving a standard-clearance vehicle, try to make it this far. It will leave only 2.8 miles to hike to the mine, through the most scenic part of this route. The other option is to hike from the main fork, which makes for a long day, most of it spent in uneventful country.

But it's worth the walk. At the Tucki Mine you'll find a great little mining camp, composed of two well-preserved wooden cabins and a tin shed lined up along the north side of the wash. One of the cabins is maintained by the Park Service; it is furnished with a table, chairs, shelves, and old magazines. The mine workings are on the opposite side. The four tanks at wash level were used to leach the gold-bearing tailings. On the rocky slope above them is the main shaft, with its ladders and old timber, headframe, part of its ore chute, and the little shack that housed the hoist machinery. This is an interesting site, so isolated it's a pleasure to come upon it after the long ride or hike.

■

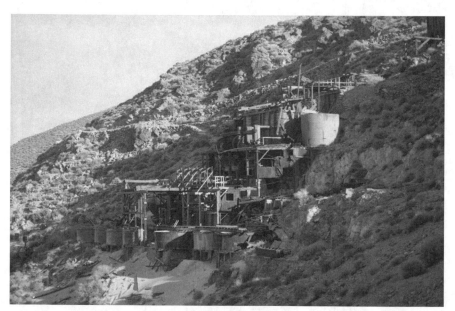

Skidoo's Quartz Mill

SKIDOO

> *During Death Valley's gold rush, Skidoo rose at the crest of the Panamints to become one of its largest gold producers and one of the area's most enduring legends. Drive to the old town site to visit Skidoo's well-preserved mill and browse through its extensive mine workings. Or better yet, hike to it up the forgotten Saddle Rock Mine trail, visiting along the way the site of the original gold discovery that sparked the rush.*

General Information

Road status: Primitive road to town site; hiking from paved road
Shortest hike: Short strolls / very easy
Longest hike: 5.2 mi, 2,450 ft one way (or more) / difficult
Main attractions: Historical Skidoo, gold mines, the Saddle Rock Mine trail, ridge hike
USGS 15' and 7.5' topo maps: Emigrant Canyon
Maps: pp. 459*, 393

Location and Access

The most popular way to reach Skidoo is to drive the unpaved Skidoo Road from Emigrant Canyon. This marked road branches off the Emigrant Canyon Road 9.4 miles south of Highway 190 (or 11.7 miles north of the Wildrose Canyon Road). It's 7.4 miles to the town site. The road is a little bumpy at places but OK with normal clearance. The alternative is to hike one of several possible routes. The one described here is the Saddle Rock Mine trail, which is one of the most interesting approaches. This trail also starts off the Emigrant Canyon Road, 4.2 miles from Highway 190 (or 5.2 miles north of the Skidoo turnoff). Don't look for the trail, which is washed out near the road, but for a narrow wash. If you are coming from the north, this wash is about 300 feet past a right bend in the road; its gravel bank is riprapped with chicken wire. The Saddle Rock Mine trail is closed to motorized traffic. Park well off the road and walk up the wash to it.

History: 23 Skidoo

Skidoo was one of the most famous and colorful mining towns in the history of Death Valley. It was started by a major gold discovery made by two prospectors, John L. Ramsey and John A. Thompson, in January 1906. Legend has it that while on their way to Harrisburg,

455

where gold had been discovered six months earlier, they got caught in a rare fog that forced them to camp in Emigrant Canyon. There they found evidence of gold, which they traced the next day to a giant lode in the hills to the east. The rich Gold Eagle claims they filed soon after attracted the attention of E. A. (Bob) Montgomery, a competent mining promoter. He had been involved in several successful mines, including the Montgomery-Shoshone Mine in the Bullfrog Mining District, whose sale had just made him a millionaire. Montgomery purchased the claims from the original discoverers, and formed the Skidoo Mines Company.

As elsewhere, the major barriers to profitable mining were poor transportation and the lack of communications and a reliable water supply. A road was soon constructed to connect the mining site to the rest of the world via Emigrant Canyon. The water problem was far more serious, as there is no large reliable spring for miles around. Montgomery enlisted Matt Hoveck, his former manager at the Montgomery-Shoshone Mine, to develop and supervise the mines. Hoveck immediately began the construction of an ambitious pipeline that would bring water from Birch Spring, located more than 20 miles away below Telescope Peak. Over the next few months, as Montgomery invested hundreds of thousands of dollars in the mine, hundreds of prospectors rushed to the site, spurred by Montgomery's reputation. Other companies were formed, in particular the Granite Contact Mine, adjacent to the Skidoo Mines, and before long most of the surrounding ground was claimed. The town of Skidoo was laid out to support the increasing population of workers and merchants attracted by the boom. Its name was derived from "23 Skidoo," a popular phrase of the time, which meant "beat it." Various reasons have been given for this choice—the 23 claims originally purchased, the discovery date of January 23, the reportedly 23-mile long pipeline—but no one knows anymore. For a while Skidoo rivaled the mining camps of Harrisburg, Emigrant Spring, and Wild Rose, but its original 23 blocks were soon sold out and the town grew to be the largest community in the Panamints. Together with Rhyolite, Nevada, on the far side of the Grapevines, it was the only real town Death Valley ever had. At its height, it had a population of 400-500, and over 100 business houses and residences. It enjoyed such amenities as a bakery, a school, several restaurants, a physician, even a bank, the *Southern California Bank of Skidoo*, and a newspaper, *The Skidoo News*. By the spring of 1907 a telephone line had been strung all the way to Rhyolite (see *Telephone Canyon*). Regular coach services ran between the two towns.

The long-awaited Telescope Peak pipeline was completed in December that year. Besides quenching the thirst of the Skidoovians, the water had plenty of pressure to power the mill's 10-stamp battery, erected on a hillside near town. The Skidoo Mill thus became the only milling plant in the desert region to be operated almost entirely by water power.

Gold production started in May 1908. The ore was hauled from the mines directly to the mill in trains of mine cars pulled by burros. Skidoo was one of the few mines in the region that produced significant amounts of gold. Its success was largely due to its water-powered mill, which made processing as inexpensive as $7 per ton. For quite some time, tens of tons were processed every day, yielding from $5,000 to as much as $18,000 a month. In 1909 the Skidoo Mine was the second largest gold producer in California after the Keane Wonder Mine. Despite several hardships, a depressed national economy, a frozen pipeline one particularly cold winter, and the destruction of the original mill by fire in 1913, Skidoo kept on churning out gold at a sizeable profit for years, while other mines faded one by one.

The great Skidoo era didn't come to an end until September 1917, when the main ore bodies either played out or became too difficult to exploit. The area still witnessed sporadic activity for many more years, and several of the old mines were reopened in 1934 after the price of gold went up, but the heyday of Skidoo was over. By the end of 1917, Montgomery's mine had produced over $1.3 million and was second behind the Shoshone Mine, the largest gold producer in the Death Valley region. Although Montgomery may have been the only investor who made a profit, Skidoo was the only mine of the Death Valley gold rush that brought back dividends to its stockholders.

Although some of the companies that mined around Skidoo fared reasonably well, many others did not do so well. The Saddle Rock Mine, Ramsey and Thompson's original Skidoo strike, may be a case in point. Through 1906 the two men filed several other claims in the area, including the Saddle Rock, Pima, and K. K. claims. Since they were bordering Skidoo, which was booming by then, the two men were able to sell them for $25,000 in cash by the end of the year. The property was active from 1906 to 1910. Ore showings were reported to be so good that plans were made to acquire water from the Skidoo pipeline, but nothing came of it. In 1929, Bob Eichbaum, who had opened the Eichbaum Toll Road over Towne Pass three years earlier, formed a new company and reopened the area as the Emigrant Springs Mine. The trail to the mine was built then, reportedly by a coalition of old-timers, including Shorty Harris. After ore that reportedly assayed a staggering $10,000 per ton was exposed, heavy milling machinery was hauled up to the site. A few other mining attempts took place under various ownerships until the 1960s. Unfortunately, no production records are available, and we don't know how any of these ventures fared. As it turns out, the deposit was fairly large but contained mostly low-grade ore. Chances are that other than a few high-grade pockets, mining was not profitable.

Route Description

The Saddle Rock Mine trail. If you love the desert and its history, you may find this route the only befitting way to get to Skidoo. From the car park on Emigrant Canyon Road, walk up the steep wash for 0.25 mile to the first trace of the old trail, on the right a few feet above the wash. The trail soon doubles back sharply to the right and climbs to a low ridge. From here to the trail's end, this is mostly a ridge walk. The trail is well-defined the whole way, never very steep, and it even levels off periodically to let you catch your breath. The views get increasingly finer—first the colorful dissected west wall of Emigrant Canyon, then the barren south face of Tucki Mountain, and finally far away Mesquite Flat.

The Saddle Rock Mine has two main sites near the end of the trail, with a few prospects, tent sites and claim monuments scattered in between. The local mineralogy is quartz monzonite and quartzite. Fractures in the quartzite are filled with gold-bearing quartz. The lower site, located on a high ridge, is marked by the ruins of a small camp—a collapsed cabin, assorted debris, and a tin shack up the wash. This is the location of the Pima and K. K. claims. The main tunnel, a short distance north, cuts through quartz monzonite. It has narrow-gauge tracks and a sizeable tailing. There are other workings down the washes on either side of the ridge. The upper site, about 0.3 mile further up the trail, has two inclined shafts, one of which still has its wooden access ladder. The trail ends shortly on a narrow saddle, near a cluster of tent sites.

The cross-country route to Skidoo. From here it's about 1.6 cross-country miles to the edge of the Skidoo area. You can actually see your destination: the square shape barely sticking out above the east-north-east horizon is the top of the Skidoo Mill. The easiest way is to go up the ridge just north of the ridge you are on. To get to that ridge, hike down

Skidoo		
	Dist.(mi)	Elev.(ft)
Emigrant Canyon Road	0.0	3,545
Trail	0.3	~3,700
Rhyolite-Skidoo Road	0.8	4,045
Saddle Rock Mine tunnels	2.2	4,840
Saddle Rock Mine shafts	2.5	~5,080
End of trail	2.7	5,110
Skidoo (closest road)	4.3	5,780
Skidoo (downtown)	5.2	5,680

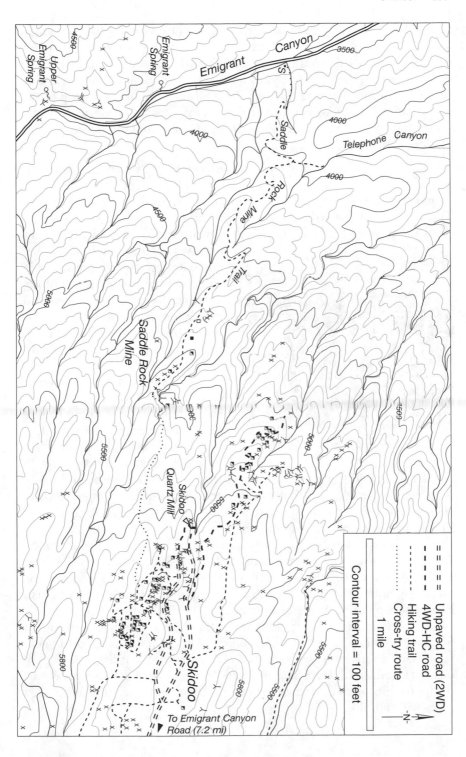

To Emigrant Canyon
Road (7.2 mi)

Skidoo

Skidoo
Quartz Mill

Saddle Rock
Mine

Saddle Rock Mine Trail

Telephone Canyon

Emigrant Canyon

Emigrant Spring

Upper Emigrant Spring

═ ═ ═ ═　Unpaved road (2WD)
▬ ▬ ▬ ▬　4WD-HC road
‑ ‑ ‑ ‑ ‑　Hiking trail
· · · · · ·　Cross-try route

‑N‑

1 mile

Contour interval = 100 feet

to the wash between them, towards the small prospects below (which are part of the Saddle Rock Mine). This 100-foot descent is steep and unstable, but it's the only tricky part. Follow the wash up about 100 yards to where the ridge on your left is fairly low, and climb to it. The rest is straightforward: follow this ridge all the way up to the top of the mountain. From there you can see Telescope Peak, the Sierra Nevada, and a network of mining roads just ahead. You have reached greater Skidoo. Downtown is less than a mile away.

   Skidoo. The town of Skidoo used to be right around the interpretive sign at the Y near the end of the Skidoo Road. Today there is not a single standing structure to attest to the glory of this legendary town. The few houses that were not dismantled and moved—an old desert tradition—are now broken boards. Only scattered debris and tent sites betray the old town site. The mines are certainly more interesting. The two main roads splitting off at the interpretive sign, and their many branches, give access to ore bins, rusted car bodies, stoped adits, and dozens of tailings and mine openings (most of which, in everyone's best interest, have been wired off). Gold was mined from quartz veins in late Cretaceous granite, which is plentiful all around. The veins were unusually thin, typically only 18 to 24 inches wide. It made mining difficult, as reflected by the many long, narrow, and impressively deep trenches scattered all over. Some of these stopes are still supported by the original timber, logged near Telescope Peak almost a century ago.

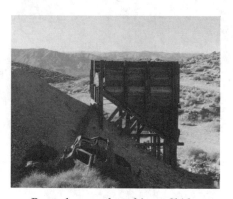

Rusted car and ore bin at Skidoo

   The two roads eventually converge at the ruins of the Skidoo Quartz Mill, the largest remains of Skidoo. With its multiple levels cascading down a steep canyon wall, overlooking the distant peaks of the Sierra Nevada, it is quite a sight, and certainly the highlight of a visit here. The top floor was restored soon after it collapsed in 1993.

   Another interesting remnant is the Skidoo pipeline, considered to be an engineering feat of early mining. Although it was unfortunately scrapped for metal at the end of 1917, its route is still marked by a cleared swath south from Skidoo across Harrisburg Flat, and a good part of the way to Birch Spring. Some of the stone structures that supported it are still standing.

■

JAYHAWKER CANYON

This canyon is named after the Jayhawkers, a group of immigrants believed to have come through here on their historical journey out of Death Valley in 1849. For most people the main destination is the spring, where a few boulders bear petroglyphs and inscriptions left by the expedition. Hard-core hikers may want to continue on and retrace the immigrants' footsteps to their presumed camp on a high pass overlooking Wildrose Canyon, then up to 7,508-foot Pinto Peak.

General Information

Road status: Roadless; hiking from paved road
Shortest hike: 2.3 mi, 1,070 ft one way / moderate
Longest hike: 9.3 mi, 4,550 ft one way / strenuous
Main attractions: Forty-niners, rock inscriptions, petroglyphs, spring
USGS 15' topo map: Emigrant Canyon
USGS 7.5' topo maps: Emigrant Canyon*, Emigrant Pass
Maps: pp. 465*, 471, 393

Location and Access

Jayhawker Canyon drains the north side of Pinto Peak, the prominent mountain forming the west side of Emigrant Canyon. The starting point is around the 3,000-foot elevation sign on Highway 190, 2.2 miles south of the Emigrant Ranger Station. The mouth of Jayhawker Canyon is at the foot of the conical butte to the southeast.

History: The Route of the Jayhawkers

This canyon and the rock inscriptions found in it are connected to the Jayhawkers, one of several parties of immigrants who stumbled into Death Valley at the close of 1849 on their way to the California gold mines. These parties had traveled together from Salt Lake City since October, breaking up into smaller parties across Nevada. The leading party entered Death Valley along Furnace Creek Wash around December 13 and camped near Travertine Springs. As they moved on to McLean Spring, north of the salt flats, other parties caught up—the Jayhawkers, the Bennett-Arcane party, the Haynes party (who probably crossed over Indian Pass), and then Reverend Brier and his family. So it was, by some cunning twist of fate, that about 100 men, women, and children had converged in Death Valley within a few days, as if drawn by some irresistible force to this final gathering place before facing what was to be the worst hardship of their historical journey.

They were probably the first white people to see Death Valley, then an unchartered place. When time came to move on and leave the valley, each party chose its own route, relying on hunches for want of anything better. These various routes have been the subject of much research, based on numerous letters, diaries, and books left by the settlers, and on historical inscriptions such as those found in Jayhawker Canyon. Many of these accounts, written years later, lack accuracy and completeness, rely on subjective descriptions to identify landmarks then unnamed, and often leave plenty of room for interpretation. Inevitably, the reconstructed story of their journey varies from author to author.

Although the Jayhawkers route is not known with certainty, the two most prominent theories involve Jayhawker Canyon. The first one contends that from McLean Spring they circled around Tucki Mountain towards the Cottonwood Mountains, then south across the fan to Jayhawker Canyon, and up this canyon to the pass below Pinto Peak. This hypothesis is supported by two dated rock inscriptions left by Jayhawker William Rood, one near the mouth of Lemoigne Canyon, the other in Jayhawker Canyon. The second theory favors a more direct route: westward up either Tucki or Blackwater wash to the Skidoo area, then up a side canyon of Emigrant Canyon (perhaps near Malapi Spring) to Jayhawker Canyon. This route, however, would not have taken them near Jayhawker Spring. It has been argued that Rood could have made his inscriptions years later, when he returned to Death Valley in search of the Lost Gunsight Lode in 1869. Seeing at the time the inscriptions left by Dr. French's 1860 party, he may have felt entitled to predate his own inscription to record his historical passage of 1849.

After their long ascent out of Death Valley, the Jayhawkers camped near the top of a mountain, presumably Pinto Peak. Often referred to as "Summit Camp," their camp is described in one account as "astride the highest rafter of the roof of hell." Two peculiar events took place here. The first one is the discovery of a sample of silver ore by one of the immigrants, somewhere on his way to Summit Camp. The sample was so pure that when he reached civilization he had a gunsight fashioned from it for his gun. He boasted that where his sample came from, "a mule could be loaded with the same kind of stuff without much work." In those times of fabulous strikes and instant fortunes, imaginations were easily inflamed, and with this simple incident the legend of the Lost Gunsight Lode was born. Of the countless rumors that lured fortune seekers to Death Valley, few had as profound and enduring an effect as the Lost Gunsight. In the following decades, several expeditions were launched from the California coast—some involving Jayhawkers—to try to locate this presumed treasure. Two of the earliest expeditions were led by Dr. E. Darwin French, in 1850 and 1860. Members of his party also left inscriptions in Jayhawker Canyon. Over time, many others gave it a try, but to this day no one knows whether the Gunsight is still lost. There is a good chance that it was relocated and exploited as one of the silver mines that sprouted in this general area years later, without ever being connected to the Lost Gunsight.

The second incident is the burial, at Summit Camp, of $2,000 to $2,500 in gold coins collected among the Jayhawkers, a burden they deemed too heavy and unimportant given the circumstances to carry along. Rood reported the coin stash was missing in 1869. Perhaps members from earlier parties in search of the Lost Gunsight had gotten to it first. Since then, many have searched for the forty-niners' gold, but again whether it ever turned up is unknown.

Route Description

The route to the spring. The mouth of Jayhawker Canyon is a little hard to see from the highway. Aim straight for the center of the base of the flat-topped, 1,000-foot-high, conical hill to the southeast, about a mile across the fan. You will first go over a low ridge, then drop down its steep far side into a shallow wash. The rest of the way is across the gently sloping fan to the canyon mouth. The main interest here is the fan itself, which is one huge field of closely spaced cobbles and small boulders deeply set in desert pavement. Made almost exclusively of basalt, they glisten with unusually dark rock varnish, a sign that they have not been disturbed in a very long time. These rocks have probably been baking in the sun essentially the way they are for millennia—perhaps since the close of the last Ice Age.

Once in the canyon, directions are easier. The only potential source of error is the fork 0.4 mile in, where you'll need to bear left. The spring is another mile up canyon.

All of Jayhawker Canyon cuts through the fanglomerate of the Funeral Formation, deposited in the Pliocene and perhaps early Pleistocene—in geological terms, just about yesterday. The accumulation of these arid-basin deposits was periodically interrupted by intense volcanic activity that covered the area under thick basaltic flows. These flows now form the long, hard ledges exposed across the canyon slopes. They have weathered to produce a few impressive volcanic screes and the many basaltic boulders stranded in the wash.

The rock inscriptions and Jayhawker Spring. The site of the rock inscriptions is marked by a large, squarish boulder, about 5 feet across, resting on a broad ledge on the west side, a few feet above the wash. The spring is on the steep canyon slope a few hundred feet behind it. The

main boulder has several groups of petroglyphs, some much older than others.
They represent different styles of sheep,
small human figures, and a variety of
abstract figures. The vertical string of tan-
gential circles on the west side of the boulder may not be random doodling. It also
occurs in Titus Canyon and Marble
Canyon, among other places, and probably has a special meaning.

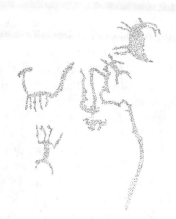

  Most of the historical inscriptions
are found on this same boulder. The two
main inscriptions, "Frank L. Weston March
27 1860" and "J. Hitchens 1860," were left by members of Dr. French's
expedition. The spring was originally called Hitchens Spring, until it
was renamed to commemorate its probable historical significance. Other
inscriptions are found on two smaller boulders next to the main boulder.
The most significant one reads "1849 W.B.R.," attributed to William B.
Rood. The other inscription reads "LI ER". Although it could have been
made by Reverend Brier, it is sufficiently incomplete to warrant caution
in identification.

  From the inscriptions site a narrow game trail leads up to
Jayhawker Spring, a cluster of cane and a thicket of dwarf mesquites just
above it. At times, a little water pools up on the edge of the mesquites,
and you may find more than the usual gang of lizards.

	Jayhawker Canyon	
	Dist.(mi)	Elev.(ft)
Highway 190	0.0	3,000
Mouth	1.0	3,350
1st side canyon	1.4	3,540
Rock inscriptions	2.3	4,030
Jayhawker Spring	(0.05)	4,100
Narrows (start)	3.0	4,340
Narrows (end)/2nd side canyon	3.3	4,500
Side canyon to Summit Camp	7.7	6,640
Probable site of Summit Camp	(0.4)	~6,900
Emigrant Pass (Pinto Peak trail)	(6.2)	5,318
Pinto Peak	9.3	7,508

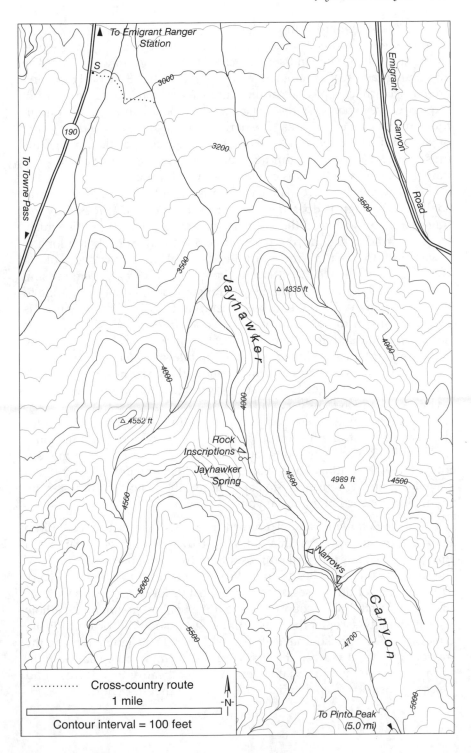

To Emigrant Ranger Station

S

190

To Towne Pass

3000

3200

3500

Jayhawker

△ 4335 ft

4000

4000

4600

△ 4552 ft

Rock Inscriptions

Jayhawker Spring

4989 ft △

4500

4560

4500

Narrows

5000

Canyon

5500

4700

Emigrant Canyon Road

3500

4000

4500

5000

To Pinto Peak (5.0 mi)

.... Cross-country route

1 mile

-N-

Contour interval = 100 feet

The upper canyon. If you have time, you can continue up canyon to retrace the presumed route of the forty-niners. The canyon deepens shortly past the spring and soon reaches its first and only narrows. The alternating layers of fanglomerate and basalt of the Funeral Formation are particularly conspicuous at the entrance to the narrows. Several full sequences are exposed on the east side, which bear witness to the tumultuous recent past of this area. The narrows are a shallow, winding gorge of shattered basaltic walls. No falls—but imagine what the immigrants must have felt, struggling through here after months of privation, wondering all along whether this canyon even went through.

Beyond the narrows, the canyon is considerably more open and shallow, although it does narrow a little further on. It forks several times, and you will need the 7.5' map to work out which fork is which. Near the head of the canyon, where it begins to curve back in a long U towards Pinto Peak, a short gully heads south to a pass overlooking Nemo Canyon. This is the probable site of Summit Camp. The missing stash of the Jayhawkers and the Lost Gunsight add a definite sparkle to this area—you may find them good incentives to hike all the way up this desolate canyon to the "roof of hell." You'll find a sprinkling of trees here, and a hiking trail, the old Pinto Peak trail, which comes all the way from Emigrant Pass. Following it right will take you to Pinto Peak and a breathtaking overlook of Panamint Valley, the crowning glory of this hike. You can also get to the peak by returning to and following Jayhawker Canyon to its very end.

Count on 2-3 hours round trip to see the spring, and 4 hours for the narrows. A strong hiker can make the return hike to Summit Camp or Pinto Peak in one long day, but most people will prefer to make it into a three day outing. For a shorter but still healthy day hike into little travelled country, return via Malapi Spring, then back to your starting point along scenic Emigrant Canyon.

The Pinto Peak trail. To return from this hike or to access Pinto Peak a different way, try this old, overgrown trail. If you start from Emigrant Pass, it is the northernmost of the two trails on the west side of the road (the other one heads down White Sage Wash to Nemo Canyon). The Pinto Peak trail crosses some of the most desolate terrain I have ever hiked—in Death Valley country, this is not a benign qualifier. The whole way it steadily ascends the long southeastern shoulder of Pinto Peak, crossing the same bush-dotted slopes, with hardly a change to break the monotony until it reaches the first conifers at timberline, near Summit Camp. It made me appreciate even more the beauty of Wildrose and Telescope peaks, which dominate the entire southeastern horizon.

■

BURNS SPRING AND JOURNIGAN'S MILL

> *The main attractions of this area are the historic ruins of two mills and the half a dozen small springs located in nameless canyons on the slope of Pinto Peak, some of which provided water to run the mills for many years. It is an easy and pleasant hike to the springs and the small creeks and oases they support.*

General Information

Road status: Essentially roadless; easy access from paved road
Shortest hike: 0.9 mi, 460 ft one way / moderate
Longest hike: 4.8 mi, 3,330 ft one way / difficult
Main attractions: Mills, springs, creeks, flora, mining history, wildlife
USGS 15' and 7.5' topo maps: Emigrant Canyon
Maps: pp. 471*, 393

Location and Access

Journigan's Mill is located in Emigrant Canyon, in the western Panamint Mountains. It is reached by driving the Emigrant Canyon Road 6.5 miles south of Highway 190 (or 2.9 miles north of the Skidoo turnoff). It is marked by two old water tanks on the west side of the road.

Except for Burns Spring, all the springs used in the past to run Journigan's Mill are located up in the nameless canyon about 250 yards north of Journigan's Mill. For the most direct route to Burns Spring and its mill, park about 0.5 mile further south on the Emigrant Canyon Road and hike the old road (now a foot trail) on the west side.

History: Journigan's Mill

For several decades the site that became known as Journigan's Mill processed gold and silver ore from nearby mines, and it witnessed some of the most exciting moments in the mining history of Death Valley. By reducing the volume of useful ore, and thus cutting down on transportation costs, local processing was an important step towards profitable mining in remote areas. Journigan's Mill thus contributed to the success of several famous mines, including Skidoo and Harrisburg. The mill's location was dictated by the proximity of springs in two near-by canyons, which provided the water needed to run it.

The area saw its first activity perhaps as early as 1909, when Skidoo, across the hills to the east, was three years old and booming. At the time, a one-stamp mill was reportedly processing Skidoo ore. The first documented activity dates from about 10 years later, when Carl Suksdorf and famed single-blanket prospector Shorty Harris ran a custom ball mill for local miners. In 1924, Harris and another renowned prospector, Shorty Borden, were said to have operated a five-stamp mill here to process ore from the Skidoo and Poppy mines. However, this site did not fully expand until 1934, when the Gold Reserve Act sent the price of gold from around $20 to $35 an ounce, prompting the revival of mines at Skidoo and Harrisburg. In March that year, Roy Journigan and a few partners filed the first claim of this site, which they called the Gold Bottom Mill Site. Later on, Journigan acquired his partners' interests and formed the Journigan Mining and Milling Company. With a capacity to treat 25 tons a day, his plant was the largest around. It had a stamp mill, a cone-type ball mill, a crusher, amalgamation plates, and cyanide treatment. Water was initially piped from one spring only. In 1937 Journigan applied for water rights and a permit for a pipeline to also tap nearby Burro, Willow, Green, and Burns springs. For several years, ore from the tunnels and old dumps of the Skidoo and Cashier mines was trucked to the plant where it was crushed and treated before being shipped out.

Roy Journigan sold his mill in April 1939. The site still remained busy for years, undergoing several changes of ownership, transfers of water rights, and renovations. The Del Norte Mining Company, which was operating in the Skidoo area, acquired it in 1943. In subsequent years the company became actively involved in gold mining at Skidoo and used the water to operate Skidoo's mill. The Journigan site was rebuilt and operated in the 1950s, then acquired in 1959 by the Argentum Mining Company, which moved the machinery to Columbia Flats, Nevada. When the mill finally closed down in the late 1960s, it had been active longer than any other in the park.

Route Description

Journigan's Mill. You may want to start this hike by browsing through the remains of the mill, which has the largest ruins of an amalgamation and cyanide plant of the 1930-1950 era in Death Valley. Closest to the road are six of the concrete cyanide tanks from Journigan's era. The extensive concrete foundations and machinery pilings on the levelled bench above them mark the location of the mill, once covered by a large wooden structure. Debris and the foundations of several residences can still be found east of the site. The two 25,000-gallon steel tanks behind the mill were used to store the spring water. From here miles of disjointed pipes, slowly filling with dust, lead up the two nearby canyons to the springs.

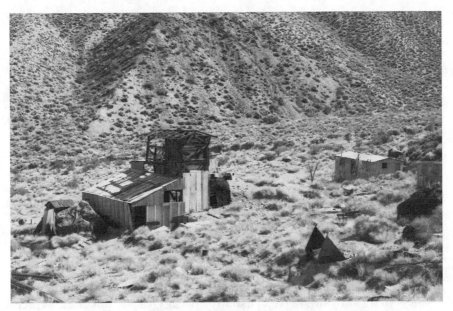

The Greene-Denner-Drake Millsite near Burns Spring

Hiking to the springs. The canyon to the main springs is mostly an open wash climbing between rounded hills, which is typical of the Emigrant Canyon drainage. The walking is fairly easy and usually comfortable at this cooler, higher elevation. Although closely spaced, the springs are very different. They attract birds, bighorn sheep and burros, whose prints and droppings are fairly common. In the winter and early spring most of the springs carry water, but in the summer and fall they often run dry. My first visit here was in February, after four consecutive dry winters, and their water level was abnormally low. I still found a small bridge of ice spanning the creek below Malapi Spring.

Burro Spring. On the way up, don't miss the massive pinnacle and sculptured walls around the first side canyon, near the end of the road. The first spring is Burro Spring, just inside the third side canyon on the east side, in a small amphitheater formed by a wide, curving, 20- to 40-foot cliff. A little water drips from the top of a fall eroded in the cliff. A tunnel was dug at the base of the cliff, perhaps for water reclamation. This spring is unusual for its setting, and its high cliff provides deep and welcome shade.

Canyon and Willow Springs. The next side canyon has two springs. Canyon Spring, a short distance in, is also a cliff spring, a patch of dampness surrounded by shrubs. Above it the side canyon squeezes through a narrow passage with short falls. It then turns to a wide open wash. In this barren land, the little creek that rises in the sandy wash a little further on comes as a surprise. Only a foot wide and 300 feet long, it nourishes green algae and patches of grass. Willow Spring is a little further, near the head of this side canyon. It normally has just a little ground moisture, yet underground water supports the largest and most scenic grove in this area, mostly willows and golden cane entangled with grapevine. Look around for typical high desert plants—Mormon tea, sage, cliffrose, and blackbrush.

From here you can loop back to your starting point by hiking over the low hill to the east (refer to Burns Spring below).

Green Spring and Malapi Spring. Back to the main canyon, at the next confluence (buried deep in alluvia) the right fork leads to Green Spring (misspelled "Greer" on USGS maps). This spring is located on a high ridge, and you'll need a map to find the right ravine or ridge to get to it. This is a more demanding hike, but the views make it worthwhile.

The main, left fork leads to Malapi Spring. The canyon cuts through reddish volcanic rock and is fairly narrow. In the cooler months it has a delightful little creek, usually the longest in this area, which starts just above the confluence. At places it flows over bedrock and produces small waterfalls. Elsewhere it vanishes, then resurfaces amidst algae and green shrubs. The narrow wash is densely crowded with brush and low trees, and you will need to bushwhack your way through or bypass this stretch along the low rim to get to the head of the spring.

Burns Spring and Journigan's Mill		
	Dist.(mi)	Elev.(ft)
Journigan's Mill	0.0	4,365
Side canyon to Burro Spring	0.8	4,670
Burro Spring	(0.1)	4,800
Side canyon to Willow Spring	0.9	4,720
Canyon Spring	(0.05)	4,750
Willow Spring	(0.8)	5,260
Burns Spring and millsite	(1.4)	~5,020
Back to starting point via trail	(2.9)	4,365
Side canyon to Green Spring	1.1	4,820
Green Spring	(0.3)	5,210
Malapi Spring	1.5	5,035
Unnamed Spring	1.7	5,205
Head	3.6	6,730
Jayhawker Canyon	3.9	6,580

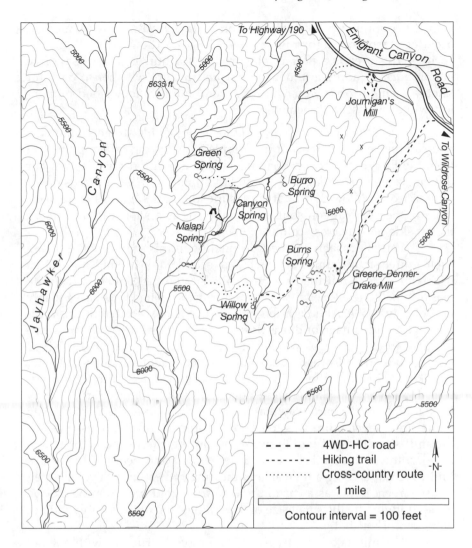

It is a peaceful spot where trees hugging a shallow overhang form a shady nook of greenery and stone. Look for a small arch in broken volcanic rock in the last bend below the spring, on the west side about 25 feet above the wash.

Shortly past Malapi Spring there is a small unnamed spring, a tangle of high shrubs clogging the open wash. From here you can take a cross-country shortcut to Willow Spring (0.5 mile) and make a loop back to Journigan's Mill. Hike up into the very short side canyon just below the unnamed spring and bear southeast across the hills to the second ravine, where Willow Spring is located. Instead, dedicated hikers may want to continue up the main canyon to Jayhawker Canyon, along a broader wash and high rolling hills. Far from the road and close to springs, this area is a perfect playground for burros. I once saw five young burros huddling under the sun and unsure whether to dash for safety. Their curiosity won, and for several minutes they stood motionless while we observed each other.

Burns Spring and the Greene-Denner-Drake Mill. To get to this site, you can hike either cross-country from Willow Spring or along the trail from the Emigrant Canyon Road 0.5 mile south of Journigan's Mill. For the first route (~0.6 mile), look for an old mining trail 50-100 yards down canyon from Willow Spring. It climbs mostly east to a low saddle overlooking the next canyon south. Burns Spring is a short distance down the far side (mostly cross-country).

This is probably the best destination in this area. Not the spring itself—three small clumps of vegetation, scattered on the hillside, with a trickle of water—but the forgotten mill located just below it. The site was originally developed by a prospector named Thad Greene, probably in the early 1950s. Although the mill was probably erected at this location to take advantage of Burns Spring's water, there are no mines nearby, and what ore it was processing remains a mystery. In 1952-1953 Greene located and prospected some tungsten claims about 4 miles up the Skidoo Road, and his mill may have been connected to this operation. However, the claims were never fully developed—Greene may have found out the hard way that here as elsewhere in the Death Valley region the tungsten ore was too poor to process on site. Subsequently, the mill site changed hands twice, becoming the property of Erwin Denner, then John Drake. At the time, Skidoo and nearby Journigan's Mill were undergoing a revival, and the new owners may have intended to use Greene's mill as a custom mill to treat gold ore from the Skidoo mines. Judging by the small size of the tailings, the mill probably did not witness much activity.

The mill itself is a two-story, tin-roofed structure with a small ore bin, custom-built settling tanks, and covered loading area. There is a fairly large concrete house nearby, with a home-made coal-burning stove, a few shelves and beds, and a bathroom with a tub. The residents enjoyed hot water, generated by a wood-fired heater just outside the house. The nearby junkyard is well stocked with car parts, which were used for welding. This is a delightful site, quite interesting yet often overlooked. The foot trail below the mill returns down the wide open canyon to the Emigrant Canyon Road.

■

PART IX

EUREKA, SALINE,
AND
PANAMINT VALLEYS

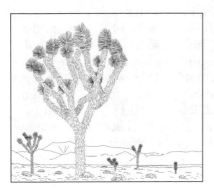

THE REGION COVERED in this last section is the three valleys on the west side of Death Valley. Like the latter, they are not true valleys but grabens, narrow, northwest-southeast trending tectonic sinks defined by fault-block mountains. Eureka Valley is the northernmost valley. Bounded by the Sylvania Mountains and the Last Chance Range to the east, by the Inyo Mountains and the Saline Range to the west, it extends further north than the northernmost tip of Death Valley. Saline Valley, the next one south, has roughly the same length as Eureka Valley, about 27 miles. It is sandwiched between the Saline Range and the Last Chance Range to the east, and the Inyo Mountains to the west. Panamint Valley, the southernmost of the three valleys, is by far the largest. Nearly 50 miles long, it parallels the southern part of Death Valley. It is flanked on its eastern side by the high Cottonwood and Panamint mountains. Its western boundary is formed by several lower ranges, from north to south: the Nelson Range, the southern tip of the Inyo Mountains, the Argus Range, and the Slate Range.

Not all of this region belongs to Death Valley National Park, and it is not completely uninhabited, but almost. The southern two thirds of Eureka Valley, all of Saline Valley, and the northern third of Panamint Valley are part of the park. The largest permanent center of human activity in this vast area is the small resort of Panamint Springs, on the edge of Panamint Valley. The only other human settlements are isolated private properties in Saline Valley and the small towns of Darwin, Indian Ranch, and Ballarat just outside the park. Panamint Springs is the only place that offers services—food, lodging, camping, showers, and gas. The closest towns are Big Pine, Lone Pine, Olancha, and Trona, all of them a good 40-minute drive from the park boundary. There is no water available in Eureka Valley or Saline Valley—at least no tap water.

This area, particularly Saline and Eureka valleys, ranks amongst the most remote in the California desert. To get to the heart of either valley takes a couple of hours of driving on dusty graded roads. Isolation is certainly a strong ingredient of their charm. I hope you will not encounter too many people when you go there, since being alone to explore it is what makes the experience unique. The downside, as usual, is that isolation can be dangerous. When you are in the middle of Saline Valley, you are far from help. A vehicle breakdown or physical injury a few miles from a road could leave you stranded for hours, if not days, without any human contact. Be prepared to handle such emergencies. Bring plenty of water and food, enough for a couple of days more than your intended stay, and a first aid kit. This is also true for winter, in the event a snow storm cuts you off overnight from a main highway. Bring tire chains, even if the forecast is favorable. Take warm clothes and sleeping gear with you, even if you are not planning to stay overnight. Again, Saline Valley has a few residents. Respect their privacy, and contact them only in case of an emergency. If possible, check Saline Valley's Lower Warm Springs first; the warden who is sometimes based there has a radio telephone.

Weather

In all three valleys the weather is comparable to that of Death Valley, although not as extreme. The first reason is their location, further north and west, which means slightly higher precipitation. The second one is their higher elevation—the low points are 2,870' in Eureka Valley, 1,060' in Saline Valley, and 1,040' in Panamint Valley—which means slightly lower temperatures. In Saline Valley and Eureka Valley, another factor is the Inyo Mountains, which are high enough to create their own weather. In the winter and spring, they can capture a lot of moisture brought in from the Pacific Ocean, and they are often covered with thick clouds that cool down the air significantly. But it is still desert weather, quite dry and usually only a few degrees cooler than Death Valley. In the summer, that's still plenty hot. Daytime temperatures are commonly above 100°F, and nights can still be a little too hot for comfortable sleeping. In the winter, it gets cold, even on the valley floors. At such times you may want to take advantage of Death Valley's few extra degrees.

Access and Backcountry Roads

The main access road to Eureka Valley is the Big Pine Road, which starts from Highway 168, 2.3 miles east of Big Pine, and ends after about 72 miles near Ubehebe Crater. It is a very scenic road, and one of the most lonesome backcountry roads this desert has to offer. From its start at the western foot of the Inyo Mountains, it climbs through forested slopes to a pass near 7,600', then drops along the east side of the mountains to the dense Joshua tree forest of Joshua Flats. After losing several thousand feet of elevation, it comes out of the range on the edge of Eureka Valley and glides down across it on long empty desert slopes. On the far side of the valley, before continuing over the Last Chance Range to Death Valley, the road crosses the North and South Eureka Valley roads. These two roads give access to some of the most scenic places in and around Eureka Valley, including Cucomungo Canyon and the Eureka Dunes.

The Saline Valley Road, the main graded artery through Saline Valley, is equally scenic. Starting from Highway 190 just west of the park boundary, it wanders across the colorful rolling terrain of Santa Rosa Flat, then crosses the low Santa Rosa Hills. On the other side of the hills is Lee Flat, a narrow high desert valley hosting one of the most impressive Joshua tree forests in the northern Mojave Desert. Some of the trees reach over 30 feet and have exceptionally dense branched crowns. You may want to take a side trip on the good graded road up Lee Flat, or a random walk through the largest Joshua tree forest in the park. Past Lee Flat, the Saline Valley Road ascends the southwestern slope of Hunter Mountain. Over the next few miles everything changes rapidly. Joshua trees are replaced by barren desert slopes, then by one of the thickest pine forests in the park. The junction with the Hunter Mountain Road is just past the high point of this southern approach into Saline Valley (near 6,200'), locally referred to as South Pass. Stop here to enjoy the magnificent views of Panamint Valley down steep-walled Mill Canyon, especially the pale dunes resting on the sweeping fan below. From here the road winds down along spring-dotted Grapevine Canyon into Saline Valley. After traversing the valley northward, it climbs steeply up through Whippoorwill Canyon to forested North Pass (~7,300'), then drops into Marble Canyon. From here it climbs again to eventually reach the pavement at the Big Pine Road (~7,500') about 15.7 miles east of Big Pine.

Both the Big Pine and Saline Valley roads are mostly graded but they are long, and driving them should not be undertaken lightly. The closest services are at Scotty's Castle, Big Pine, and Panamint Springs. In the summer, the high temperatures and the long stretches of rattling washboards may trigger an unexpected car breakdown. A robust, preferably high-clearance, vehicle will reduce the chance of running into trouble. This is not meant to discourage you from coming here without one, however. Every year in the dry season many people make it

Suggested Hikes around Eureka, Saline, and Panamint Valleys					
Route/Destination	Dist. (mi)	Elev. change	Mean elev.	Access road	Pages
Short hikes (under 5 miles round trip)					
Arcane Meadows	2.4	1,510'	8,880'	P/1.6 mi	518-520
Big Dodd Spring	2.5	2,120'	~4,300'	Graded	325-326
Craig Canyon (lower cyn)	1.5	1,480'	2,260'	P/1.5 mi	496
Darwin Falls (first fall)	1.1	220'	2,650'	Graded	506-507
Darwin Falls (highest fall)	1.3	~310'	2,680'	Graded	506-508
Eureka Dunes (sand mtn)	1.3	650'	3,200'	Graded	482
Hummingbird Spring	1.0	910'	6,860'	H/1.8 mi	516
Hunter Canyon (sixth fall)	1.3	1,200'	2,120'	P/1.0 mi	497-500
Lippincott Mine Road	2.5	1,230'	3,170'	P/4.4 mi	325
Little Hunter Canyon spr.*	0.5	440'	1,710'	P/1.0 mi	489-490
Monarch Mine	2.0	1,110'	5,000'	Paved	512-513
Mud Spring	2.1	960'	3,590'	Graded	516
Saline Valley Dunes	0-2	<300'	1,160'	Graded	490
Saline Valley salt lake	1.5	60'	1,070'	Graded	489
Upper Warm Spring	2.4	360'	1,650'	P/0.6 mi	491
Intermediate hikes (5-12 miles round trip)					
Bighorn Mine trail (summit)	4.4	4,620'	3,800'	P/1.0 mi	500
Bighorn Spr. (Hunter Cyn)	3.9	3,430'	3,310'	P/1.0 mi	497-500
Bighorn Spring (via trail)	5.2	5,580'	4,110'	P/1.0 mi	500
Blue Jay Mine from Saline V.	6.0	1,410'	2,050'	Graded	322
Craig Canyon (narrows)	2.9	2,600'	2,890'	P/1.5 mi	496-497
Craig Canyon (to spring)	4.7	4,110'	3,650'	P/1.5 mi	496-497
Darwin Canyon (rd to rd)	2.6	~700'	2,850'	Graded	506-510
Eagle Spring	5.2	1,820'	9,210'	P/1.6 mi	518-520
Eureka Dunes (south dunes)	4.9	~1,300'	3,160'	Graded	482
Hidden Dunes	3.4	530'	3,170'	P/2.4 mi	484
Mohawk Mine and Tuber Pk	3.9	2,610'	5,610'	Paved	512-514
Panamint Valley Dunes	3.9	~1,100'	2,120'	Graded	501-504
Salt Tram first control station	~3.5	2,600'	2,040'	Graded	488-489
Wildrose antimony mines*	4.8	2,490'	5,450'	Paved	512-514
Wildrose Peak	4.2	2,160'	8,000'	Graded	517-518
Long hikes (over 12 miles round trip)					
Bighorn Mine (Hunter Cyn)	5.3	5,060'	3,970'	P/1 mi	497-500
Bighorn Mine (via trail)	6.6	7,280'	4,470'	P/1 mi	500
Burgess Mine via Craig Cyn	8.5	8,200'	5,500'	P/1.5 mi	496-497
Burgess Mine (via trail)	12.7	11,520'	6,210'	P/1 mi	500

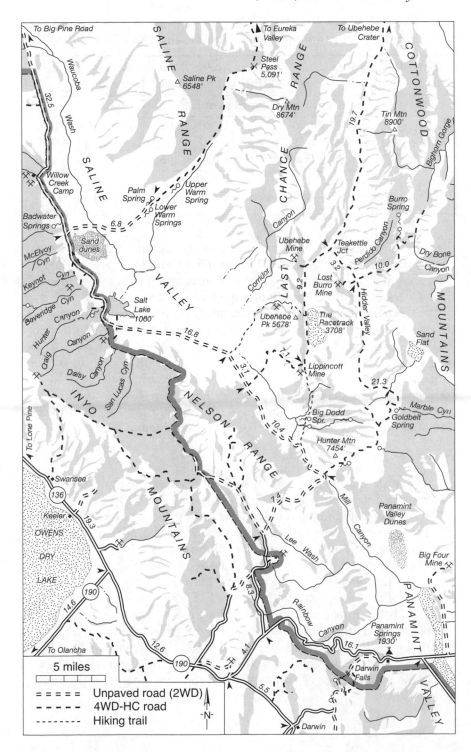

To Big Pine Road

Waucoba

32.5

SALINE RANGE

Saline Pk
6548'

To Eureka
Valley

Steel
Pass
5,091'

Dry Mtn
8674'

To Ubehebe
Crater

COTTONWOOD

Tin Mtn
8900'

Bighorn Gorge

LAST CHANCE RANGE

19.7

Palm
Spring

Upper Warm
Spring

Lower
Warm
Springs

Willow
Creek
Camp

Badwater
Springs

6.8

McElvoy
Cyn

Sand
dunes

Keynot
Cyn

Boveridge Cyn

Hunter
Canyon

Craig Canyon

Salt
Lake
1060'

Daisy Canyon

San Lucas Cyn

SALINE

VALLEY

Canyon

Corridor

Ubehebe
Mine

Teakettle
Jct

Perdido Canyon

Burro
Spring

Dry Bone
Canyon

3.2

10.0

9.2

Lost
Burro
Mine

Hidden Valley

MOUNTAINS

Ubehebe
Pk 5678'

The
Racetrack
3708'

Sand
Flat

16.8

7.1

Lippincott
Mine

21.3

INYO

3.7

NELSON RANGE

Big Dodd
Spr.

Marble Cyn

Goldbelt
Spring

To Lone Pine

10.4

Hunter Mtn
7454'

Swansea

136

Keeler

193

MOUNTAINS

7.4

Mill Canyon

Panamint
Valley
Dunes

OWENS

DRY

LAKE

190

146

To Olancha

12.6

8.3

Lee Wash

Rainbow Canyon

190

4.1

5.5

16.1

Panamint
Springs
1930'

Big Four
Mine

PANAMINT

VALLEY

Darwin
Falls

Darwin

5 miles

===== Unpaved road (2WD)
- - - - 4WD-HC road
- - - - - - Hiking trail

-N-

Suggested Hikes around Eureka, Saline, and Panamint Valleys					
Route / Destination	Dist. (mi)	Elev. change	Mean elev.	Access road	Pages
Long hikes (over 12 miles round trip) (Cont'd)					
The Corridor from Saline V.	9.6	1,780'	1,990'	Graded	310
Telescope Peak Trail	6.5	3,150'	9,570'	P/1.6 mi	518-522
Ubehebe Peak from Saline V.	8.9	4,300'	2,780'	Graded	322
Key: P=Primitive (2WD) H=Primitive (HC) * =Total distance and elevation change (ups + downs) for all loops					

through with standard-clearance sedans. Just come prepared for an emergency. In the winter, North Pass and South Pass, especially the former, are often closed because of snow, sometimes for several weeks at a time. Check current road conditions at a ranger station.

Panamint Valley, in contrast, is most accessible, being crossed by paved roads along its length (the Panamint Valley and Trona-Wildrose roads) and width (Highway 190). However, the northern part of the valley, within the park boundaries, is essentially roadless. The short, primitive spur to the Big Four Mine is the only road there. In the southern part of Panamint Valley, the Indian Ranch Road, Ballarat Road, and Wingate Road are the main access routes to the spectacular canyons and mines on the west side of the Panamint Mountains.

Hiking

To pare down the wealth of three vast and magnificent desert valleys to a few pages was, to say the least, difficult. By necessity, the few hikes suggested in the following pages represent but a limited sample. I have tried to cover not so much the most spectacular places as a wide cross section of destinations, mainly to give a flavor of the variety of settings one can experience here. Just remember that there is much more—such as the dozen or so canyons that slice down the precipitous east side of the Panamint Mountains. All of them are steep, long, deep, delightfully unknown, and tough even for the best trained hikers. Or the twisted canyons that plunge into the north arm of Panamint Valley—hardly ever visited places like Mill Canyon, Lee Wash, or Dolomite Canyon. What about climbing Hunter Mountain? Or a leisure walk across the pristine floor of Eureka Valley? Your imagination is the limit.

■

THE EUREKA DUNES

> *If I had to choose one place to show a friend how beautiful the Great Basin is, I might well pick the Eureka Dunes. Towering more than 650 feet above pristine Eureka Valley, framed by imposing desert ranges, they are a desert fantasy. Walking on this spellbinding mountain of sand, with its unusual flora and fauna, is a unique experience you'll remember for years.*

General Information

Road status: Roadless; easy access from 44-mile graded road
Shortest hike: 1.3 mi, ~650 ft one way/moderate
Longest hike: ~11 mi, ~1,500 ft loop (or more)/difficult
Main attractions: Spectacular high dunes in a remote desert valley
USGS 15' topo map: Last Chance Range
USGS 7.5' topo maps: Last Chance Range SW, Hanging Rock Canyon
Maps: pp. 483*, 289

Location and Access

The Eureka Dunes are located in the southern part of Eureka Valley. To get there, starting from the paved road at Ubehebe Crater, drive the Big Pine Road about 33.8 miles to the South Eureka Valley Road. Take this road 9.8 miles to the primitive campsites at the northwest corner of the dunes and park. Although it's a long, dusty drive, standard-clearance vehicles can make it without difficulty. You can also drive and start hiking from further along this road, which continues past a group of walk-in campsites to the east side of the dunes. This part is usually sandy and needs 4-wheel drive with good clearance.

Natural History

Like most dunes in the region, the Eureka Dunes are located in a dry lake bed, near the bottom of a valley that has no outlet to the sea. They were formed after the lake that filled Eureka Valley dried up at the end of the Pleistocene. All that is left of the lake today is Eureka Dry Lake, the playa northwest of the dunes.

Unique for their striking beauty, the Eureka Dunes are also special in many other ways. Some 650 feet high, they are among the tallest sand dunes in the Great Basin. No one knows why they are so high. By preventing the sand from spreading out, the relatively abundant plants that live on the dunes may help them to stay that way. How does the vegetation get its water? Although they do not look like it, compared to most dunes the Eureka Dunes are wet. Being close to the Last Chance Range, they receive some of the moisture captured by these high mountains and have stored a huge reserve of water. It is this underground water which, as it slowly percolates to the surface, feeds the plants.

The Eureka Dunes are home to over 50 species of plants, including common dune vegetation like creosote and indigo bush. Several plants are also endemic to these few square miles of sand. The most common is a dune grass (*Swallensia*) uniquely adapted to survival in shifting sands. It is more abundant around the foot of the dunes, and helps to stabilize the dunes by holding sand together. Another endemic is a species of locoweed (*Astragalus*), which bears striking white and purple flowers. The Eureka evening primrose, more rare, blooms only in the spring after a wet winter, producing large, white showy flowers.

The fauna is as unusually rich as the flora. Dozens of species of birds and mammals, nine species of reptiles, and countless species of insects, including four endemic beetles, inhabit the dunes. Most of the mammals are rodents, like the kangaroo mouse and rat, which have adapted to the hot and arid dune environment by living in burrows and metabolizing their own water from fats. Rodents prefer to burrow in the sheets of sand surrounding the dunes. At places the density of burrows is so high that it is almost impossible to walk without breaking through the sand. If you run into one of these rodent condos, turn around and look for another way through—no need to force the little creatures to remodel.

Another unusual feature of the Eureka Dunes is that they are one of the very few singing dunes in North America. Under the right circumstances, the dunes produce a low humming vibration that has been compared to the sound of a distant airplane or a bass viol. The noise is thought to be generated by wind-blown grains of sand rubbing against each other. However, it is not clear what triggers it—people walking on the dunes, wind blowing over a particular surface, or sand cascading down a steep slope. One thing is clear: the sound itself, which is quite striking.

Topographic maps show that back in the 1950s, the Eureka Dunes were about 65 feet taller than they are today. Although this could be the result of erroneous mapping or natural evolution, a more likely reason is human abuse. Up until the late 1970s, this area witnessed increasing use by dune buggies, motorcycles, and even trucks, which slowly broke down the dunes and killed the plants that hold them together. Two decades after the off-road ban, the dunes, seemingly impervious to external forces, may still be slowly getting back to their former height. Since this area is bound to witness increasing visitation, unruly foot traffic may ultimately cause the same problems. Tread lightly on the dune world: walk on the stronger ridges, and stay away from unstable steep slopes and plants.

Route Description

As you approach the Eureka Dunes along the road, they rise tall and sharp above the flat valley floor, shimmering white and strangely precarious against the background of rugged desert mountains. The contrast between sand and the spectacularly banded range is stunning. When you reach their base you realize they are not really dunes but a mountain of sand, hundreds of feet high. The north face is truly a sand wall, chiseled by the wind into long arcuate ramps that snake up gracefully to the keen edge of the distant summit. In the winter, the ranges are sometimes covered with snow, and the mind struggles to adjust to yet another incongruous element.

The Eureka Dunes cover an oblong area pointing north, about 3.5 miles by 1 to nearly 2 miles wide. The sand mountain occupies roughly the northern half (about 2.2 square miles). The southern half is composed of smaller dunes, and an extensive sheet of sand almost completely surrounds the dunes. Consider the following possible hikes and destinations, in increasing level of difficulty.

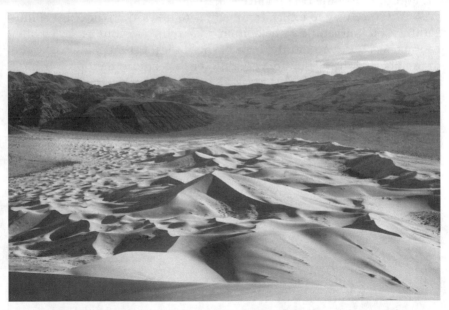

The southern part of the Eureka Dunes, seen from the sand mountain

Climbing the sand mountain. The top of the sand mountain is a popular destination for a short day hike. With slopes exceeding 45% at places, the abrupt northern and western walls make uphill progress almost hopeless, and hiking here is visually damaging. Please stay away from them. Instead, climb the more moderate northwestern ridge. It is still hard going, and slipping one step down for every few steps up can be frustrating, but the rewards match the effort. The soft sand underfoot, the rhythmic patterns of the dunes, and the shifting horizon all add up to a rare experience. If it isn't too hot, try going barefoot, at least part way. Take a break here and there to study the many imprints left in the sand by the locals—rodents, lizards, snakes, birds, and sometimes larger mammals. In the early morning when the tracks are clearest, it is a delight to follow them up and down hills of sand and try to reconstruct their owners' nocturnal activities.

From the highest ridge, the views of the pristine valley and desert ranges are truly awe-inspiring. The sand mountain has four summits, three at about the same elevation, the fourth one a little lower. At the south end of the Eureka Dunes, where the Saline Range and the Last Chance Range converge and the valley floor tapers down to a V, they break down into a sea of basins and swales. The sand seems to flow out of the V, as if the dunes were spawned by the mountain. Bring binoculars, and try to spot the shoreline of the old Pleistocene lake northwest of the dunes. Or visually "hike" into some of the tortuous canyons draining the abrupt face of the Last Chance Range.

A nice way to return from here is to hike down the ridge south-southwest to the saddle at the bottom, then return to your car by circling counterclockwise around the base of the dunes. If time allows, explore the southern dunes. They are very different, oceanic in their proportions, and even less crowded. This area is a photographer's paradise, particularly early and late in the day when the dunes are enhanced by long shadows.

The Eureka Dunes		
	Dist.(mi)	Elev.(ft)
Road	0.0	~2,870
Top of sand mountain	1.3	~3,525
Saddle	2.7	~3,050
South end of dunes	(2.2)	~3,040
Return via east side	~6.4	2,871

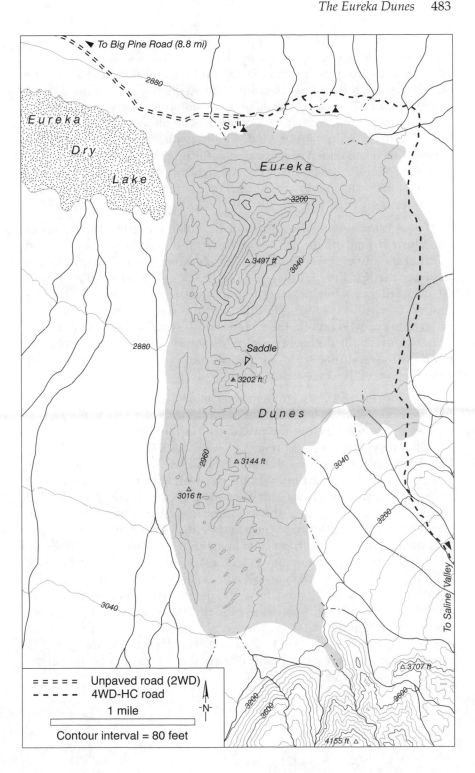

To Big Pine Road (8.8 mi)

2880

Eureka

Dry

Lake

Eureka

3200

S ▪

△ 3497 ft

3040

Saddle

2880

▲ 3202 ft

Dunes

2960

△ 3144 ft

3040

△ 3016 ft

3200

3040

△ 3707 ft

To Saline Valley

===== Unpaved road (2WD)
- - - - - 4WD-HC road

1 mile -N-

Contour interval = 80 feet

3200

3600

3600

4155 ft △

Eureka Dry Lake. For a little more diversity, walk to the dunes across the valley's dry lake. Park by the road 1.5 miles before the dunes (about 8 miles from the Big Pine Road), and hike south to and across the lake bed (~1.3 miles), then southeast towards the saddle mentioned above (another 2.3 miles). This hike offers an opportunity to sample the unusual surface of the dry playa, as well as an almost surreal approach to this unlikely mountain of sand. The playa is sometimes filled with water. It then becomes a great mirror, reflecting the dunes in one direction, the Saline Range in the other. At such times, or if the playa is still drying, don't walk on it to avoid marring it with unsightly and long-lasting footprints.

A canyon route. For a longer day hike featuring the dunes as your turn-around point, try hiking down the nameless major canyon north of the dunes. Start from the Big Pine Road about 26.3 miles from the Ubehebe Road (or 7.5 miles east of the South Eureka Valley Road), where it reaches a low point at a wash crossing and makes a sharp U-shaped bend (Elev. 4,570'). The hiking route goes down this wash 3.7 miles to the canyon mouth, then 3 miles down the fan to the road by the dunes (Elev. 2,871'). The canyon, wide and open at first, eventually winds through a nice little gorge. The fan part of the hike features superb views of the dunes from above.

The Hidden Dunes. If you prefer your dunes completely people-free, you may want to try the other main dunes in Eureka Valley, about 9 miles to the west, below the mouth of Marble Canyon. To minimize walking, drive the South Eureka Valley Road 3.45 miles from the Big Pine Road (or 6.35 miles north from the Eureka Dunes) to a road on the west side, and drive it 2.4 miles to the dry well at its end. This side road is usually passable with a standard-clearance vehicle. The Hidden Dunes are on the far side of the long sprawling ridge to the west—you can see them poking through a gap in the ridge. It's 3.2 miles to this gap, a lonesome desert walk almost clear across Eureka Valley. The dunes are just beyond the gap, where they extend a couple of miles along the back side of the ridge. From the gap it's an exhilarating 160-foot scramble to the nearby sand summit, then down the nearly 100-foot bowl south of it. At their south end, swirls of wind-blown sand festoon the high, rocky slopes, creating a desolate landscape one would only expect to find on some far away desert planet. This is a wonderful site, delightfully remote, seemingly forgotten on the edge of this long valley hidden at the confluence of two mountain ranges.

∎

SALINE VALLEY

> *Saline Valley is a world in itself, with enough to offer that an entire book could be dedicated to it. In many ways it is a parallel incarnation of Death Valley, complete with salt flats, sand dunes, towering mountains, precipitous canyons, waterfalls, springs, forgotten mines, silence, and solitude. Secluded, miraculously free of commercial enterprises, spared the humiliation of asphalted roadways, it is a perfect target for lonesome adventures in the desert.*

General Information

Road status: Graded road to and through the valley
Shortest hike: Strolls and short walks/easy
Longest hike: 3.5 miles, 2,600 ft one way (or more)/strenuous
Main attractions: Little traveled valley, dunes, salt lake, springs, solitude
USGS 15' topo maps: Waucoba Wash*, New York Butte*, Dry Mountain, Ubehebe Peak
USGS 7.5' topo maps: Pat Keyes Canyon,* Lower Warm Springs*, Craig Canyon*, West of Ubehebe Peak, West of Teakettle Junction
Maps: pp. 493*, 491, 477

Location and Access

Saline Valley is located west of north-central Death Valley, between the southern Last Chance Range and the Inyo Mountains. It is traversed approximately north-south by the Saline Valley Road, which connects Highway 190 to the Big Pine Road. It is graded and generally suitable for standard-clearance vehicles. Refer to *Eureka, Saline, and Panamint Valleys* for a description of this wild route. Two other roads lead into Saline Valley. The first one, the Lippincott Road, connects the Racetrack Valley Road to the Saline Valley Road near its south end. The second road is the continuation of the South Eureka Valley Road over Steel Pass, which joins the Saline Valley Road near its midpoint, at the dunes. These two roads require 4-wheel drive and high clearance.

History: The Salt Tram

Of the entire Death Valley region, Saline Valley witnessed what was one of the grandest and perhaps most unexpected mining enterprises. Unlike most, this venture was not interested in precious metals or gems but a dirt-cheap commodity known as halide—table salt. It all started in 1874, when the first discovery of borax in California was made on the floor of Saline Valley. The following year two men by the names of Conn and Trudo started a small borax operation near the northwest corner of the salt lake. It was quite a success: in the early 1890s they were the largest single borax producers in the country. They produced continuously until 1895, and more sporadically until 1907. The main driving force behind salt mining was an attorney named White Smith, who came here to work as a teamster for the borax mine. Smith became fascinated not by borax but by the vast halide fields surrounding the lake. He and others filed dozens of claims, but it was not until around 1911 that Smith organized the Saline Valley Salt Company and became serious about it.

Although a rough road led up the valley to Big Pine, the company somehow decided to go all out and set up a contract for the construction of a 13.5-mile aerial tramway clear across the Inyos. It would climb some 7,700 feet across the deep chasm of Daisy Canyon to a control station at the 8,740-foot crest of the mountains, then drop 5,100 feet on the far side to a railroad terminal on the shore of Owens Lake. Crossing one of the highest, steepest, and roughest ranges in this desert, subjected to extreme temperature variations, it was, to say the least, a tremendous engineering challenge. It called for two terminals, four control stations, 21 rail structures and 12 anchorage-tension stations. Around lower Daisy Canyon, the terrain was so rough that a temporary tramway had to be erected to transport supplies and water. The project took 1.3 million board feet of lumber, 650 tons of nuts and bolts, and 54 miles of cable. Construction was completed in 1913, and in July the first salt was delivered at Tramway, the discharge terminal by Owens Lake.

The salt was mined using a system of dikes to flood selected areas of the salt playa with fresh water from nearby Hunter Canyon. The water was allowed to evaporate, leaving behind nearly pure salt crystals. The salt was shoveled into 2-foot piles, then loaded into special half-ton capacity buggies with foot-wide steel wheels. The buggies were winched back to shore, where wooden cars transported the ore to the tramway terminal. The salt was finally loaded into one of the tramway's 286 buckets, which were hauled away at a rate of about one bucket per minute. By the end of the year, 5,000 tons of salt had been delivered.

Mining was straightforward, but operating the tramway was another matter. Due to an engineering flaw, the grips that clamped the buckets on the tramway cable slipped when the buckets were more than two thirds full. It took two years and several attempts to solve the problem. In the meantime, the tramway had to be operated at partial capacity. Perhaps as a result, and in spite of steady delivery, the company was in financial trouble. It was forced to lease its salt claims and tramway to the Owens Valley Salt Company, with the arrangement that profits were evenly split between them. By 1916, with the grip problem fixed, the

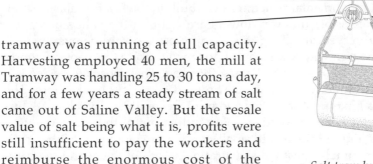

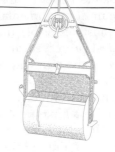

tramway was running at full capacity. Harvesting employed 40 men, the mill at Tramway was handling 25 to 30 tons a day, and for a few years a steady stream of salt came out of Saline Valley. But the resale value of salt being what it is, profits were still insufficient to pay the workers and reimburse the enormous cost of the tramway. In 1920 the company that had erected the tramway repossessed it, and the two salt companies went under.

Salt tram bucket

But Smith did not give up. While salt mining stood idle, he convinced the county to construct a road out of Saline Valley south via San Lucas Canyon to Owens Valley. The road took two years to complete. In May 1926 the salt fields, then owned by Smith and a partner, George Russell, were reactivated under the newly formed Sierra Salt Company. Trucks hauled 10-ton loads of salt over the new road to the railroad at Tramway. Smith died in 1927, and never saw his tramway come back to life. But it did the following year, when the Sierra Salt Company decided to acquire it, revamp it, and put it to use again. By December 1928, the salt tram was delivering 60 to 100 tons every day. It did so for a few years, until prices plummeted in the Depression and production was discontinued, this time forever, around 1933. For all its unlikeliness, Smith's dream had come true: for about 12 years salt was successfully mined out of Saline Valley, most of it via his fabulous tramway.

Route Description

Saline Valley is a very special place. It is in many ways a scaled-down replica of Death Valley, made of the same building blocks, only strangely disarranged. A Death Valley of years ago, with no paved roads, no towns, next to no road signs, and few visitors. From almost anywhere you will not see a single light at night. Such places are rare. Saline Valley is in fact one of the largest essentially uninhabited desert valleys in North America. Framed between tremendous mountain ranges, it is also a spectacular place, with so much hiking to offer that it is impossible to do justice to it in a few pages. This and the following section on the Inyo Mountains cover only a few common destinations, just to get you started.

The salt tramway and evaporators. The most spectacular legacy of the Saline Valley Salt Company is the tramway itself, one of the two or three most monumental structures ever built in the Death Valley region. The most accessible tramway towers are right on the valley floor, and the best preserved are along the short access road to the evaporators. Three of the tramway towers and two smaller poles (perhaps telegraph or telephone poles) still stand along the road. Their obsolete design is a delightful testimony of the past. The road ends at the lakeshore. The ground is a mixture of salt brine and mud, generally too wet to walk further. The long rows of wooden stakes jutting out of the lake were used to partition the salt fields into small ponds for evaporation. Other remnants are minimal—mostly disintegrating shreds of metal and salt-saturated wood illustrating the powerful corrosive action of salt. With binoculars you'll be able to spot remains of the salt stacks on the lake's playa.

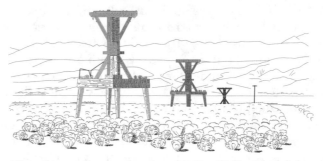

The salt tramway on the edge of Saline Valley's salt lake

As usual the best is beyond the end of the road, in this case perched high on a steep ridge of the Inyo Mountains directly south of the evaporators. To get there, drive the Big Silver Mine Road (which starts across from the road to the evaporators) about 0.4 mile to a faint road on the left and park. This was the tramway maintenance road. It is now closed to motor vehicles, so continue on foot. It passes by quite a few tower ruins and bits of cable lying on the ground before ending at the collapsed ruins of a huge anchorage-tension station, on the edge of the deep wash of Daisy Canyon. To hike the tramway trail, walk south of the tower, down into the wash, then across the wash to the ravine just east of Daisy Canyon. The faint trail climbing east at the mouth of the ravine is the Salt Tramway Trail. Over the next 8.3 miles it ascends about 7,000 feet to the crest of the Inyos, bypassing the spectacular tramway towers. Though the trail is now wiped out at the Daisy Canyon crossing, it is still in good shape up to that point. This is also one of the most spectacular trails in the Mojave Desert, and the hike is well worth it.

To reap the full benefit from this strenuous climb, go as far as the fifth and much larger structure. This is the first control station, a long and imposing wooden trestle designed to change the direction of the cable. It is surprisingly well-preserved, reminiscent of early railroad bridges. Anchored precariously on a sloping ledge 2,500 feet above the valley, it is a breathtaking sight, and an enduring testimony of early desert mining. There are five more towers further on before the trail ends at the sheer edge of Daisy Canyon, but this is a good place to stop.

The salt lake. The salt lake can be accessed at the evaporators (see previous section) or at the marsh at the west end of the lake. This area was fenced off for protection against wild burros, but it was unfortunately left open for humans to drive in. The soft salt-laden ground within the "protected" area is now crisscrossed with vehicle tracks. Until this situation is rectified, if it ever is, a walk here is somewhat pointless.

For an easy walk by the lake away from cars, drive the Saline Valley Road to the north end of the fence, which is just across the turnoff to Hunter Canyon, and park. Walk down the short road spur that follows the fence towards the lake. You'll get some good views of the marsh and its thick belt of mesquite and reeds. The gray-green plant growing along the road is arrowweed. Closer to the lake, it is replaced by dark blue-green, more salt-tolerant pickleweed. After 0.3 mile the road ends at an old turnout, close to the lakeshore. Look for a faint foot trail to the left and follow it north as it parallels the lake, along salt-encrusted ground covered with small pinnacles. The size and shape of the lake depend greatly on the time of year and on how wet the last winter has been. The trail is generally not right up against the water, yet you may see sandpipers and stilts a short distance away—sea birds usually encountered along the seashore. After about 0.4 mile, the trail reaches a long ramp made of mud, salt, and decaying boards, which is part of one of the 1880-1910 borax operations. A little further on, if the lake is low enough, you can walk out onto the salt pan. Small seeps pool up at the very edge of the pan. The water originates in Hunter Canyon to the west and flows underneath the fan before resurging here, at the valley's lowest point. The salt pan is often covered with large polygons (see *The Badwater Basin*). Tread lightly throughout this area.

Little Hunter Canyon spring. The lush, well-watered spring at the mouth of Little Hunter Canyon, just west of the salt lake, is one of the largest and most interesting springs in Saline Valley. The starting point of this hike is the same as for the Bighorn Mine trail (see *Inyo Mountains*). At the T at the end of the Hunter Canyon Road, make a left to the signed trail (Lonesome Miner Trail) on the edge of the spring. For a short walk through the spring and back the same way, take this trail. To hike the more eventful loop described below, take the other, fainter trail, which starts up the road cut on the right about 10 yards before the spring.

From the road, hike the trail up the hillside to the rim of Little Hunter Canyon, where you'll get your first bird's eye view of the sprawling spring in the canyon below. The trail follows the rim for a while, then drops to the canyon wash and disappears. Walk down the wide wash towards the spring a few hundred yards. The trail resumes on the south side of the wash, where it winds through a thick stand of arrowweed before entering the spring. What I like about this place is its wildly different mood. In just a few steps the desert leaves the stage to a dense oasis of willow and mesquite trees, entangled in thick mats of grapevine. A little creek runs through it, wandering silently in the deep shade, forking several times and flooding the trail at places. In the summer the high evaporation rate and the canopy of trees create a microclimate, a small pocket of steamy tropical jungle far away from the desert you just left. The luxuriant plants, the heady smells of wet earth, and the sound of the creek, all conspire to fool your senses. Bird watching is good—I spotted wrens, hummingbirds, swifts, ravens, and hawks. The re-entry into the desert is equally sudden: the trail joins the road on the searing edge of the desert, a short distance from your starting point.

The dunes. Saline Valley's dunes are not very extensive. They cover only approximately 2.2 square miles, a good portion of it made of whaleback dunes (see *The Death Valley Sand Dunes, Geology*). Nor are they very high. The tallest humps of sand rise only a few tens of feet above their surroundings. But they possess all the wonderful attributes of dunes, plus one: they are delightfully, almost miraculously pristine. On my few visits here I did not see a single human footprint. It was even a little painful to leave my own tracks on such immaculate terrain.

The Saline Valley dunes draw much of their beauty from their spectacular setting, almost right up against the formidable escarpment of the Inyo Mountains. Their uniqueness lies in this stunning juxtaposition of sand and stone: light against dark, smoothness against ruggedness, ripples against towering heights. It is a tranquil place, easier to walk than other dunes, with generous space to wander aimlessly. Start from the short road that cuts off the Saline Valley Road, 5.9 miles north of the evaporators turnoff. You will find a different association of plants here than at other dunes, including arrowweed, bursage, desert holly, cattle spinach, mesquite trees, inkweed, and sandpaper plant. A strange kind of beetle lives here—only a quarter inch in size, almost round, black with delicate gold trim around their heads. Although they spend a good part of their time lying immobile, they will suddenly start madly scurrying up steep slopes, as if their life depended on it, only to stop seconds later, at no particular place. They are fun to watch.

The warm springs. Saline Valley's warm springs can be reached by road, which makes them a popular destination and camping spot, if not a good hiking goal. In the 1960s and 1970s a small hippie community squatted here part of the year, and over time the springs were altered and developed. The road to the springs, which starts off the Saline Valley Road just north of the dunes, is in decent shape up to Lower Warm Springs, the largest and most developed of the three main springs. The spring water is diverted to rock-rimmed concrete tubs where visitors can enjoy a hot bath in a serene oasis of fan palms and mesquite trees. The self-appointed caretakers who take turns living here keep the place clean and in good shape. On long weekends, however, it has all the charm of a busy parking lot. Regulations are likely to change in the future as the popularity of this place continues to increase.

Past Lower Warm Springs the road continues eastward 0.6 mile to Palm Spring, smaller and almost equally developed, then 2.4 more miles to Upper Warm Spring. High clearance is mandatory about half a mile before getting there. Upper Warm Spring is the least disturbed. It has a large, deep pool of blue-green, lukewarm water, surrounded by arrowweed and grasses. It was fenced off years ago for protection against wild burros (which abound throughout this area) and to prevent it from becoming another drive-in spa. The creamy white rock abundantly exposed around all three springs is travertine. For a longer walk, check out the smaller springs on the fan to the south.

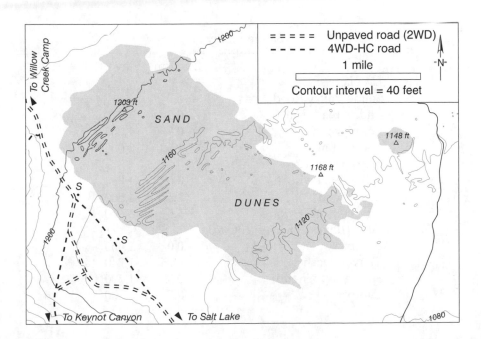

From here the road continues many rough miles to Steel Pass and eventually down into Eureka Valley, bisecting what was until recently the largest roadless area in the country outside of Alaska. This road was created illegally by irresponsible drivers. It should have been obliterated long ago, or at least when this land was added to the park. It still may be in the future. Road or no road, you may want to consider an overnight trip up the Steel Pass corridor, which gives access to remote west central Last Chance Range and the Saline Range.

The mines (no map). At the time of writing, several mining claims are still active around Saline Valley. Most of them are located along the foot of the Inyos—around Lead Canyon, Willow Creek Camp, and Beveridge Canyon. The White Eagle and the Grey Eagle mines behind Willow Creek Camp, and the Snow Flake Mine above Beveridge Canyon, are talc mines. They were started by Gilbert Price "G. P." Rogers, who gave up his real estate career in the 1920s to mine in Saline Valley. The mines have been in the family ever since. A Timbisha Shoshone named Johnny Hunter helped him develop the Grey Eagle Mine. Its ore chute, still in use eight decades later, was constructed with recycled parts from the salt tramway. G. P. Rogers' grandson David Rogers worked here with his wife in the 1970s, "a time," he recalls, "when one would not see a single visitor in a whole month." Rogers still periodically hauls out a few tons of talc under the label of International Talc and Steatite. The unusually high-quality ore, very different in tone

Saline Valley		
	Dist.(mi)	Elev.(ft)
Lakeshore		
Saline Valley Road	0.0	1,115
End of road (trail)	0.3	1,070
Borax works	0.75	1,065
End of trail	1.5	1,060
The salt tramway		
Saline Valley Road	0.0	1,094
Leave road	1.5	1,500
First control station	~3.5	3,690
Little Hunter Canyon spring loop		
Camp	0.0	1,600
Canyon wash	0.25	1,740
Spring (upper end)	0.35	~1,700
Camp	0.5	1,600

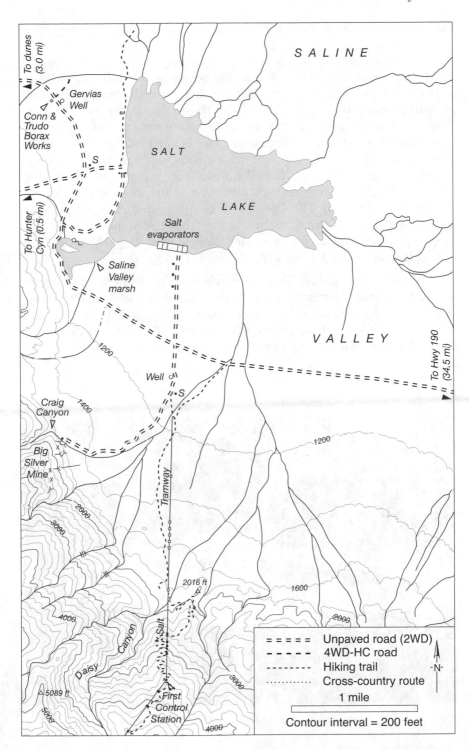

To dunes (3.0 mi)

SALINE

Gervias Well

Conn & Trudo Borax Works

SALT

S

To Hunter Cyn (0.5 mi)

Salt evaporators

LAKE

Saline Valley marsh

VALLEY

1200

To Hwy 190 (34.5 mi)

Well

S

Craig Canyon

1400

Big Silver Mine

1200

Tramway

2000

3000

2016 ft

1600

Salt Canyon

2000

4000

3000

Daisy

3000

5089 ft

First Control Station

4000

5000

= = = = =	Unpaved road (2WD)
- - - - -	4WD-HC road
- - - - -	Hiking trail
· · · · · ·	Cross-country route

-N-

1 mile

Contour interval = 200 feet

from mine to mine as indicated by their names, is shipped to the Inuits who use it to carve elaborate statues.

Today, mining here is stifled by the designation of the Inyos as a BLM Wilderness Area. In the future, the access roads to the Snow Flake and the White Eagle mines, rebuilt by Rogers in the mid-1990s, will either become public or continue to be closed to vehicle traffic. Either way you can use them for foot travel to access the Inyo Mountains or visit the mines. The road to the Snow Flake is particularly scenic. In less than 1.5 miles it ascends to a breathtaking viewpoint 1,400 feet above the valley floor. From here you can hike down into well-watered Beveridge Canyon, thus bypassing the high waterfalls in the lower canyon (there are more up canyon). The Grey Eagle is still periodically active; stay away from it. Mining may resume at the other two mines as well. If it does, respect the owners' privacy and obey posted signs. To be on the safe side, check with the caretaker at Willow Creek Camp.

Other destinations. There is much more to do here. Try a walk around the lake, or climbing the huge volcanic mass of Saline Peak. Starting from the Saline Valley Road, hike to Corridor Canyon, the Blue Jay Mine, or the Lippincott Mine, all described elsewhere in this book. Or explore one of the many tremendous canyons of the Inyos.

■

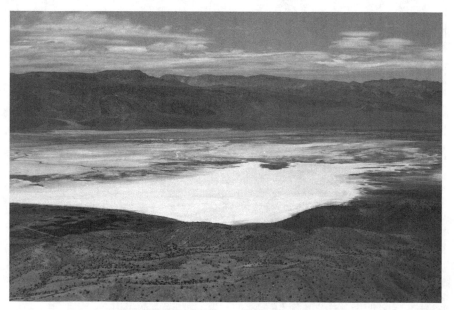

Saline Valley from the Lonesome Miner Trail

THE INYO MOUNTAINS

> *Preserved as a wilderness area adjacent to the park, the Inyo Mountains are included here because they rank among the most majestic ranges in the region and offer some of the greatest hiking out of Saline Valley. The spectacular ridge trail and the two rugged, fall-ridden gorges described below are wonderful illustrations of the potential of this immense stone wilderness. Perfect for well-trained hikers with a taste for treasure hunts à la Indiana Jones.*

General Information

Road status: Roadless; access via Saline Valley Road
Shortest hike: 0.3 mi, 220 ft one way / easy
Longest hike: 8.5 mi, ~8,200 ft one way / grueling
Main attractions: Spectacular canyons and trails, falls, waterfalls
USGS 15' topo maps: Waucoba Wash, New York Butte
USGS 7.5' topo maps: Craig Canyon*, New York Butte*, Pat Keyes
   Canyon*, Waucoba Canyon
Maps: pp. 499*, 493, 477

Location and Access

The portion of the Inyos covered here includes Craig Canyon, Hunter Canyon, and the ridge trail between them, all located just west of Saline Valley's salt lake. Craig Canyon is easily accessed by the Big Silver Mine Road, a short primitive road that branches off the Saline Valley Road just south of the tramway towers. This road ends in 1.5 miles at a small dugout below the Big Silver Mine. It's a little rocky, but not too steep, and with some care a passenger car with normal clearance can make it without scraping off vital parts. The mouth of Craig Canyon is a short distance up the steep, rocky wash to the northeast.

The Hunter Canyon Road starts 1.9 miles north of the salt evaporators turnoff. It is slightly better than the road to Craig Canyon, though not by much. Drive this road 1 mile to its upper end at the Little Hunter Canyon spring. A short spur road leads south to the edge of the spring, and another spur road goes right to a wide cleared area where you can park. A small camp was located here until early 1999, when it was dismantled at the request of the BLM. To get to Hunter Canyon, walk up the short fan to the north. To get to the Bighorn Mine trail, which the BLM has renamed the Lonesome Miner Trail, walk up the spur road to the edge of the spring where the signed trailhead is located.

Route Description

From around 1,600 feet at the floor of Saline Valley, the Inyo Mountains rise abruptly, reaching over 11,000 feet in less than 6.5 air miles. Very few places in the desert are this steep over such distances. The canyons, needless to say, are equally formidable. Because the Inyos are young, they have risen faster than they have eroded. Most canyons draining their sheer eastern slopes are strewn with massive taluses, boulder jams, and impassable falls. Being the furthest north and west, the Inyos are also much wetter than the other ranges in the park. Many of the canyons have streams and waterfalls. Water can be a problem, this time because there is too much of it. Not surprisingly, this coalition of obstacles makes for some of the roughest canyoneering around. In most canyons, a 3-hour hike may only take you a few miles in. To reach the crest of the mountain may take several days.

The two canyons and trails described below are just a sampler. There are 15 named and several unnamed canyons draining the east side of the Inyos. The few I have tried are rugged, wild, and beautiful, well worth extensive exploration. Willow Creek is covered by private water rights, and for this one you should ask permission from the caretaker in residence at Willow Creek Camp at the mouth of the canyon. Try any one of them. You will be well rewarded. Just about everywhere you go, you could swear you are the first human visitor.

Craig Canyon. Steep, deep, and fall-ridden are perhaps the best qualifiers for Craig Canyon. Almost right away, and for several miles, its fairly narrow wash is deeply entrenched in very steep walls rising up to 2,000 feet. On a bright November day, I spent a whole day here and only saw the sun twice. I felt dwarfed by immense sweeps of stone that just never seemed to come to an end.

Hiking here is strenuous. The average slope exceeds 15%, and the wash is often one huge field of boulders. At places, you go over high obstructions and gain 50 or 100 feet at a time. But the climbing is a good part of the fun. To get to the central narrows, about 2.7 miles in, you'll have to climb or bypass 13 falls and boulder jams, two of which are essentially impassable. The first one, about 60 feet high, has a slick recessed chimney. The canyon above it is even deeper and more impressive. A little further on there are some short, good narrows—a long corridor between high polished walls reminiscent of the narrows in lower Marble Canyon. There are some nice climbs and hard traverses to try in this area. The second impassable fall is a dark grotto stacked with huge chockstones, totalling nearly 80 feet in height. Both falls are bypassed by short trails on the left side. The other falls are not to be sneered at either: some of them reach 40 feet and also need to be circumvented.

The central narrows are at the end of all of this. About 300 yards long, only 6 feet wide at their narrowest point, they are deep, dark, and tight. You'll pass by a deep undercut and a huge overhang. At their upper end, the passage is occluded by the third impassable fall, a pile of chockstones reaching 60 feet up.

This is where most people turn around. There is a possible bypass route on the left side, just downhill from the undercut, but it looks like it would take some work. After climbing two and a half hours, I was still looking up at craggy peaks several thousand feet higher, which were not even the crest of the range. It was still 1.8 miles and 1,500 feet to the first spring, which is itself about halfway to the Burgess Mine. I had run out of time and turned around. To go significantly farther and return before dark (down climbing the falls at night would be foolish, and not very much fun) come here when the days are longer, and start at the crack of dawn.

Hunter Canyon.   Although just a couple of miles away, Hunter Canyon is fairly different from its southern neighbor. It is just as deep and narrow, as is made obvious by the impressively tight gorge you enter right away. But the main difference is the little stream that comes out of the canyon mouth. It carries enough water to flow part way out onto the fan, a rare event in greater Death Valley. Although the stream is not continuous, it goes on uninterrupted for long stretches in the lower canyon. The difference water makes is stunning. What would normally be a rocky wash is here a lush creek, dry falls are turned to tropical waterfalls, and desert bushes are supplanted by thickets of willows too dense to cross.

The downside is that although the walking is a little easier than in Craig Canyon, the water will slow you down, and the waterfalls all need to be bypassed. The first two falls, located back to back a short distance in, are a good example of what to expect. They are covered with green mats of moss and fern, sometimes grapevine, so thick that the waterfall itself gets lost in them. The first one is easy to bypass, the second one, about 40 feet high, a little harder. The third one, a little further, is far worse, and stops a lot of people. It needs to be circumvented on the left side, along a tilted ledge that climbs and circles around a steep, curving wall. It definitely gets a high mark on the scare meter! It's a technical climb, about 5.4, high above the canyon floor, and I would not have tried it without climbing shoes.

Past this fall, things ease up for a while. There is another waterfall (this one not as difficult), then a short stretch of polished narrows, and the canyon opens up on to a lush oasis of willows and cottonwoods. Here walking gets tricky again. To avoid the impenetrable vegetation clogging the wash, you'll have to clamber over huge taluses that have come down from the steep canyon walls. They can be so enormous that they fill up a good part of the canyon floor, leaving just enough room for the stream. You may discover minor mineral treasures along these natural dumps, including a rich assortment of granitic rocks. Thick plutonic veins known as dikes run through the nearby limestone walls. These granite-like veins intruded the original rock, and at the contact zone between them the limestone has been metamorphosed into white marble. At places you'll be forced to cross the stream. At others, the wash opens up, and you'll walk along a bank flushed with Mojave thistle, wild rose, willow shoots, and cane. The true treasure here is to be immersed in two wildly different landscapes, closely intertwined. In a short walk you can absorb the essence of both of them, one a lush wash animated by a stream, the other waterless desert slopes.

The Inyo Mountains		
	Dist.(mi)	Elev.(ft)
Craig Canyon		
End of road	0.0	1,520
Mouth	0.1	1,600
60-ft fall	1.5	3,000
80-ft fall	2.2	3,600
Central narrows (start)	2.7	3,950
60-ft fall (end)	2.9	4,120
Spring	4.7	5,630
Divide	7.9	9,300
Burgess Mine	8.5	~9,630
Hunter Canyon		
Camp	0.0	1,600
Mouth	0.1	1,600
40-ft waterfall (#2)	0.3	~1,820
50-ft waterfall (#5)	1.2	2,590
50-ft waterfall (#6)	1.3	2,780
Bighorn Spring	3.9	5,030
Bighorn Mine trail		
Camp	0.0	1,600
Upper springs	0.6	2,110
Summit	4.4	6,100
Bighorn Spring	5.2	5,030
Bighorn Mine	6.6	~6,600
Burgess Mine	12.7	~9,640

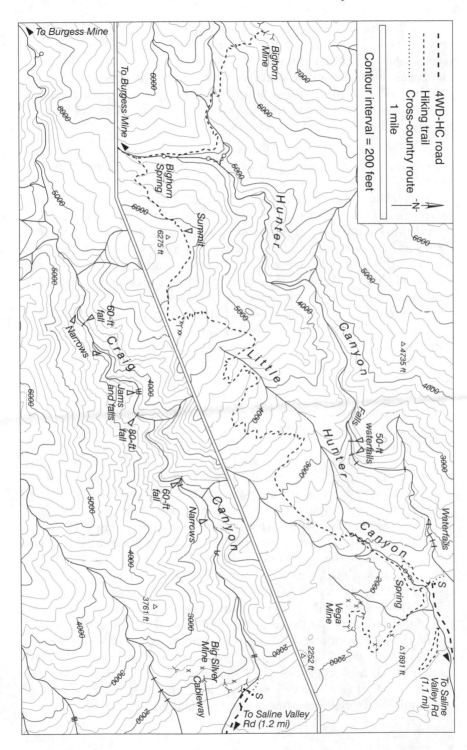

The next two waterfalls are nearly 50 feet high each. This is as far as I went. Going around the first one was not too difficult, but the second one looked like it would take some effort. But it is not impossible: I was told there are at least five more waterfalls beyond. The map suggests several more miles of spectacular gorge. Again, progress through this canyon is surprisingly slow. To go only as far as Bighorn Spring would take a good part of a day.

The Bighorn Mine trail. From the end of the road the trail crosses the spring, then continues up the wash of Little Hunter Canyon. It vanishes for a short while, then resumes just before some short and shallow narrows (about 0.4 mile). The trail bypasses the narrows on the left, then returns to the wash, crosses it, and forks. This is the first tricky part. The straight fork climbs up to the bench just west of the Vega Mine. The right fork, the one you want, is very easy to miss. Look for it climbing the steep, dusty hillside on the right. After a few minutes you will get to two small clumps of mesquite, and to the second tricky part: the trail is hidden in the narrow opening on the left just past the second clump.

From here on up, the trail is hard to lose, thanks to occasional BLM posts and many small cairns. Although not always in great condition—rocky, narrow at places, and slanting the wrong way—it is a lot better than most old trails. It keeps on climbing the ridge to a distant summit overlooking Hunter Canyon, then drops to Bighorn Spring and climbs again to the Bighorn Mine. The trail's innumerable switchbacks nicely pace the climb, but it's still tough and slow going—4,500 feet in under 5 miles just to the summit, which is not even half way to the crest of the Inyos.

The rewards certainly match the hard work. The flower show, for one thing, can be awesome. Because of the large elevation change, anytime between early spring and late summer you'll see plenty of flowers along the way. Another bonus is the impressive spring and the little mine beyond it, which are rarely visited, this trail being the easiest access to them. My favorite part was the views from the trail, which are Saline Valley's replica of Dante's View. The center of focus is Saline Valley's little salt lake, which is not all that little after all. As you gain elevation it slowly expands, revealing its eastern shore, twisted like a fractal, fringed with shades of pink, until it eventually fills a good portion of the landscape. At the summit you'll be standing on the brink of a bright abyss, almost a mile above an immense valley floor cocooned between alien ranges. Few views in the desert are as awe-inspiring. That there is a trail here to give us such an experience is a true wonder. We should silently thank the unknown miners who toiled to construct it, and hope that the Bighorn Mine rewarded them for their efforts.

■

THE PANAMINT VALLEY DUNES

> *Lost at the far end of the valley, ringed by desolate mountains, the Panamint Valley Dunes are among the most remote dunes in the park. It's close to 4 level desert miles to get there, but unless this is your unlucky day you'll be all alone to discover them.*

General Information

Road access: Roadless; access from graded road
Shortest hike: 3.4 mi, 750 ft one way / moderate
Longest hike: 4.5 mi, ~1,470 ft one way (or more) / moderate
Main attraction: Isolated dunes, valley floor hiking
USGS topo maps: Panamint Butte (15'), The Dunes (7.5')
Maps: pp. 503*, 333, 477

Location and Access

The Panamint Valley Dunes are at the north end of Panamint Valley, at the foot of Hunter Mountain. The easiest way to get to them is to hike from the Big Four Mine Road. This road starts 4.5 miles east of Panamint Springs, which is about 0.25 mile east of the dry lake's eastern edge. Drive it about 5.8 miles to where it makes a right bend and park. It's a good graded road up to that point. On the way there you'll drive by Lake Hill, an island of Tin Mountain Limestone that probably slipped down the side of Panamint Butte to the east by detachment faulting.

Route Description

The approach. This is a pure desert walk, across sandy, sparsely vegetated flats. Your target is in full view the whole time, but it is far away and it gets closer very slowly. The most common bushes along the way are the ubiquitous creosote, and bursage, the low gray-green bushes responsible for the spiny burs you'll be periodically plucking off your socks. Most of them, as well as smaller plants, are covered with tangles of bright orange threads, a parasite known as dodder—or devil's guts. Hard to guess it's a plant: it has no leaves, no chlorophyll, and no roots at maturity. After growing as a normal seedling, it attaches itself via tiny suckers to a plant, then lives off the juices of its host, often dehydrating it to death. Dodder is fairly common in the desert, but it does not often occur so densely over such a vast area as it does here.

In the spring, quite a few flowering plants add vibrant strokes of color to the landscape, including evening primrose and desertgold, but none is as striking as the prickle poppy. You'll have to be patient: it's just about the last plant you'll see before all vegetation finally gives out, where the sand first swells into dunes. When in bloom, this blue-green, thistle-like plant graces the sandy slopes with a dazzling belt of large white flowers, their papery petals fluttering in the slightest breeze.

Wildlife is fairly abundant, if you are willing to think small. You may even spot a few animals you have never seen before, like the sand-dwelling bees that live in the dunes. Their burrow openings are just wide enough for a single bee to crawl through. They swarm over large areas, aimlessly it seems, producing an unceasing drone. They have left me alone so far, but I have often wondered whether they are always this complacent. At least three species of grasshoppers also manage to live here, each one beautifully matched to its surrounding. Near the road, where the fan material is mostly brown to black cobbles of lava, they are brownish. Much larger grasshoppers, up to 2 inches long, live a little further out. When on the ground they are mottled gray and white, matching the dominant granitic rocks of the fan. In flight, their wide blue wings merge with the sky. In the dunes the grasshoppers are smaller and the color of sand.

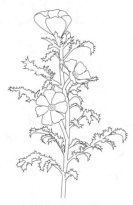

Desert prickle poppy

Other locals blend in remarkably well. Once in a while a zebra-tailed lizard will dart out of nowhere, scared silly by what may be its first encounter with a human being. They must hold some sort of lizard record for speed. They run with such amazing swiftness, and their skin is so pale against the sand, that it's hard to follow them. You may even wonder whether you actually saw anything moving. If you manage to track one for long enough, you'll see that they run on stretched legs, sometimes only on their hind feet, their black and white tail curled high over their back. They stop almost as swiftly—literally on a dime.

Larger animals, too, inhabit or visit these hostile flats: wrens, sparrows, ravens, cottontail rabbits, snakes, even an occasional coyote or wild burro. One day in early summer I was checked out on several occasions by Costa's hummingbirds. While I was crouched in the meager shade of a creosote, one of them parked in midair 3 feet from my face, hovered for a few seconds, then proceeded to describe a half circle around me, in those sudden little skips hummingbirds like to do, slowly inspecting the red trim of my pack. Then it landed on the high branch of a nearby creosote and kept me company for several minutes.

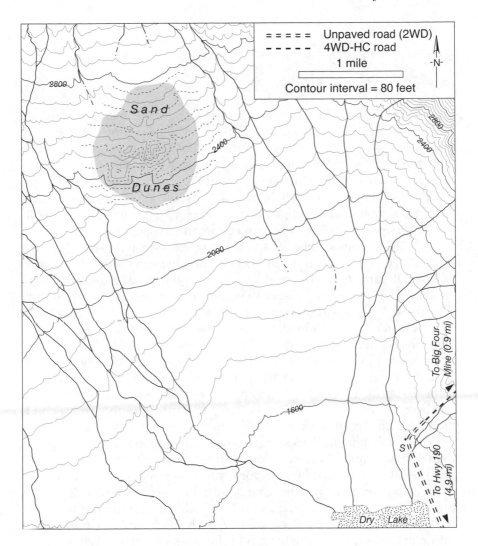

Legend	
= = = = =	Unpaved road (2WD)
– – – – –	4WD-HC road

1 mile

Contour interval = 80 feet

-N-

The Panamint Valley Dunes

	Dist.(mi)	Elev.(ft)
Big Four Mine Road	0.0	1,570
Edge of dunes	3.4	~2,320
Summit of highest dune	3.9	~2,670
Summit of furthest dune	4.5	~2,650

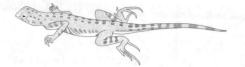

Zebra-tailed lizard

The dunes. The sand sheet surrounding the dunes is extensive; you'll be walking on it a good part of the way. On a summer day, it may even seem like a good fraction of forever. But the dunes are worth the wait, the heat, the sweat, and the lukewarm water. Besides their aesthetic appeal, there is something special about the Panamint Dunes. Perhaps it is their improbable location, high up against the fan. Or their isolation, miles from asphalt and steel, at the far end of a lonesome valley. Or is it the virgin sand, often free of human beings and footprints?

This enormous pile of sand resting precariously, it seems, on the steep curve of the fan, is an unlikely sight. One can't help wondering where it all came from. The main source of sand is probably quartz monzonite, which makes up most of the crescent of mountains surrounding the dunes. A good part of the north valley fill is also made of chunks of this rock, shed by the mountains over the last few million years. The slipface of a dune is the side that's the steepest, the side facing away from the dominant wind. Here, all the slipfaces face north. As in Death Valley, the wind blows dominantly from the south, picking up speed as it travels up the long floor of Panamint Valley. For thousands of years it has been relentlessly abrading the fan rocks into quartz particles and blowing them uphill, back towards the mountain they came from.

The Panamint Dunes are relatively small in extent, covering less than 1 square mile. There are four main dunes, surrounded by a few much smaller ones. The highest dune, the easternmost one, is linked to its neighbor by two saddles. One saddle is a razor sharp ridge with unusually deep and steep sinks on both sides of it. Walking it is like being on a tight rope—a deep void on both sides, and not much substance in the middle. At the bottom of the sinks I felt like I was in a well of sand. The other saddle is dusted with black sand. It gives it a strange look, almost too artistic for nature, perhaps what it would look like if Georgia O'Keefe had put it on canvas. The views from the top extend straight down the length of Panamint Valley, overlooking its oddly shaped lake of dry mud. The highest summit visible on the east side of the valley is Telescope Peak, nearly 30 miles away and 8,400 feet higher. Across from it stands the Argus Range, and to the north of this range volcanic Rainbow Plateau, utterly barren and desolate. Turn around and you'll be looking up at Hunter Mountain, crowned with green pines and junipers.

■

DARWIN FALLS

> *Punctuated with idyllic waterfalls and irrigated by a lovely perennial creek, the deep narrows of Darwin Canyon are among the most lush and beautiful in the park. The short walk to the lower waterfall is a wonderful illustration of the miracle of water in the desert. The challenging climb through the serene upper narrows to China Garden Spring is a gem for the experienced hiker.*

General Information

Road access: Graded road in lower and upper canyon
Shortest hike: 0.9 mi, 220 ft one way / easy
Longest hike: 2.4 mi, ~700 ft one way / difficult, with rock climbing
Main attractions: Lush narrow canyon with waterfalls, flora, birds, rock
    climbing
USGS 15' and 7.5' topo maps: Darwin
Maps: pp. 509*, 477

Location and Access

This magical little place is at the north end of the Argus Range, just a few miles west of Panamint Springs. Like the nearby town and several geographical features, it is named after Dr. Darwin French, who established a base camp here when he led his first prospecting expedition to Death Valley in 1850 (see *Jayhawker Canyon*).

The easiest access to Darwin Falls is via the lower canyon. From Panamint Springs, drive Highway 190 west 1 mile to a graded road on the left (or 7.2 miles east of the turnoff to Father Crowley Point). This road was part of Bob Eichbaum's original Death Valley Toll Road to Stovepipe Wells (see *Golden Canyon*), which used to go through Darwin. This good graded road follows the wide bed of Darwin Wash for 2.5 miles and forks. Make a right and park 200 feet further at the turn-out just above the wash.

To access the upper canyon, make a left at the fork. Continue 3.9 winding miles up along the side of Zinc Hill, then back down into the canyon wash. Follow the road down canyon 1.1 miles to its end at China Garden Spring. Most of this road is good, except around its high point where some soft spots require high clearance. The alternative is to go through the colorful town of Darwin. Make a left at the stop sign in town and go 7.5 miles down a paved, then graded road to China Garden Spring.

Natural History

One of the pleasures of this well-watered canyon is the diversity of its vegetation. In the spring, many kinds of wild flowers can be found along the more open lower and upper parts of the canyon. The flowering plants you are most likely to see are prince's plume, globemallow, golden evening primrose, Mojave aster, and phacelias, but also the showy desert prickle poppy, spotted langloisia, and bright yellow monkeyflower. The main trees growing here are willows; there are very few cottonwoods. At places they are in fierce competition for space with tamarisk, an exotic plant that has become a pest throughout much of the North American desert. In the darker narrows, the creek bed is lined with watercress and rushes. Deep in the narrows, I was fortunate to find a cluster of beautiful orchids (stream orchis) along the creek bank.

Darwin Canyon is also a haven for birds, and heaven for bird lovers. Many species inhabit this small ecological island, and during the spring migration other birds, like warblers, use this place as a rest area. A bird enthusiast I met here spotted about 20 species just along the short stretch of wash below the narrows, including goldfinches, wrens, Costa's hummingbirds, swifts, sparrows, prairie falcons, and red-tailed hawks. Even if you cannot identify them, you can look forward to their lively songs and chirps echoing against the canyon walls.

Route Description

The lower canyon. From the road, hike down to the broad wash and follow the developing trail 0.2 mile up canyon to a metal barricade. Beyond it, the trail wanders up the open wash, mostly on the left side. It is faint at places, but follow it carefully to avoid creating new tracks, as this place is heavily visited. The pipeline running along the west side of the wash has been here for decades, diverting a portion of the perennial creek flow further up canyon down to Panamint Springs. In the colder months, the creek from Darwin Canyon usually flows through this area, but in the summer you will have to hike some distance to find it.

The wash gradually narrows; rabbitbrush and indigo bush leave the way to thickets of willows, tamarisk, cattail, and rushes. As you approach the narrows, stay on the left side of the wash. After about 0.8 mile, there is a second barricade where the canyon turns to narrows. The main trail continues on the left side, right up against the canyon wall. To avoid damaging the vegetation and getting wet, do not use the trail on the other side, which dead-ends shortly in a tangle of trees.

The narrows and the falls. The next stretch is the most pleasant part of this canyon. For a few hundred yards, the trail winds along the creek under a dense canopy of tall willows, deep beneath the vertical, high-rising walls of the narrows. In the pure tradition of riparian desert creeks, this cool and shaded oasis is a very special place. After a few hot days in the desert, it strains your credulity. The vegetation is so dense that you may not see the first waterfall until the last moment. Here the creek leaps over a slanted wall and plunges 18 feet into a shallow pool. Moss and maidenhair fern cling to the wet rock. The surrounding high walls and tall trees block the view in all directions but upward, creating a secluded environment, divorced from the nearby parched desert.

Although most visitors turn around at this point, this is just the beginning. The rest of the narrows, about half a mile long, has nine main waterfalls and a few smaller ones. Getting through obviously requires some climbing and is physically demanding, but it can be done without getting wet!

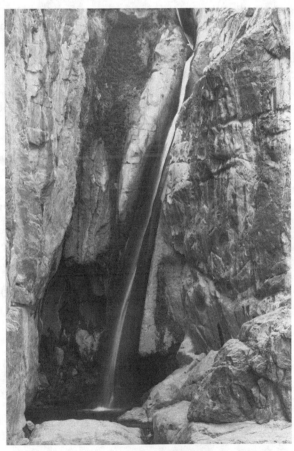

Darwin Falls, the highest of many waterfalls
along Darwin Canyon

To circumvent the first waterfall, climb the east canyon wall starting from just downstream of the pool, and go high enough to find a safe passage around the sheer wall overlooking the waterfall. This route calls for scrambling over a series of hard rock ledges, at places only a foot wide, and it should not be attempted if you have a fear of heights. In about 150 yards, you will be able to climb back down to the creek, within earshot of the next waterfall. Only 5 feet high, it plunges into a deep and narrow pool pinched between the canyon walls. The third waterfall, just behind it, tumbles 12 feet over the overhanging lip of a circular grotto. A short distance beyond, the narrows' walls loom vertically well over 100 feet, hiding from view the fourth and highest waterfall.

The route continues up the steep talus on the right side just before the second waterfall. After gaining 40 or 50 feet in elevation, you'll be level with a gap in the canyon wall to your left. Walking through this gap will put you in the middle of a majestic well of slick-rock at the foot of the thundering fourth waterfall. From about 60 feet overhead, the water glides down a long narrow groove in the sheer wall before plunging into a deep dark pool. The canyon walls, as well as the sturdy ledges you have been climbing, are made of a pretty granite-like rock called monzonite, formed about 180 million years ago. Because it contains biotite, hornblende, and quartz in varying proportions, its aspect changes markedly throughout the narrows.

To circumvent this fall, return to the talus and climb it another 60 feet or so, then cross the talus towards the creek on a narrow foot trail and down into the canyon bed. The trail soon enters the thick creek-side vegetation and ends below the fifth waterfall, only a few feet high but wedged in a short stretch of flooded narrows. You could wade through it and get very wet but there is little point, as the next two waterfalls are

	Darwin Falls	
	Dist.(mi)	Elev.(ft)
Parking (gate)	0.0	2,540
1st waterfall	1.1	2,760
2nd and 3rd waterfall	1.2	~2,790
4th waterfall (60-ft)	1.3	~2,820
5th waterfall	1.4	~2,890
6th and 7th waterfall	1.45	~2,900
8th waterfall	1.55	2,970
9th waterfall	1.6	2,990
Spring head	1.9	3,060
China Garden Spring	2.6	3,150

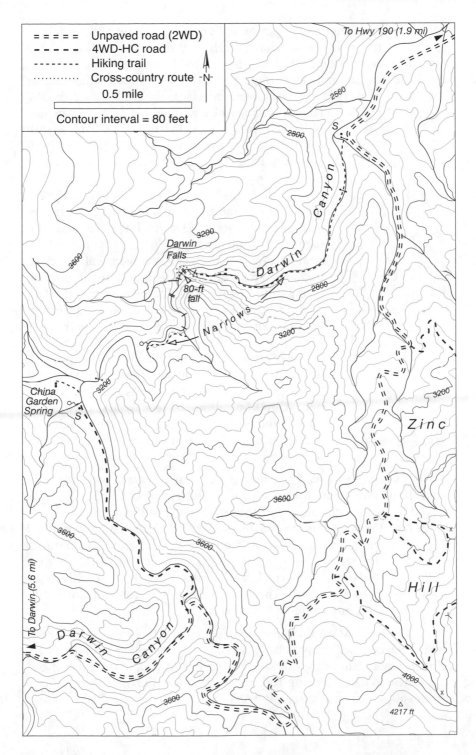

= = = = =	Unpaved road (2WD)
- - - - -	4WD-HC road
- - - - - -	Hiking trail
··············	Cross-country route -N-

0.5 mile

Contour interval = 80 feet

To Hwy 190 (1.9 mi)

2560

2800

3200

Darwin
Falls

Darwin

80-ft
fall

2800

Narrows

3200

3200

China
Garden
Spring

S

Zinc

3200

3600

3600

Hill

3600

3600

To Darwin (5.6 mi)

Darwin Canyon

4000

3600

4217 ft

just around the corner and impassable. Bypassing this set of three falls is the crux of this hike. People have obviously tried scrambling up the steep talus some distance back on the west side, but this route is quite unsafe. The easiest and safest route I found is on the east side, starting about 20-30 yards below the fifth waterfall. Here the wall is only about 7 feet high, topped by a broad ledge, and there is a wide, slanted crack to its right. This climb requires a technical move (low 5s), and you should not attempt it alone if you are not an experienced climber.

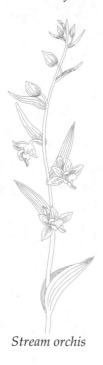

Past this wall things are comparatively easier. After scrambling up a series of short ledges and taluses of large rocks, you'll reach a high vantage point at the next bend in the canyon and look straight down at the next two waterfalls. Back to back, they total about 30 feet, and are as impressive as the lower falls. The next waterfall (#8), past a more open stretch of slickrock, is a 6-8 foot cascade along a narrow funnel clogged with trees. The route crosses the creek just above it, continues on slickrock benches, then crosses again (back to the east side) at the head of the final waterfall, a 6-foot ribbon of clear water splashing into a deep pool. Climbing about 70 feet up the ravine just outside the tree cover will put you on a high trail

Stream orchis

that goes around the rest of the tree-choked narrows to the more open upper canyon.

The upper canyon. From here the dry canyon wash winds around a couple of loose meanders before reaching China Garden Spring, marked by a thick cluster of old cottonwoods. The large tin house, ore bin and loading platform behind the spring are the remains of a small mill, which may have been used as a custom mill when the local mines were active. The trees at the spring provide shade for what used to be a small residential area, a tiny creek, and a pond of cool water with colorful and unexpected residents. This is a lovely spot to rest, and a nice conclusion to a short but action-packed hike.

Caution. More than ever, please respect this rare oasis. In the heavily visited lower canyon, stay on the trail. Do not step on the vegetation. If other visitors are sharing this place with you, respect their need for silence. When climbing to bypass the falls, make sure no one is underneath you in case you dislodge a rock.

■

WILDROSE CANYON

> *Wildrose Canyon is a broad, high-desert valley framed by lofty forested peaks, an ideal place to escape from the summer heat and hike or camp in the high country. The graded canyon road provides easy access to the historic charcoal kilns, one of Death Valley's early mining wonders. Hikers can explore trails to the old antimony mines that first put this area on the map, to several springs, or to one of the surrounding peaks.*

General Information

Road status: Paved/graded road through canyon
Shortest hike: Short strolls/very easy
Longest hike: 5.2 mi, ~2,500 ft one way/difficult
Main attractions: Charcoal kilns, pine forest, springs, peak climb, mines
USGS 15' topo maps: Emigrant Canyon, Telescope Peak
USGS 7.5' topo maps: Emigrant Pass*, Jail Canyon*, Wildrose Peak,
   Telescope Peak*
Maps: pp. 515, 519, 521, 393

Location and Access

Wildrose Canyon is one of the largest canyons draining into Panamint Valley. A road runs through its entire length up to the crest of the Panamints at Mahogany Flat. It is partly paved, partly graded up to the kilns, and generally suitable for passenger cars.

History: Antimony Mining

Wildrose Canyon was one of the first places to be named around Death Valley, and probably the earliest one to be mined. Antimony was discovered here in 1860, more than 40 years before Death Valley's major gold strikes. This discovery is credited to a party of fortune seekers led by Dr. Samuel George, who came to Death Valley in search of the Lost Gunsight Lode (see *Jayhawker Canyon*). While camped at Wildrose Spring, George and one of his partners, William Henderson, discovered thick veins of silver-like ore around what is now Antimony Canyon. It was the 25th of December, and they optimistically named their lode the Christmas Gift. But when samples were later assayed, the silver-like ore appeared to contain little silver. It was rich antimony ore, a metal then too cheap to mine in such a remote location. They still returned the following April for further prospecting and to stake more claims, and incidentally, to climb and name Telescope Peak. In July, convinced that silver would eventually show up in spite of additional disappointing assays, they formed the Combination Gold and Silver Mining Company and proceeded to develop their claims. For two years Henderson managed a small team that opened a couple of tunnels and shafts in the most promising veins. But after over 100 feet had been exposed they still had found no silver—only antimony. Bloody skirmishes with local Indians, combined with this failure, forced them to stop in the spring of 1864.

Ten years later George, lured by the hype of a new silver bonanza in nearby Surprise Canyon, came back with yet another party. They prospected the area for a year, but again all they kept turning up was—you guessed it—antimony. George eventually gave up, but over the next four decades others relocated his claims, somehow insisted on looking for silver, and failed to find any.

It was not until metal prices skyrocketed in World War I that the area was finally mined for what it was worth. In January 1915, a mining engineer acquired some of the claims and formed the Western Metals Company. The company patented and operated the Monarch, Combination, and Monopoly claims, near Antimony Ridge on the south side of Wildrose Canyon, and the Kennedy Quartz claims on the north side. On Antimony Ridge many of the veins had already been opened up by earlier prospectors, and a lot of ore was just lying around waiting for the picking. The ore was packed by burro to a chute that dropped it at the upper end of the road. It was treated at a small concentrating smelter in Wildrose Canyon and trucked to the railroad in Trona. Later on, the market value of antimony increased enough that the inefficient on-site smelter was discontinued and the raw ore was shipped to the company's smelter in San Pedro, California. Most of the production occurred in 1915 and 1916. The company shipped 4,000 tons of ore that reportedly produced around 1,000 tons of antimony, about half of the US war-years production. The operations stopped around 1918. Other than a small-scale effort in 1937 and 1938 to screen the old Monarch dumps and exploit high-grade pockets on the Kennedy Quartz claims, the mines were never reactivated. But the old Christmas Gift had finally produced its own bonanza—close to a million dollars in antimony.

Route Description

The antimony mines and Tuber Peak. Wildrose Canyon's main antimony mines are located in two short side canyons known in the past as Jones and Antimony canyons. Although their physical remains are minimal, they are historically significant as probably the earliest mines in Death Valley. The road to the mines is on the south side of the Wildrose Canyon Road, 0.8 mile east of the ranger station. It ends in 1.3

miles just inside Antimony Canyon. This road is very rough and you'll likely have to walk it. Instead, you can drive the Wildrose Canyon Road 0.9 mile further and walk southwest across the fan 0.6 mile to the mining road. This is shorter, but the fan's dense cover of blackbrush and thornbush is harsh on human legs. The foot trail to the Monarch Mine splits off on the east side just before the end of the mining road.

Most of the rocks exposed near the mines (and along Wildrose Canyon) belong to the Kingston Peak Formation. There are also small exposures of gneiss and schists, like on the west side of Antimony Canyon, and amphibolite, around the mines on Antimony Ridge. The schists vary greatly in composition, containing mainly quartz and biotite, chlorite and/or actinolite (green schists), amphibolite (dark schists), with occasional inclusions of tourmaline and rutile. The antimony deposits occur mostly in brecciated amphibolite (usually low grade), but also in schists and quartz veins (higher grade). The primary mineral is stibnite (antimony sulfide). It was deposited in the Tertiary or Quaternary, probably by solutions rising along fissures from igneous sources. Stibnite is known to occur near hot springs. The more recent travertine deposits found in the area may have been formed by hot springs that rose along the same fissures.

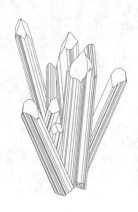

Stibnite

To get to the Monarch Mine, follow the mining trail (overgrown but discernable) into Jones Canyon and up to Antimony Ridge (0.8 mile). Formerly known as the Wildrose Antimony Mine, the Monarch Mine yielded most of the 1915-1916 production. It was worked by several adits and an open cut. The lower adit, at the end of the trail, had 200 feet of tunnels and narrow drifts in brecciated amphibolite. The open cut is just beyond it. The yellow ore coating some of the rocks on the mine tailings is antimony oxide, formed by weathering of exposed stibnite. It prevailed in the shallow deposits mined in the past.

The other mines are similar and smaller, and this is a good turning point, unless you want to climb Tuber Peak, which is really the best part of this hike. At the east end of the open cut, a worn-out foot trail winds up Antimony Ridge. It bypasses the Combination Mine, which exploited a system of parallel quartz veins about 400 yards long. It had four shafts, the main one 70 feet deep, all of which are now partly filled. The trail continues to Tuber Ridge, then follows the ridge for 0.3 mile. Although the slope is steep, the trail makes the ascent relatively easy. Tuber Peak is just west of the highest peak. Both peaks offer good views

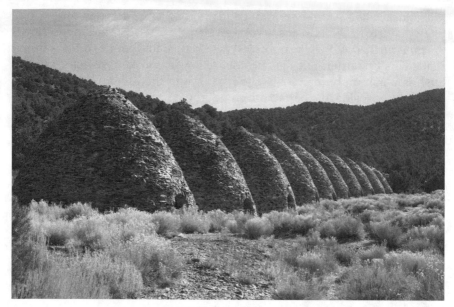

The charcoal kilns

of Panamint Valley's salt pan, the high Panamints, Wildrose Canyon, and the auburn face of Pinto Peak. The Mohawk Mine is just south of the peaks, overlooking Tuber Canyon. Its main tunnels, below the highest peak, contained stibnite in a quartz vein near a small fault. The Monopoly Mine is on the northeast ridge of the highest peak. From Tuber Peak you can climb down along that ridge to its two main tunnels, then continue down to the west fork of Antimony Canyon to the mining road, which completes the loop. Look for the large travertine exposure just uphill of the two forks of Antimony Canyon.

If this is not enough, try the Kennedy Quartz Mine, on the north side of Wildrose Canyon. Look for the road to it 0.4 mile east of the ranger station, and for fluorite when you get there (1.2 miles, 660 feet).

The charcoal kilns. The kilns, high in the forested upper canyon, are the main destination of most visitors to this canyon. These impressive structures are one of the wonders of early desert mining. Their existence is connected to a silver strike that took place in 1875 in the Argus Range, on the west side of Panamint Valley. The ore, which also contained lead and gold, was promising enough that in just a few months several mines had sprung up and a new district was formed, centered around the camp of Lookout. Charcoal was needed to operate two smelters near the mines, and wood was needed to produce charcoal. The closest wood supply was the scant forest up in Wildrose Canyon, nearly

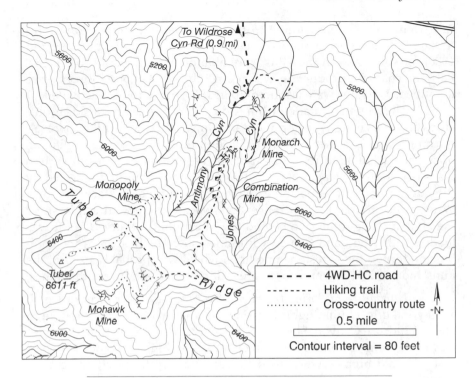

Wildrose Canyon Antimony Mines		
	Dist.(mi)	Elev.(ft)
Wildrose Canyon Road	0.0	4,495
Junction with mining trail	1.2	5,100
Monarch Mine	2.0	5,520
Combination Mine	2.2	~5,740
Tuber Ridge	2.9	~6,440
Mohawk Mine	(0.4)	~6,380
Tuber Peak	3.5	6,611
Monopoly Mine	3.9	~6,440
Mining trail	4.8	5,100

25 miles away, but this did not stop the enterprising mine managers. By the spring of 1877 the ten huge furnaces had been erected and were ready to produce. They were loaded with 4-foot pinyon and juniper logs, which were left to burn for several days until the wood had turned to charcoal. The operation probably employed only a small crew to cut the wood, stack, fire, and tend the kilns, and haul the charcoal by mule team to the Modock smelters. It looked so promising that for a while a

rail tramway was envisioned to take the charcoal across Panamint Valley. But although the Lookout District remained active until around 1900, for some reason the kilns were abandoned after only two years. Perhaps charcoal production was too costly, or cheaper sources were identified. The kilns were last fired up in 1879, never to be reactivated.

The kilns are made of limestone blocks quarried at local out-crops and cemented by a mortar of sand, lime, and gravel. Like charcoal-burning ovens at other mines of that era, they were designed like an opera house, so as to reflect as much heat—which behaves in certain ways like sound—as possible. The faintest sound is audibly reflected by the curved walls. The portholes in the back served to stack the logs. When fired, the arched entranceways were closed with crude sheet metal doors. The stone ruin behind the fourth kiln is a lime kiln. It was loaded with wood and topped with limestone. The heat from the com-bustion turned the limestone into lime, which was probably used in the kilns' mortar, and maybe also for ore milling and cyaniding at the mines.

Hummingbird Spring (no map). To probe another facet of Death Valley, hike to Hummingbird Spring, located in the thick forest high above Wildrose Canyon. Start at the primitive road on the right 3.6 miles east of the ranger station. You can either drive (high clearance helps) or walk this old high-crowned road to just before a sharp left switchback (about 1.8 miles). The spring is up the canyon on the right, once known as Hummingbird Canyon. Its wash is steep and cluttered with talus debris and fallen trees, and walking is tedious, but it is a shaded and fra-grant place, quite pleasant in hot weather. It is about 1 mile and 910 feet up to Hummingbird Spring, located near the head of a right fork in the canyon, on a steep slope above the wash (the 7.5' topo comes in handy). It is a restful place, often livened, like much of this area, by colorful hummingbirds. The stone basin was built to provide water for the superintendent's house, when this was a national monument and its summer headquarters were in Wildrose Canyon. The house was located on Pinyon Mesa, at the end of the access road, 0.2 mile past the switch-back. Today, what is left is its incongruous towering chimney and beau-tiful flagstone terrace, a low stone wall, and the old water tank.

Mud Spring (no map). This small spring is located in Nemo Canyon, a side canyon that branches into Wildrose Canyon on the north side just above its mouth. The wide wash will take you past impressive high walls of fluted conglomerate and a few narrow side draws. The spring is about 2.1 miles in on the left, where the canyon makes a sharp right. It is marked by low clumps of mesquite trees, and an unusual water hole hidden behind a screen of cane.

■

WILDROSE PEAK AND TELESCOPE PEAK

> *These are two of the best peak hikes in Death Valley, rivaling with Dante's View and Chloride Cliff. The trail hike to Telescope Peak, the highest summit in the park, is on the strenuous side, but the awesome views from over two miles above the salt pan more than make up for it. On the shorter hike to Wildrose Peak you will enjoy similar views, although not quite as spectacular, for a fraction of the effort.*

General Information

Road status: Hiking on trails from graded or primitive road
Shortest hike: 1.7 mi, 780 ft one way / moderate
Longest hike: 6.5 mi, 3,150 ft one way / strenuous
Main attractions: Trail hikes to high forested peaks
USGS 15' topo maps: Emigrant Canyon*, Telescope Peak*
USGS 7.5' topo maps: Wildrose Peak*, Telescope Peak*
Maps: pp. 519*, 521*, 427, 433, 393

Location and Access

The two trails described here start from upper Wildrose Canyon, on the west side of the Panamints. To get to the Wildrose Peak Trail, drive the Wildrose Canyon Road up to the charcoal kilns and park. This is 6.8 miles east of the ranger station. The trailhead is near the west end of the kilns. For Telescope Peak, drive to the trailhead at the Mahogany Flat Campground, at the end of the Wildrose Canyon Road (1.6 miles past the kilns). The road is a little rough past the kilns, but generally manageable with a standard-clearance vehicle.

Route Description

The Wildrose Peak Trail. If you don't want to tackle Telescope Peak, or if you want to acclimate yourself to the high elevation first, start with Wildrose Peak, which is a shorter and easier version. Except near the summit, the maintained trail to Wildrose Peak lies in the midst of the green pygmy forest that covers the high Panamints. Surrounded on all sides by dry desert, this ecological island is a rare treat that provides a pleasant mixture of sun and shade in the summer. The vegetation is largely mixed stands of single-leaf pinyon pines (the ground is covered with fragrant pine cones) and Utah junipers (most of which are infested with mistletoe). You will also find plants that thrive only at higher elevations, including big sagebrush, cliff rose, wild cabbage, tansybush,

517

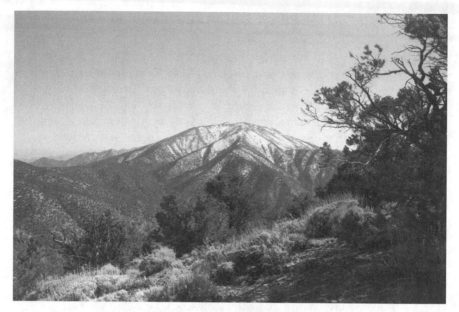

Snow-sprinkled Telescope Peak

Panamint eriogonum, phlox, and the grizzly bear pricklypear cactus, recognized by its long and thin spines. The 100-year-old stumps along the trail are remains from early logging operations when the kilns were active (see *Wildrose Canyon*).

After about 2.1 miles the trail reaches the divide at a saddle overlooking Death Valley Canyon. If your time is limited, this is a good turning point. The trail climbs on along the crest and soon reaches a second saddle. The last mile, most of it switchbacks, is the steepest and most strenuous part, but it offers increasingly spectacular views of the south fork of Trail Canyon and Death Valley.

For a great overnight trip, use this trail as the first leg of a longer hike to the Aguereberry Point Road. Most of this route is on old mining roads. From the second saddle on the Wildrose Peak Trail, hike down the steep ridge to the Morning Glory Mine, then follow the switchbacks of the mining road down to the south fork of Trail Canyon. The next stretch is along the old road down this fork to the confluence, then up the north fork of Trail Canyon to the Aguereberry Point Road (see *Trail Canyon* and *South Fork of Trail Canyon*). This is about 13 miles, with an elevation gain of 3,900 feet and an elevation loss of 4,900 feet.

The Telescope Peak Trail. Telescope Peak is "the roof of Death Valley," and one of the highest mountains in the deserts of California. Two ways to climb it are suggested in this book: the hard way, up

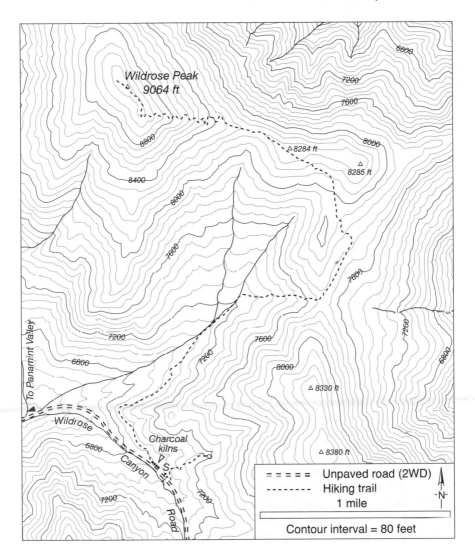

Wildrose Peak Trail

	Dist.(mi)	Elev.(ft)
Trailhead	0.0	6,900
Divide (1st saddle)	1.7	7,740
2nd saddle	3.1	8,220
Wildrose Peak	4.2	9,064

Hanaupah Canyon, and the easier way, up the trail from Mahogany Flat. The latter is one of Death Valley's classics, tackled every year by many visitors. The Hanaupah Canyon route is brutal, but the trail is not a stroll either: 6.5 miles and 3,150 feet up, one way, which for most people is a long, demanding day hike.

The Telescope Peak Trail is one of the few maintained foot trails in the park. The first part of the trail circles the east side of Rogers Peak, under a thick canopy of trees—mostly pinyon pines, with some junipers and scattered mahogany. From time to time, you will cross a giant slide of small colorful slabs. This is slate from the Johnnie Formation, a Proterozoic formation brought all the way up here by the same forces that pried Death Valley apart. In the summer, flowering plants grow right between the slabs, in essentially humus-free ground. This somewhat steep stretch ends at Arcane Meadows, a barren, often wind-swept pass offering the first glimpse of the Argus Range on the west side.

The next few miles are essentially along the high spine of the Panamints and fairly level. The trail swings back and forth over the crest, offering alternating views of the east and west sides. You will be continuously rewarded by awe-inspiring views of Death Valley, Panamint Valley, and several deep canyons—the three forks of Hanaupah Canyon on the east side, and Tuber and Jail canyons on the west side. Consider this: if you were transported to the same elevation in the Sierra Nevada, only 100 air miles away, you would be in the deep shade of a temperate forest, dwarfed by trees more than a hundred feet high. But as the Sierra robs all the moisture from the Pacific, precipitation here is too scant, even this far up, to support such a luxuriant forest. The tree cover gradually thins to a scarce forest of limber pines and grizzled bristlecone pines. Towards the end of this stretch, a side trail on the right drops a few hundred feet into the drainage of Jail Canyon to Eagle Spring, the highest spring in the park.

The last segment of this hike is up the steep north ridge of Telescope Peak. Oxygen becomes a pretty scarce commodity up here,

Telescope Peak		
	Dist.(mi)	Elev.(ft)
Trailhead	0.0	8,120
Arcane Meadows	2.4	~9,630
Fork to Eagle Spring	4.1	9,500
Eagle Spring (dry)	(1.1)	~9,300
Telescope Peak	6.5	11,049

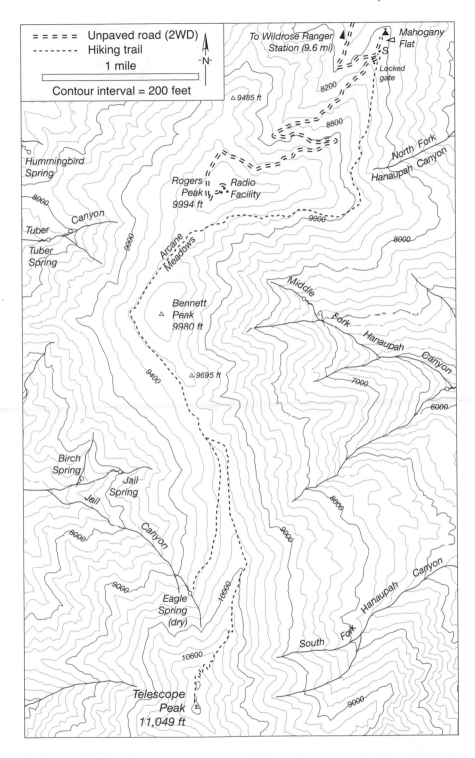

= = = = = Unpaved road (2WD)
- - - - - - - Hiking trail
1 mile
Contour interval = 200 feet

-N-

To Wildrose Ranger
Station (9.6 mi)

Mahogany
Flat

S

Locked
gate

North Fork
Hanaupah Canyon

8200

8800

△ 9485 ft

Hummingbird
Spring

Rogers
Peak
9994 ft

Radio
Facility

9000

8000

8000

Canyon

Tuber

Tuber
Spring

Arcane
Meadows

Bennett
△ Peak
9980 ft

Middle

Fork

Hanaupah

Canyon

9400

△9695 ft

7000

6000

Birch
Spring

Jail
Spring

Jail

Canyon

8000

9000

8000

9000

Eagle
Spring
(dry)

10000

9000

South

Fork

Hanaupah

Canyon

10600

9000

Telescope
Peak
11,049 ft

and if you are not used to this elevation you will grope for air and progress very slowly. Pause often to quiet your heart and smell the roses. Some of the largest trees in the park are found along here, impressive specimens several feet in diameter at the base and towering tens of feet overhead. Even late in the spring you may well find high snow drifts along the tight switchbacks.

The ultimate rewards of this climb are the stunning views from Telescope Peak, which encompass much of the surrounding desert, from the hazy valley of Las Vegas to the distant Sierra Nevada. From the rocky summit it is more than two vertical miles down to the eerie swirls of Death Valley's salt pan—to get higher above ground in the lower 48 states, you'll have to fly.

The best time to be here (and on the Wildrose Peak Trail) is May or June. Later in the summer the temperature is still fine, but heat haze often fills the valley and spoils the views. Between November and May snow on the ground is likely, at least part of the way. In the late spring it may be a bonus if you don't want to carry too much water. In the dead of winter the trail is often treacherous with ice.

■

BIBLIOGRAPHY

Traveller's Guidebooks

Bryan, T. S., and B. Tucker-Bryan. *The Explorer's Guide to Death Valley National Park*. Niwot, Co.: University Press of Colorado, 1995.

Ganci, D. *The Basic Essentials of Desert Survival*. Merrillville, Ind.: ICS Books, Inc., 1991.

Gebhardt, C. *Backpacking Death Valley*. 2nd edition. Michigan: Bookcrafters, 1985.

——. *Inside Death Valley*. Michigan: Bookcrafters, 1973.

Foster, L. *Adventuring in the California Desert*. San Francisco: Sierra Club Books, 1987.

Kirk, R. *Exploring Death Valley*. Stanford University Press, 1956.

Krist, J. *50 Best Short Hikes in California Deserts*. Berkeley, Ca.: Wilderness Press, 1995.

Lawson, C. *A Traveler's Guide to Death Valley National Park*. Los Olivos, Ca.: Cachuma Press for Death Valley Natural History Association, 1996.

Olsen, L. D. *Outdoor Survival Skills*. Provo, Ut.: Brigham Young University Press, 1984.

Wiseman, J. *ASA Survival Guide*. Glasgow, Scotland: HarpersCollins Publishers, 1993.

Geology

Blanc, R. P., and G. B. Cleveland. "Pleistocene Lakes of Southeastern California—I." *Cal. State Div. Mines* 14, No. 4 (1961): 1-7.

——. "Pleistocene Lakes of Southeastern California—II." *Cal. State Div. Mines* 14, No. 5 (1961): 1-6.

Collier, M. *An Introduction to the Geology of Death Valley*. Death Valley, Ca.: Death Valley Natural History Association, 1990.

Curry, H. D. "Turtlebacks in the Central Black Mountains, Death Valley, California." *Cal. Div. Mines Bull.* 170 (1954): 53-59.

Dorn, R. I., M. J. Deniro, and H. O. Ajie. "Isotopic Evidence for Climatic Influence on Alluvial-Fan Development in Death Valley, California." *Geol.* 15, No. 2 (1987): 108-110.

Dorn, R. I., A. J. T. Jull, D. J. Donahue, T. W. Linick, and L. J. Toolin. "Accelerator Mass Spectrometry Radiocarbon Dating of Rock Varnish." *Geol. Soc. Am. Bull.* 101, No. 11 (1989): 1363-1372.

Drewes, H. "Geology of the Funeral Peak Quadrangle, California, on the East Flank of Death Valley." *U. S. Geol. Survey Prof. Paper* 413 (1963): 1-78.

Evans, J. R., G. C. Taylor, and J. S. Rapp. "Mines and Mineral Deposits in Death Valley National Monument, California." *Cal. Div. Mines and Geol. Spec. Rept.* 125 (1976): 1-61.

Fiero, B. *Geology of the Great Basin*. Reno, Nev.: University of Nevada Press, 1986.

Hall, W. E. "Geology of the Panamint Butte Quadrangle, California." *U. S. Geol. Survey Bull.* 1299 (1971): 1-67.

Hall, W. E., and H. G. Stephens. "Economic Geology of the Panamint Butte Quadrangle and Modoc District, Inyo County, California." *Cal. Div. Mines and Geol. Spec. Rept.* 73 (1963): 1-39.

Hamilton, W. B. "Detachment Faulting in the Death Valley Region, California and Nevada." In *Geologic and Hydrologic Investigations of a Potential Nuclear Waste Disposal Site at Yucca Mountain, Southern Nevada*, M. D. Carr and J. C. Yount, eds. *Geol. Survey Bull.* B 1790 (1988): 51-85.

Hildreth, W. *Death Valley Geology*. Death Valley, Ca.: Death Valley Natural History Association, 1976.

Hill, M. L., and B. W. Troxel. "Tectonics of Death Valley Region, California." *Geol. Soc. Am. Bull.* 77, No. 4 (1986): 435-438.

Holm, D. K., R. J. Fleck, and D. R. Lux. "The Death Valley Turtlebacks Reinterpreted as Miocene-Pliocene Folds of a Major Detachment Surface." *J. of Geol.* 102, No. 6 (1994): 718-727.

Hunt, C. B. *Death Valley: Geology, Ecology, Archaeology*. Berkeley, Ca.: University of California Press, 1975.

Hunt, C. B., and D. R. Mabey. "Stratigraphy and Structure, Death Valley, California." *U. S. Geol. Survey Prof. Paper* 494-A (1966).

Hunt, C. B., T. W. Robinson, W. A. Bowles, and A. L. Washburn. "Hydrologic Basin, Death Valley, California." *U. S. Geol. Survey Prof. Paper* 494-B (1966).

Labotka, T. C., A. L. Albee, M. A. Lanphere, and S. D. McDowell. "Stratigraphy, Structure, and Metamorphism in the Central Panamint Mountains (Telescope Peak Quadrangle), Death Valley Area, California: Summary." *Geol. Soc. Am. Bull.* 91, No. 3 (1980): Part I, 125-129, Part II, 843-933.

McAllister, J. F. "Geology of the Furnace Creek Borate Area, Death Valley, Inyo County, California." *Cal. Div. Mines and Geol.* Map Sheet 14 (1970).

———. "Rocks and Structure of the Quartz Spring Area, Northern Panamint Range, California." *Cal. Div. Mines Spec. Rept.* 25 (1952): 1-38.

Miller, J. M. G. "Glacial and Syntectonic Sedimentation: The Upper Proterozoic Kingston Peak Formation, Southern Panamint Range, Eastern California." *Geol. Soc. Am. Bull.* 96, No. 12 (1985): 1537-1553.

———. "Tectonic Evolution of the Southern Panamint Range, Inyo and San Bernardino Counties." *Cal. Geol.* 40, No. 9 (1987): 212-222.

Miller, R. R. "Correlation Between Fish Distribution and Pleistocene Hydrography in Eastern California and Southwestern Nevada, with a Map of the Pleistocene Waters." *J. of Geol.* 54, No. 1 (1946): 43-53.

Noble, L. F. "Structural Features of the Virgin Spring Area, Death Valley, California." *Geol. Soc. Am. Bull*, 52, No. 7 (1941): 941-999.

Reynolds, M. W. "Geology of the Grapevine Mountains, Death Valley, California: A Summary." In *Guidebook: Death Valley Region, California and Nevada*, Shoshone, Ca.: Death Valley Pub. Co., 1974: 91-97.

————. *Stratigraphy and Structural Geology of Titus and Titanothere Canyons Area, Death Valley (Inyo County), California.* Doctoral thesis, Berkeley, Ca.: University of California, 1963.

Snow, J. K. *Cordilleran orogenesis, extensional tectonics, and geology of the Cottonwood Mountains area, Death Valley region, California and Nevada.* Doctoral thesis, Cambridge, Mass.: Harvard University, 1990.

Stewart, J. H. "Extensional Tectonics in the Death Valley Area, California: Transport of the Panamint Range Structural Block 80 km Northwestward." *Geol.* 11, No. 3 (1983): 153-157.

Stock, C. "Titanotheres From the Titus Canyon Formation, California." *Nat. Acad. Sci. Proc.* 22, No. 11 (1936): 656-661.

————. "Mammalian Fauna From the Titus Canyon Formation, California." *Carnegie Institute of Washington Pub.* 584 (1949): 229-244.

Stock, C., and F. D. Bode. "Occurence of Lower Oligocene Mammal-Bearing Beds Near Death Valley, California." *Nat. Acad. Sci. Proc.* 21, No. 11 (1935): 571-579.

Taylor, G. C. "Mineral Land Classification of the Eureka-Saline Valley Area, Inyo and Mono Counties, California." *Cal. Div. Mines and Geol. Spec. Rept.* 166 (1992).

Troxel, B. W. "Geologic Guide to the Death Valley Region, California and Nevada." In *Guidebook: Death Valley Region, California and Nevada,* Shoshone, Ca.: Death Valley Pub. Co., 1974: 2-16.

————. "Guide to Selected Features of Death Valley Geology." In *Geologic Guide to the Death Valley Area, California, Annual field trip guidebook.* Sacramento, Ca.: Geol. Soc., 1970: 40-55.

Wells, J. W. "Coral Growth and Geochronometry." *Nature* 197, No. 4871 (1963): 948-950.

White, D. E. "Antimony Deposits of the Wildrose Canyon Area, Inyo County, California." *U. S. Geol. Survey Bull.* 922-K (1940): 307-325.

Wills, C. J. "A Neotectonic Tour of the Death Valley Fault Zone, Inyo County." *Cal. Geol.* 42, No. 9 (1989): 195-200.

Wright, L. A. "Geology of the Superior Talc Area, Death Valley, California." *Cal. Div. Mines and Geol. Spec. Rept.* 20 (1952): 1-22.

————. "Talc Deposits of the Southern Death Valley-Kingston Range Region, California." *Cal. Div. Mines and Geol. Spec. Rept.* 95 (1968):1-79.

Wright, L. A., J. K. Otton, and B. W. Troxel. "Turtleback Surfaces of Death Valley Viewed as Phenomena of Extensional Tectonics." *Geol.* 2, No. 2 (1974): 53-54.

Wright, L. A., and B. W. Troxel. "Geology of the Northern Half of the Confidence Hills 15-minute Quadrangle, Death Valley Region, Eastern California: The Area of the Amargosa Chaos." *Cal. Div. Mines and Geol.,* Map Sheet 34 (1984).

Wright, L. A., B. W. Troxel, E. G. Williams, M. T. Roberts, and P. E. Diehl. "Precambrian Sedimentary Environments of the Death Valley Region, Eastern California." *Cal. Div. Mines and Geol. Spec. Rept.* 106 (1976): 7-15.

Native American History

Clements, T. D., and L. Clements. "Evidence of Pleistocene Man in Death Valley." *Geol. Soc. Am. Bull.* 64, No. 10 (1953): 1189-1204.

Coville, F. V. "The Panamint Indians of California." *Am. Anthropologist* 5, No. 4 (1892): 351-362.

Crum, S. J. *The Road On Which We Came: A History of the Western Shoshone.* Salt Lake City: University of Utah Press, 1994.

Dutcher, B. H. "Piñon Gathering Among the Panamint Indians." *Am. Anthropologist* 6, No. 4 (1893): 377-380.

Grosscup, G. L. "Notes On Boundaries and Culture of the Panamint Shoshone and Owens Valley Paiute." *Contrib. Univ. of California, Berkeley, Arch. Res. Facility* 35 (1977): 109-147.

Hunt, A. "Archaeology of the Death Valley Salt Pan, California." *Anthropology Papers* 47, Dept. of Anthropology, University of Utah, 1960.

Kerr, M. *The Shoshoni Indians of Inyo County, California: The Kerr Manuscript.* Philip J. Wilke and Albert B. Elsasser, eds. Publications in Archaeology, Ethnology and History, No. 15. Menlo Park, Ca.: Ballena Press, 1980.

Kirk, R. E. "Where Hungry Bill Once Lived." *Desert Magazine* 16 (March 1953): 15-18.

Sennett, B. "Wage Labor: Survival for the Death Valley Timbisha." In *Native Americans and Wage Labor: Ethnohistorical Perpectives.* Alice Littlefield and Martha C. Knack, eds. Norman, Okla.: University of Oklahoma Press, 1996: 218-244.

Thomas, D. H., L. S. A. Pendleton, and S. C. Cappannari. "Western Shoshone." In *Handbook of North American Indians* 11, W. C. Sturtevant and W. L. D'Azevedo, eds. Washington, D.C.: Smithsonian Institution, 1986: 262-283.

Wallace, W. J., and E. S. Taylor. "Early Man in Death Valley." *Archaeology* 8, No. 2 (1955), 88-92.

Wallace, W. J., and E. Wallace. *Ancient Peoples and Cultures of Death Valley National Monument.* Ramona, Ca.: Acoma Books, 1978.

————. *Desert Foragers and Hunters: Indians of the Death Valley Region.* Ramona, Ca.: Acoma Books, 1979.

Wheat, C. I. "Hungry Bill Talks." *Westways* 31 (May 1939): 18-19.

History

Belden, L. B. "The Battle of Wingate Pass." *Westways* 48 (Nov. 1956): 8-9.

Caruthers, W. *Loafing Along Death Valley Trails.* Palm Desert, Ca.: Desert Magazine Press, 1951.

Chalfant, W. A. *Death Valley: The Facts.* Stanford, Ca.: Stanford University Press, 1953.

Corle, E., and A. Adams. *Death Valley and the Creek Named Furnace.* Los Angeles: The Ward Richie Press, 1941.

Coolidge, D. *Death Valley Prospectors.* New York: E. P. Dutton and Co., 1937.

DeDecker, M. *White Smith's Fabulous Salt Tram.* Morongo Valley, Ca.: Sagebrush Press for the Death Valley '49ers, Inc., Keepsake No. 33, 1993.

Ellenbecker, J. G. *The Jayhawkers of Death Valley*. Marysville, Kans., 1938.

Farnsworth, H. "Dolph Nevares of Death Valley." *Desert Magazine* 21 (Dec. 1958): 16-18.

Greene, L. W. and J. A. Latschar. *Historic Resource Study: A History of Mining in Death Valley National Monument*. Denver, Co.: National Park Service, 1981.

Hanna, P. T. "The Origin and Meaning of Some Place Names of the Death Valley Region." *Touring Topics* 22 (Feb. 1930): 42-43, 54.

Harris, F. "Half a Century Chasing Rainbows." as told by Philip Johnston, *Touring Topics* 22 (Oct. 1930): 12-20, 55.

Johnson, L. and Johnson J. *Escape from Death Valley*. Reno, Nev.: University of Nevada Press, 1987.

Johnston, P. "In Quest of the Lost Breyfogle." *Touring Topics* 21 (Feb. 1929): 18-21, 56-57.

———. "Skidoo Has 23'd." *Westways* 28 (Feb. 1936): 8-10.

Koenig, G. *Beyond this Place There Be Dragons*. Glendale, Ca.: The H. Clark Company, 1984.

———. *Death Valley Tailings*. Morongo Valley, Ca.: Sagebrush Press, 1986.

Lee, B. *Death Valley Men*. New York: Macmillan, 1932.

Lingenfelter, R. E. *Death Valley and the Amargosa: A Land of Illusion*. Berkeley, Ca.: University of California Press, 1986.

Lingenfelter, R. E., and R. A. Dwyer. *Death Valley Lore: Classic Tales of Fantasy, Adventure, and Mystery*. Reno, Nev.: University of Nevada Press, 1988.

Majmundar, H. H. "Borate Mining History in Death Valley; Inyo and San Bernardino Counties." *Cal. Geol.* 38, No. 8 (1985): 171-177.

Manly, W. L. *Death Valley in '49*. Bishop, Ca.: Chalphant Press, 1977.

Palmer, T. S. *Place Names of the Death Valley Region in California and Nevada*. Morongo Valley, Ca.: Sagebrush Press, 1980.

Putnam, G. P. *Death Valley and its Country*. New York: Duell, Sloan and Pierce, 1946.

Spears, J. R. *Illustrated Sketches of Death Valley and Other Borax Deserts of the Pacific Coast*. Chicago and New York: Rand McNally, 1892.

U. S. Borax. *The Story of Pacific Coast Borax Co., Division of Borax Consolidated, Limited*. Los Angeles: The Ward Ritchie Press, 1951.

Weight, H. O. *Twenty Mule Team Days in Death Valley*. Twentynine Palms, Ca.: The Calico Press, 1972.

Natural History

Annable, C. R. *Vegetation and Flora of the Funeral Mountains, Death Valley National Monument, California-Nevada*. Nat. Park Service/University of Nevada, Las Vegas, Contrib. No. CPSU/UNLV 016/07, 1985.

Coville, F. V. "Botany of the Death Valley Expedition." *U. S. Dept. Agric., U.S. Natl. Herbarium, Contrib.* 4, 1893.

DeDecker, M. *Flora of the Northern Mojave Desert, California*. California Native Plant Society, Spec. Pub. No. 7, 1984.

Ferris, R. S. *Death Valley Wildflowers*. Death Valley, Ca.: Death Valley Natural History Association, 1962.

Grinnel, J. "Further Observations Upon the Bird Life of Death Valley." *The Condor* 36, No. 2 (1934): 67-72.

————. "Observations Upon the Bird Life of Death Valley." *Proc. Cal. Acad. Sci.* 13, 4th ser., No. 5 (1923): 43-109.

————. "The Mammals of Death Valley." *Proc. Calif. Acad. Sci.* 23, 4th ser., No. 9 (1937): 115-169.

Hunt, C. B., and L. W. Durrell. "Plant Ecology of Death Valley, California: With a Section on Distribution of Fungi and Algae." *U. S. Geol. Survey Prof. Paper* 509, 1966.

Jaeger, E. C. *A Naturalist's Death Valley*. Palm Desert, Ca.: Desert Magazine Press, 1957.

————. *Desert Wildflowers*, Stanford, Ca.: Stanford University Press, 1950.

————. *Desert Wildlife*. Stanford, Ca.: Stanford University Press, 1950.

Kurzius, M. A. *Vegetation and Flora of the Grapevine Mountains, Death Valley National Monument, California-Nevada*. Nat. Park Service/University of Nevada, Las Vegas, Contrib. No. CPSU/UNLV 017/06, 1981.

Miller, R. R. "The Cyprinodont Fishes of the Death Valley System of Eastern California and Southwestern Nevada." University of Michigan, Museum of Zoology Misc. Pub. 68, 1948.

Moore, M. *Medicinal Plants of the Mountain West*. Santa Fe, New Mex.: Museum of New Mexico Press, 1979.

Norris, L. L. *A Checklist of the Vascular Plants of Death Valley National Monument*. Death Valley, Ca.: Death Valley Natural History Association, 1982.

Norris, L. L., and W. Schreier. *A Checklist of the Birds of Death Valley National Monument*. Death Valley, Ca.: Death Valley Natural History Association, 1982.

Parson, M. E. *The Wild Flowers of California*. New York: Dover Publication, Inc., 1966.

Peterson, P. M. *Flora and Physiognomy of the Cottonwood Mountains, Death Valley National Monument, California*. Nat. Park Service/University of Nevada, Las Vegas, Contrib. No. CPSU/UNLV 022/06, 1984.

Randall, D. C. *An Analysis of Some Desert Shrub Vegetation of Saline Valley, California*. Doctoral thesis, Davis, Ca.: University of California, 1972.

Rothfuss, E. L. "Death Valley Burros." In *Proceedings, Third Death Valley Conference on History & Prehistory*. J. Pisarowicz, ed. Death Valley, Ca.: Death Valley Natural History Association (1992): 182-206.

Schramm, D. R. *Floristics and Vegetation of the Black Mountains, Death Valley National Monument, California*. Nat. Park Service/University of Nevada, Las Vegas, Contrib. No. CPSU/UNLV 012/13, 1982.

Wauer, R. H. "A Survey of the Birds of Death Valley." *The Condor* 64, No. 3 (1962): 220-233.

Welles, R. E., and F. B. Welles. "The Bighorn of Death Valley." In *Fauna of the National Parks of the United States*, Fauna Series No. 6, Washington, D. C.: U. S. Gov. Print. Office, 1961.

INDEX